The Orbit

Editor

STEPHEN A. SCHENDEL

ORAL AND MAXILLOFACIAL SURGERY CLINICS OF NORTH AMERICA

www.oralmaxsurgery.theclinics.com

Consulting Editor
RICHARD H. HAUG

November 2012 • Volume 24 • Number 4

ELSEVIER

1600 John F. Kennedy Blvd. ● Suite 1800 ● Philadelphia, PA 19103-2899

www.oralmaxsurgery.theclinics.com

ORAL AND MAXILLOFACIAL SURGERY CLINICS OF NORTH AMERICA Volume 24, Number 4
November 2012 ISSN 1042-3699, ISBN-13: 978-1-4557-4963-8

Editor: John Vassallo; j.vassallo@elsevier.com
Developmental Editor: Teia Stone

Oral and Maxillofacial Surgery Clinics of North America (ISSN 1042-3699) is published quarterly by Elsevier Inc., 360 Park Avenue South, New York, NY 10010-1710. Months of issue are February, May, August, and November. Business and Editorial Offices: 1600 John F. Kennedy Blvd., Suite 1800, Philadelphia, PA 19103-2899. Periodicals postage paid at New York, NY and additional mailing offices. Subscription prices are $355.00 per year for US individuals, $522.00 per year for US institutions, $159.00 per year for US students and residents, $414.00 per year for Canadian individuals, $621.00 per year for Canadian institutions, $476.00 per year for international individuals, $621.00 per year for international institutions and $216.00 per year for Canadian and foreign students/residents. To receive student/resident rate, orders must be accompanied by name or affiliated institution, date of term, and the *signature* of program/residency coordinator on institution letterhead. Orders will be billed at individual rate until proof of status is received. Foreign air speed delivery is included in all *Clinics* subscription prices. All prices are subject to change without notice. **POSTMASTER:** Send address changes to *Oral and Maxillofacial Surgery Clinics of North America,* Elsevier Periodicals Customer Service, 11830 Westline Industrial Drive, St. Louis, MO 63146. Tel: 1-800-654-2452 (U.S. and Canada); 314-447-8871 (outside U.S. and Canada). Fax: 314-447-8029. E-mail: journalscustomerservice-usa@elsevier.com (for print support); journalsonlinesupport-usa@elsevier.com (for online support).

Reprints. For copies of 100 or more, of articles in this publication, please contact the Commercial Reprints Department, Elsevier Inc., 360 Park Avenue South, New York, NY 10010-1710. Tel.: 212-633-3812; Fax: 212-462-1935; Email: reprints@elsevier.com.

Oral and Maxillofacial Surgery Clinics of North America is covered in *MEDLINE/PubMed (Index Medicus), Science Citation Index Expanded (SciSearch®), Journal Citation Reports/Science Edition,* and *Current Contents®/Clinical Medicine.*

Printed and bound by CPI Group (UK) Ltd, Croydon, CR0 4YY

Transferred to digital print 2012

Contributors

CONSULTING EDITOR

RICHARD H. HAUG, DDS
Carolinas Center for Oral Health,
Charlotte, North Carolina

GUEST EDITOR

STEPHEN A. SCHENDEL, MD, DDS, FACS
Professor Emeritus, Stanford University
Medical Center; Adjunct Clinical Professor of
Neurosurgery, Stanford University Medical
Center, Menlo Park, California

AUTHORS

R. BRYAN BELL, DDS, MD, FACS
Medical Director, Oral, Head and Neck Cancer
Program, Providence Cancer Center;
Attending Surgeon, Trauma Service/Oral and
Maxillofacial Surgery Service, Legacy Emanuel
Medical Center; Affiliate Professor, Oregon
Health and Science University, Portland,
Oregon

AARON J. BERGER, MD, PhD
Resident, Division of Plastic and
Reconstructive Surgery, Stanford Hospital
and Clinics, Stanford, California

JOSEPH A. BROUJERDI, MD, DMD
Aesthetic Plastic Surgery Institute, Beverly
Hills, California

ERIC J. DIERKS, MD, DMD, FACS
Affiliate Professor, School of Dentistry,
Oral and Maxillofacial Surgery, Oregon
Health and Science University; Director,
Fellowship in Head and Neck Oncologic
and Microvascular Reconstructive Surgery;
Head and Neck Surgical Associates,
Portland, Oregon

EDWARD ELLIS III, DDS, MS
Professor and Chairman, Department of Oral
and Maxillofacial Surgery, University of Texas
Health Science Center at San Antonio, San
Antonio, Texas

G.E. GHALI, DDS, MD
Professor and Chairman, Department of Oral
and Maxillofacial Surgery, Louisiana State
University Health Sciences Center at
Shreveport, Shreveport, Louisiana

BRENT A. GOLDEN, DDS, MD
Assistant Professor, Department of Oral
and Maxillofacial Surgery; Adjunct
Assistant Professor, Department of Pediatrics,
University of North Carolina, Chapel Hill,
North Carolina

DAVID C. HATCHER, DDS, MSc, MRCD(c)
Adjunct Professor, School of Dentistry,
Department of Orthodontics, University of
Pacific, San Francisco, California; Clinical
Professor, School of Dentistry, University of
Southern Nevada, Henderson, Nevada; Clinical
Professor, Orofacial Sciences, School of
Dentistry, University of California, San Francisco,
California; Private Practice, Diagnostic Digital
Imaging, Sacramento, California

MATTHEW J. HAUCK, MD
Oculofacial Plastic and Reconstructive Surgery
Fellow, Casey Eye Institute-Marquam Hill,
Oregon Health and Science University,
Portland, Oregon

DAVID KAHN, MD
Clinical Associate Professor, Division of Plastic
and Reconstructive Surgery, Stanford Hospital
and Clinics, Stanford, California

MICHAEL MALMQUIST, DDS
Resident, Department of Oral and Maxillofacial
Surgery, Baylor College of Dentistry, Texas
A&M Health Science Center, Dallas, Texas

MICHAEL R. MARKIEWICZ, DDS, MPH, MD
Resident in Training, Department of Oral and
Maxillofacial Surgery, Oregon Health and
Science University, Portland, Oregon

JUSTINE MOE, DDS
Surgical Resident, Division of Oral and
Maxillofacial Surgery, Emory University School
of Medicine, Atlanta, Georgia

LARRY MICHAEL OVER, DMD, MSD
Maxillofacial Prosthodontist, Private Practice,
Prosthodontics and Maxillofacial Prosthetics,
Eugene, Oregon; School of Dentistry, Adjunct
Professor, Oregon Health and Science
University, Portland, Oregon

CELSO F. PALMIERI Jr, DDS
Assistant Professor, Department of Oral and
Maxillofacial Surgery, Louisiana State
University Health Sciences Center at
Shreveport, Shreveport, Louisiana

JASON K. POTTER, MD, DDS
Clinical Adjunct Professor, Department of
Plastic Surgery, University of Texas
Southwestern Medical Center, Dallas, Texas

JOEL POWELL, DDS, MD, MSc
Private Practice, Dartmouth, Nova Scotia,
Canada

JU YON SOPHIE YI, MD, DDS
Oral and Maxillofacial Surgery Resident,
School of Dentistry, Oral and Maxillofacial
Surgery Resident, Oregon Health and Science
University, Portland, Oregon

MARTIN B. STEED, DDS
Associate Professor and Residency Program
Director, Division of Oral and Maxillofacial
Surgery, Emory University School of Medicine,
Atlanta, Georgia

TIMOTHY A. TURVEY, DDS
Professor and Chairman, Department of Oral
and Maxillofacial Surgery, University of North
Carolina, Chapel Hill, North Carolina

Contents

ORAL AND MAXILLOFACIAL SURGERY CLINICS OF NORTH AMERICA

THE CLINICS ARE NOW AVAILABLE ONLINE!
Access your subscription at:
www.theclinics.com

Preface

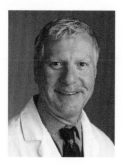

Stephen A. Schendel, MD, DDS, FACS
Guest Editor

In reference books the orbit is defined as the cavity in the skull in which the eye and its appendages are situated. It is often also thought of as a bony socket. In reality this does not begin to describe the complexity and importance of this structure in the human face. This bilateral 4-sided pyramidal structure is composed of 7 bones and forms the structural boundary between the facial skeleton and jaws and the cranium. Surgery or fractures of the jaws frequently involve the orbit and the surgical approaches and reference points aligned accordingly. Skull trauma especially of the frontal bone also involves the orbit. As Paul Tessier first demonstrated, the best approach to the midface may be intracranially through the orbits. By this deduction, the fields of cranial and facial surgery were forever united, creating a cascade of new techniques and possibilities.

The contents of the orbit, the eye and associated nerves, muscles, and glands, are extremely intricate. This adds to the complexity in the diagnosis and treatment of this area. In this text we have set forth the anatomical foundation and principles to diagnose and treat a number of conditions of the orbit and eye. Obviously this is not a complete treatise on the subject but is meant to be of practical use for the surgical specialist. Thus, the articles have been written by specialists with special expertise in the orbit and its contents.

Stephen A. Schendel, MD, DDS, FACS
Face Center Los Angeles
881 Alma Real Drive, Suite 204
Pacific Palisades, CA 90272, USA

E-mail address:
Etienne@stanford.edu

Oral Maxillofacial Surg Clin N Am 24 (2012) ix
http://dx.doi.org/10.1016/j.coms.2012.09.001
1042-3699/12/$ – see front matter © 2012 Elsevier Inc. All rights reserved.

Orbital Anatomy for the Surgeon

Timothy A. Turvey, DDS[a],*, Brent A. Golden, DDS, MD[a,b]

KEYWORDS

- Surgical anatomy • Orbit • Eyelids • Suspensory ligaments • Muscles • Arterial and nerve supply

KEY POINTS

- The orbits are conical structures dividing the upper facial skeleton from the middle face and surround the organs of vision.
- The walls, apex, and base of the orbit are curvilinear and are perforated by foramina and fissures, which have several irregularities where ligaments, muscles, and capsules attach.
- When considering the size and shape of the orbit, it is a well-designed and protective structure, which shields the ocular globes.
- The floor of the orbit is most vulnerable to fracture when there is direct force exerted on the ocular globe because it is thin and unsupported.
- The orbit and its contents have a rich blood supply coming from both the internal and the external carotid systems.
- Access to the orbital contents without osteotomy can proceed from the anterior orbit using either transcutaneous or transconjunctival approaches.

INTRODUCTION

The purpose of this article is to review the anatomy of the orbit from a surgical perspective. The content focuses on the skeletal and soft tissue architecture and does not include a description of the ocular globe, which is beyond the intention of this article and can be found in most anatomy texts.

SIZE, SHAPE, AND PURPOSE

The orbits are conical structures dividing the upper facial skeleton from the middle face and surround the organs of vision. Although the orbit is commonly described as pyramidal in shape, it is not an angular structure, and the walls are not regular. Rather, its walls, apex, and base are curvilinear and are perforated by foramina and fissures, and they have several irregularities where ligaments, muscles, and capsules attach.

The apex is located proximally, whereas the base opens onto the facial skeleton. The apex and base of the orbit are composed of thick bone, whereas the walls are thinner. The height of the orbit is usually 35 mm, whereas the width is approximately 40 mm as measured at the rims. The child's orbit is rounder, but with age the width increases. The widest circumference of the orbit is inside the orbital rim at the lacrimal recess. From the medial orbital rim to apex, the orbit measures approximately 45 mm in length, whereas from the lateral orbital rim to the apex, the measurement is approximately 1 cm shorter.[1,2]

When considering the size and shape of the orbit, it is a well-designed and protective structure, which shields the ocular globes (extensions of the

This work was supported in part by NIDCR R01 DE005215.

The authors have nothing to disclose.

[a] Department of Oral and Maxillofacial Surgery, University of North Carolina, 149 Brauer Hall, CB#7450, Chapel Hill, NC 27599-7450, USA; [b] Department of Pediatrics, University of North Carolina, 149 Brauer Hall, CB#7450, Chapel Hill, NC 27599-7450, USA

* Corresponding author.

E-mail address: tim_turvey@dentistry.unc.edu

Oral Maxillofacial Surg Clin N Am 24 (2012) 525–536

http://dx.doi.org/10.1016/j.coms.2012.08.003

brain). The thickened rim is able to resist fracture forces more than the weaker walls, especially the medial wall and floor. Similarly, the thicker bone at the apex shields the brain and the optic nerve from direct force. Pressure to the eye is dispersed to the walls, which absorb the forces and fracture easily. This structural feature reduces the force dispersed to the deeper orbital contents.

The medial walls of the orbits are parallel to the sagittal plane and extend forward on the facial skeleton. The lateral walls are shorter, convergent, and more recessed, which facilitate peripheral vision (a greater projection of the orbit toward the midline of the face with gentle loss of projection laterally).

The conical design of the orbit maintains the position of the globe with acceleration; however, this design is not protective of deceleration injuries. Although the widest diameter of the orbit is inside the rim, which helps maintain ocular position during deceleration, it is not always preventative of injury, especially with high-speed injuries (**Fig. 1**).

OSTEOLOGY

The orbit is composed of 7 bones. The lateral wall is formed by the greater wing of the sphenoid apically and the frontal and zygomatic bones facially. The floor is formed from the sphenoid, the orbital process of the palatine bone, and the orbital process of the maxillary bone. The medial wall is formed from the lesser wing of the sphenoid, the ethmoid bone, the lacrimal bone, and the frontal process of the maxilla. The roof of the orbit is derived from the sphenoid and the frontal bones (**Fig. 2**).

In general, the bone is thickest at the apex, thins as the walls diverge anteriorly, and then thickens again at the rims on the surface of the face.

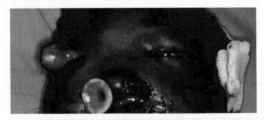

Fig. 1. Avulsion of the eye occurred as a result of a deceleration injury in which the patient also sustained severe midfacial fractures. This is an example of deceleration forces exceeding the strength of the lid retractors, suspensory and check ligaments, and the natural shape of the orbit where the internal diameter exceeds the diameter of the orbital rims. (Patient treated at Parkland Memorial Hospital, Dallas, TX, under the direction of Dr R.V. Walker.)

Although the bone of the medial orbital wall is thinnest, followed by the bone of the floor of the orbit, in actuality the medial wall is strengthened by the perpendicular septa of the ethmoid sinuses. The floor of the orbit is most vulnerable to fracture when there is direct force exerted on the ocular globe because it is thin and unsupported. When orbital cellulitis occurs, its most likely source is direct extension from the ethmoid sinuses because the thin bone of the medial wall is easily penetrated by expanding masses from the sinus. The floor of the orbit is thicker and offers more resistance to maxillary sinus abnormality.

None of the walls of the orbit are flat; they are curvilinear in shape, and their purpose is to maintain the projection of the ocular globe and to cushion it when subjected to blunt force.[1-5]

FLOOR OF THE ORBIT

From the inferior orbital rim, the floor dips inferiorly while maintaining the same cephalo-caudad position for approximately 15 mm, past the inferior orbital fissure. It then gently curves cephalically to the superior orbital fissure. This anatomic subtlety is important when repairing orbital floor fractures because re-creating this gentle curvature will restore normal anatomy and will help prevent enophthalmos.

MEDIAL ORBITAL WALL

The medial orbital walls are parallel to the sagittal plane and have the greatest degree of superioinferior curvature. The medial orbital rim is less defined than the other rims. The entire wall is thin from the base to the apex, but it is strengthened by the perpendicular septa of the ethmoid sinus. The wall separates the ethmoid sinuses and nose from the orbit. The superior aspect of the medial rim is the most prominent and blends into the forehead, curving anteriorly toward the midline.

ROOF AND LATERAL ORBITAL WALL

The roof of the orbit curves cephalically in the lateral aspect to accommodate the lacrimal gland. The bone of this wall separates the anterior cranial fossa from the orbit. It is generally thin and becomes thinner with age. The superior orbital rim has a notch on the medial third through which the supraorbital nerve runs and supplies sensation to the forehead. Sometimes this notch is calcified and forms a distinct foramen.

The lateral orbital rim is the least projected and this facilitates lateral vision. The zygomatic portion of the lateral orbital wall is thin, but the wall

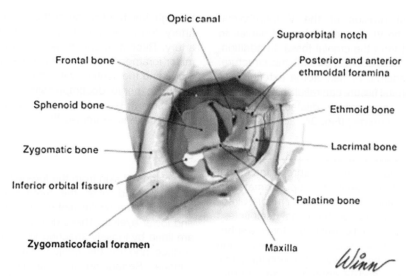

Fig. 2. The 7 bones of the orbit. (*From* Rougier J, Tessier P, Hervouet F, et al. Chirurgie plastique orbito-palpébrale. Paris: Elsevier Masson SAS; 1977. Copyright © Société Française d'Ophtalmologie. All rights reserved; with permission.)

thickens considerably in the sphenoid, where it borders the superior orbital fissure.

FORAMEN, FISSURES, TUBERCLES, AND CRESTS
Nasolacrimal Canal

The inferomedial orbital wall is penetrated by the nasolacrimal canal, which houses the nasolacrimal duct. Just anterior to the canal and on the frontal process of the maxilla lie the anterior lacrimal crests, which are elevated prominences to which attaches the anterior portion of the medial canthus. Just posterior to the canal is a smaller and less obvious prominence, the posterior lacrimal crest, which is part of the lacrimal bone and to which attaches the deeper fibers of the medial canthus and orbicularis oculi (Horner's muscle, pars lacrimalis).[6,7]

Anterior and Posterior Ethmoidal Foramen

Approximately 15 mm behind the medial orbital rim at the level of the junction of the frontal bone with the ethmoid bone, the anterior ethmoidal foramen exits into the orbit. This canal houses the anterior ethmoidal artery. Approximately 1 cm further posteriorly is the posterior ethmoidal foramen through which the posterior ethmoidal artery exits. These arteries can be the source of epistaxis and/or orbital bleeding.[1–5]

Whitnall's Tubercle

No discussion of orbital anatomy would be complete without the mention of this anatomic landmark. Located on the lateral orbital wall just inferior to the frontozygomatic suture and approximately 1 cm posterior to the lateral orbital rim is a protuberance that Whitnall indicated was present in 96% of the specimens he dissected. He further indicated that this protuberance was the attachment of the lateral canthus and other globe suspensory ligaments of significance.[8,9]

Inferior Orbital Fissure

Approximately 1 cm posterior to the inferior-lateral orbital rim lies the fissure, which connects the pterygo-palatine fossa with the floor of the orbit. The fissure is composed of the zygomatic and sphenoid bones on the lateral side and the zygoma and maxilla on the medial side. In the anterior portion of the fissure, a small canal runs anteriorly through the floor of the orbit and exits on the facial side of the maxilla approximately 5 mm inferior to the rim. Through this canal runs the infraorbital nerve, which also gives off small dental branches (anterior, superior alveolar, and middle superior alveolar nerves) before exiting facially. The artery, a terminal branch of the internal maxillary artery, and vein, which drains into the pterygoid plexus, run with this sensory-only extension of the second division of the trigeminal nerve.

Superior Orbital Fissure

Located near the apex of the orbit lies a club-shaped fissure, where the greater and lesser wings of the sphenoid meet the maxilla. This fissure serves as the conduit for the III (oculomotor), IV (trochlear), 1st division of the V (ophthalmic branch), and the VI (abducens) cranial nerves to enter the orbit from the cranial fossa. In addition, the ophthalmic vein courses through this structure.

Fractures, edema, or hematoma extending to the superior orbital fissure can result in ophthalmoplegia, ptosis, or pupillary dilatation (superior orbital fissure syndrome) (**Fig. 3**).

Optic Canal

Medial to the superior orbital fissure at the orbital apex lies the optic canal. It is approximately 5 mm in diameter and runs in a superior medial direction into the cranial fossa. The canal itself is less than 1 cm in length and lies entirely within the sphenoid. The walls of the canal can be thinned by the proximity of the sphenoid sinus. Through this canal run the optic nerve and the ophthalmic artery. Fractures extending to the optic canal can result in blindness in addition to the findings of superior orbital fissures syndrome (orbital apex syndrome).

Cranio-orbital Foramen

Just anterior to the superior orbital fissure, located on the medial orbital wall, lies a small foramen through which a branch of the middle meningeal artery forms an anastamosis with the lacrimal artery. Recent attention has been called to this minor foramen because of the potential of hemorrhage and the sentinel value it has when performing optic nerve decompression or deep orbital dissection. It is present in approximately 55% of the specimens examined.[10]

EYELIDS

Extensions of skin from the forehead and cheeks, which spread over the inferior and superior aspects of the ocular globe, represent the upper and lower eyelids. These uniquely designed folds are lined by loosely attached skin on the external surface and by the conjunctiva on the internal surface. Separating the internal and external surfaces of the eyelids are several rows of hair-bearing lines at the eyelid margin (eyelashes) and the openings of the tarsal glands. The purposes of the eyelids include protection of the globes, lubrication, cleansing, and drainage of the region. The separation of the 2 lids is called the palpebral fissure, which is widest at the midpoint of the pupils; the fissure tapers medially and laterally.

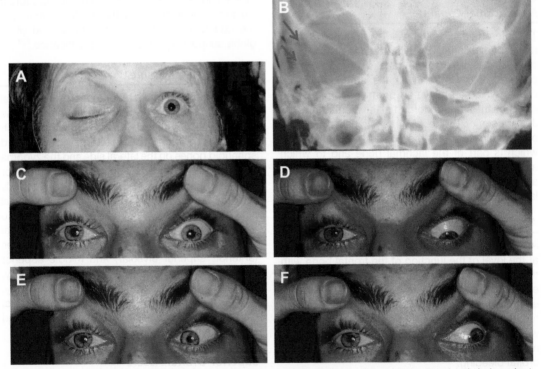

Fig. 3. Superior orbital fissure syndrome consists of ptosis, proptosis, pupillary dilation, and ophthalmoplegia. (*A*) Ptosis associated with the condition. (*B*) Radiograph demonstrating a fracture extending into the superior orbital fissure (*arrows* demonstrate orbital fracture). (*C*) Pupillary dilation of the right eye in another patient with superior orbital fissure syndrome. (*D, E, F*) Ophthalmoplegia. (Patient treated at John Peter Smith Hospital, Ft. Worth, TX, under the direction of Drs Bruce Epker and Larry Wolford.)

The medial and lateral extensions of the eyelids and tarsus are anchored by the medial and lateral canthal (palpebral) tendons.[1,6–9,11]

MEDIAL CANTHUS

The medial canthal anatomy has been described in detail by Robinson and Stranc.[7] The upper and lower eyelids on the medial canthus do not contact the globe, but rather form a lake that collects tears. When the eyelids are everted, small punata can be visualized in the upper and lower lids, which represent the beginning of the lacrimal drainage system. The lateral fissure contacts the ocular globe and under normal circumstances tears flow from lateral to medial to the lacrimal lakes, through the lacrimal puncta, into the canaliculi, and into the lacrimal sac.

The medial canthus consists of a tendonous attachment of the orbicularis oculi muscle and a ligmamentous attachment to the tarus. The attachment is primarily at the anterior lacrimal crest, which is located on the frontal process of the maxilla. The posterior or minor contributor to the attachment is the posterior medial canthus, known as pars lacrimal or Horner's muscle. This posterior limb also represents the attachment of the orbicularis oculi muscle to the posterior lacrimal crest. Located between the lacrimal bone and wedged between the anterior and posterior tendons is the nasolacrimal canal. Just above the canal is the lacrimal sac, which receives contributions from the lacrimal canaliculi to the nasolacrimal duct. It is postulated that the contracture of the orbicularis oculi muscle results in closure of the eyelids, and the movement also squeezes the lacrimal sac, which results in emptying tears into the nasolacrimal canal and eventually drainage into the nose (**Fig. 4**).

SEPTUM ORBITALE

Covering the orbicularis oculi muscle is a loosely attached layer of skin. Just extending back to the orbicularis oculi muscle is an extension of the periorbita that runs into the eyelid called the septum orbitale. This septum orbitale is a consistent feature of both the upper and the lower eyelids, and it separates the orbital contents from the lid contents. Its major purpose is postulated to be to contain the spread of infection. It also contains the extraconal fat that is reduced during blepharoplasty. The septum orbital extends from the tarsus to the orbital rim, where it then attaches to the bone and becomes the periorbita inside the orbit and periosteum outside the orbit.

TARSAL PLATES

Extending back to the septum orbital are multiple muscles surrounded by fat and connective tissue.

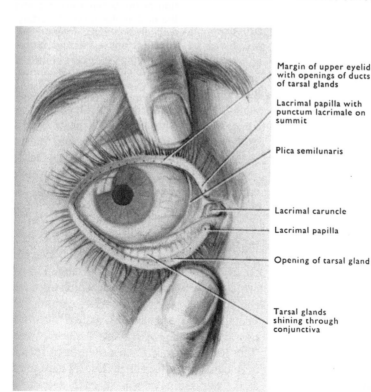

Fig. 4. The anatomy of the medial aspect of the palpebral fissure. (*Reprinted from* Romanes GJ. Cunningham's textbook of anatomy. 10th edition. Oxford Press; 1962. Fig. 957, p. 803; with permission.)

Margin of upper eyelid with openings of ducts of tarsal glands

Lacrimal papilla with punctum lacrimale on summit

Plica semilunaris

Lacrimal caruncle

Lacrimal papilla

Opening of tarsal gland

Tarsal glands shining through conjunctiva

In the lid margins are thick pads of dense connective tissue called tarsal plates. The tarsal plates add rigidity to the lids and also accept attachments of multiple muscles and membranes. Within the tarsal plates are large sebaceous glands (Meibomian glands). The plates are curvilinear in shape and extend away from the lid margins approximately 1 cm in the upper lid and approximately 5 mm in the lower lid.

MUSCLES AND ACTIONS

The orbicularis oculi muscle is present in the superior and inferior lids (palpebral portion) and lies just below the skin. The muscle has a palpebral and an orbital component. The septum orbitale is the next layer. Under it are other muscles connecting to the tarsus. In the upper lid is the aponeurosis of the levator muscle, which attaches to the tarsus toward the lid margin. In the lower lid, the fascia of the inferior rectus attaches to the inferior tarsus, into the orbicularis oculi muscle, and into the subcutaneous tissues of the lid. Attached to this is a small, smooth muscle, the inferior tarsal

muscle (Mueller's muscle), which rises from the posterior fascia and inserts into the tarsus. The deep surface of the levator aponeurosis also contains a layer of smooth muscle known as Whitnall's muscle (also known as Mueller's muscle). Both of these smooth muscles are innervated by the sympathetic fibers coming from the superior cervical ganglion via the lacrimal nerve (**Fig. 5**). Actions of the inferior rectus include retraction of the lower lid in addition to elevation of the globe.

During normal opening and closing, the upper lid does most of the movement. With closure of the lid, contraction of the orbicularis oculi muscle is necessary, and this contraction requires VII cranial nerve activity. Opening of the eyelids requires contracture of the levator superioris muscle, which is innervated by the third cranial nerve, which enters the orbit through the superior orbital fissure and sends branches to most of the muscles of extraocular movement. Reflex closure of the eyelids occurs via the sympathetic pathways traveling to the smooth muscles of the upper and lower eyelids.

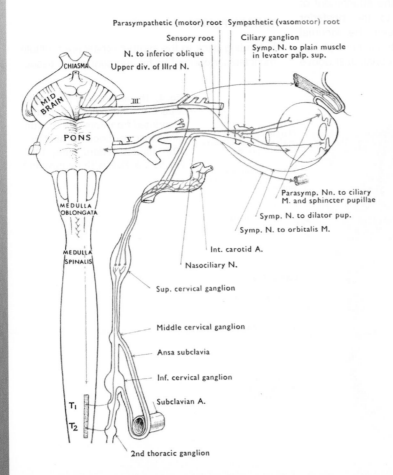

Fig. 5. Sympathetic innervation of the orbital contents arising from the superior cervical ganglion and entering the orbit via the first division of the trigeminal nerve and the oculomotor nerve. A., artery; div., division; Inf., inferior; M., muscle; N., nerve; palp. sys., palpabrae superioris; Sup., superior; Symp., sympathetic. (*Reprinted from Romanes GJ. Cunningham's textbook of anatomy. 10th edition. Oxford Press; 1962. Fig. 56, p. 692; with permission.*)

CONJUNCTIVA

The deepest layer of the eyelid is the conjunctiva, which is a modification of the skin layer, and forms the inner surface of the lid. The inner surface of the lid is a smooth layer, which folds onto itself from the eyelid and covers the outer surface of the eyeball. Where the conjunctiva reflects on itself at the inner aspect of the eyelid is the fornix. Sensory innervation of this tissue comes from the first division of the trigeminal nerve (ophthalmic branch).

The conjunctiva is attached to the deep layer of the tarsus and also covers the fascia of the inferior rectus in the lower lid and the fascia of the levator superioris and superior rectus muscle in the upper lid.

LATERAL CANTHUS

The lateral canthus anchors the tarsus of both lids laterally to the zygomatic bone at the tubercle on the lateral wall (Whitnall's tubercle). Also attaching to this tubercle are the aponeurosis of the levator and the check ligament of the lateral rectus. This structure extends to the septum orbital, whereas the fusion of the upper and lower orbicularis oculi occurs superficial to the septum (lateral paleplral raphe), which becomes confluent with the temporoparietal fascia.

THE PERIORBITA

As the optic nerve traverses the optic canal, it is surrounded by dura, which then attaches to the bone of the orbit. Similarly, anywhere the cranium comes in contact with the orbit (superior orbital fissure, anterior and posterior ethmoidal foramina, and the cranio-orbital foramen), the dura becomes continuous with the underlying bone. This underlying bone becomes the periorbita, which is loosely attached to the bone compared to the periosteum of the facial bones or the superficial surface of the skull. The periorbita also extends to the eyelids as orbita septum.

On the orbital surface of the optic canal and the medial aspect of the superior orbital fissure, the periorbita thickens and gives rise to the tendenous attachments of the 4 rectus muscles, the levator superioris, and the superior oblique muscle. This tendonous ring is called the annulus of Zinn.

The eyeball is surrounded by fat, muscle, sheaths, capsules, connective tissue, and so forth. It is contained and suspended in the orbit by an elaborate labyrinth of tendenous and ligamentous attachments and interwoven capsules, which fasten it medically and laterally.[2]

BULBOUS SHEATH OR TENONS CAPSULE

The bulbous sheath or tenons capsule is a fibrous layer between the eyeball and the intermuscular orbital fat that is interspersed between the 6 muscles of extraocular movement. It attaches to the sclera on the anterior and posterior surfaces of the eyeball and becomes continuous with the fascia of the muscles posteriorly and around the inferior oblique muscle.[8,9]

LOCKWOOD'S LIGAMENT

The thickened lower part of the bulbous sheath is known as the suspensory ligament of Lockwood. This fascial sling blends with the lateral canthus and the lateral check ligament and transverses from lateral to medial, suspending the globe and resisting anterior and posterior displacement of the eye. On the medial orbital wall, the suspensory attachment is on the lacrimal crest, where it blends with the canthus and the medial check ligament. On the floor of the orbit are the inferior oblique and inferior rectus muscles, which cover the inferior orbital fissure and serve as the inferior check ligament. On the superior surface, the superior check ligament is the fascia of the levator, which is anchored laterally at Whitnell's tubercle and medially to the trochlea.

Manson and colleagues have described 4 extensions of the ligament, including an arcuate, capsulopalpebral, inferior rectus, and conjunctival fornix.

WHITNALL'S LIGAMENT

This fascial sling extends from the trochlea (orbital roof, a cartilaginous pulley that contains the tendons of the superor oblique muscle) to the lateral orbit wall. It has attachments to the levator aponeurosis and the superior rectus, as well as the conjunctiva and Tenon's capsule.

MEDIAL AND LATERAL CHECK LIGAMENTS

The medial and lateral check ligaments extend from the orbital septum and levator aponeurosis, as well as the muscle sheaths, and attach to the medial and lateral orbital walls. The medial attachment is to the lacrimal bone (posterior lacrimal crest), whereas the lateral attachment is to the lateral orbital wall at Whitnall's tubercle.[8,9]

ORBITAL FAT

The fat of the orbit consists of extraconal and intraconal disbursements. The abundance of fat facilitates the movement of muscles and maintains the projection of the eye in the orbit. It also serves as a cushion. The intermuscular portion of orbital fat contributes significantly to the maintenance of globe position. The extramuscular fat is liberally dispersed throughout the anterior orbit. This fat is contained by the periorbita. This extramuscular fat does not seem to contribute to the position of the globe, and it is this fat that is reduced during blepharoplasty.

Although it is postulated that the loss of the extramuscular fat, as occurs with orbital fractures, may result in enophthalmos, Manson and colleagues' work suggests that the loss of the interconal fat is more likely to cause enophthalmos.[8,9] Furthermore, their work suggests that the enophthalmos occurring after orbital trauma is more likely caused by inadequate restoration of orbital anatomy and subsequent changes in the shape of the orbital contents secondary to scarring and loss of support of the suspensory system (**Fig. 6**).

LACRIMAL GLAND

The lacrimal gland is located in the superior lateral portion of the orbit and is situated in the lacrimal recess of the roof of the orbit. This gland is contained with the periorbita and is suspended inferiorly by Whitnall's capsule. The gland receives innervation from the lacrimal branch of the first division of the fifth nerve and also receives secretory parasympathetic fibers coming from the zygomatic branch via the facial nerve ganglion (**Fig. 7**).[4]

MUSCLES OF EXTRAOCULAR MOVEMENT

The extraocular muscles are responsible for eye movement. These extraocular muscles include the 4 rectus muscles, the superior oblique, and the inferior oblique. With the exception of the inferior oblique, all other muscles originate at the annulus of Zinn and travel anteriorly to insert into the globe. Although the levator superioris is considered a muscle of extraocular movement and it attaches to the annulus of Zinn, its function is lid elevation, not globe movement.

LEVATOR SUPERIORIS AND SUPERIOR OBLIQUE

The levator superioris also originates at the annulus of Zinn, and its action is to elevate the upper lid. Its innervation is the oculomotor nerve (III). The superior oblique also rises at the annulus of Zinn and is unique in that it attaches via a trochlea to the orbit

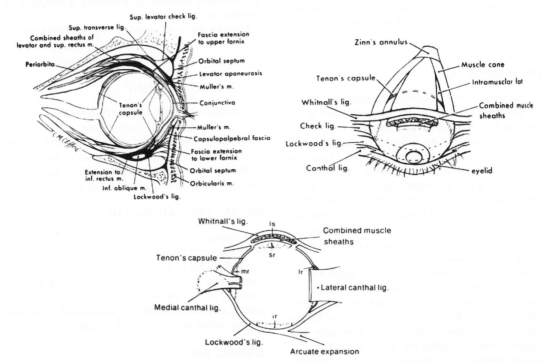

Fig. 6. The orbit and eyelids. Notice the elaborate labyrinth of muscles, tendons, ligaments, and fascia, which contribute to the movement, suspension, and containment of the ocular globe. Inf., inferior; Ir, lateral rectus; ir, inferior rectus; Is, levator superiorus; lig., ligament; m., muscle; mr, medial rectus; sup., superior. (*Reprinted from* Manson P, Clifford CM, Su CT, et al. Mechanisms of global support and posttraumatic enophthalmos: I. The anatomy of the ligament sling and its relation to intramuscular cone orbital fat. Plast Reconstr Surg 1986;77(2):193–202. Fig. 6, p. 198; with permission from Williams Wilkins Publishing Co.)

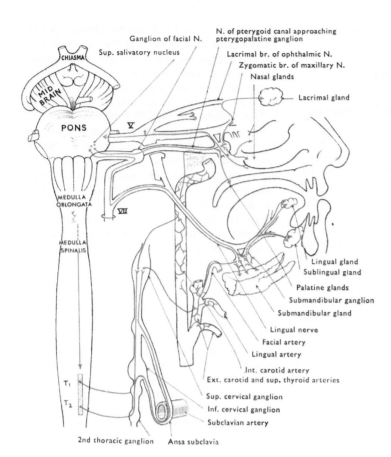

Fig. 7. The secretory innervation of the lacrimal gland via parasympathetic fibers arising from the facial nerve ganglion. br., branch; Inf., inferior; Int., internal; N., nerve; Sup., superior. (*Reprinted from* Romanes GJ. Cunningham's textbook of anatomy. 10th edition. London: Oxford Press; 1962. Fig. 868, p. 703; with permission.)

on the medial side of the roof, and its tendon extends posteriorly from the trochlea and laterally to insert on the lateral side of the posterior globe. Its action allows the globe to rotate inferiorly. Its innervation is the trochlear nerve (IV).

INFERIOR OBLIQUE

The inferior oblique is another muscle of extraocular movement whose attachment is to the medial orbital rim. It runs obliquely across the orbital floor over the inferior orbital fissure to insert into the globe behind its equator. Its action allows the eye to move superiorly. Its innervation is the oculomotor nerve (III).

RECTUS MUSCLES

The superior, medial, inferior, and lateral rectus muscles run from the annulus of Zinn anteriorly to insert into the globe. The rectus muscles function to allow the globe to move in the directions they are named for. The medial, inferior, and superior rectus muscles, as well as the inferior oblique and levator superioris, are innervated by the oculomotor nerve (III). The smooth muscle portion of the

inferior and superior lid (Mueller's muscles) is supplied by sympathetic fibers coming from the superior cervical ganglion (see **Fig. 4**). The lateral rectus is innervated by the abducens nerve (VI), which has the longest intracranial route of any of the cranial nerves. All of these nerves enter the orbit through the superior orbital fissure. The long intracranial pathway of the abducens nerve (VI) makes it the most vulnerable to injury with trauma.

BLOOD SUPPLY

The orbit and its contents have a rich blood supply coming from both the internal and the external carotid systems. In general, the globe and orbital contents are supplied from the extensions of the internal carotid via the ophthalmic artery. The ophthalmic artery gives rise to the lacrimal artery, the anterior and posterior ethmoidal arteries, the supraorbital artery, and the ciliary arteries. The eyelids are also supplied by the internal carotid system via the palpebral arteries and branches of the supraorbital artery. The anterior facial artery, an extension of the external carotid, also supplies portions of the eyelids, as does the infraorbital artery, a terminal branch of the internal maxillary artery (**Fig. 8**).[4]

VENOUS AND LYMPHATIC DRAINAGE

Venous drainage of the orbit is via the superior and inferior ophthalmic vein running through the superior orbital fissure. There are also communications with the facial vein and pterygoid plexes via the inferior orbital fissure. Of significance is the proximity of the cavernous sinus and the potential for infection to spread from the face to the intracranial contents via the venous drainage system close to the orbit.

Descriptions of the lymphatics of the orbital and periorbital region continue to evolve. The orbit has long been considered only sparsely drained, which is in contrast to the rich lymphatics of the eyelids and bulbar conjunctiva. More contemporary review now supports the presence of some orbital lymphatics, particularly in the lacrimal gland. The eyelids drain laterally into the preauricular nodes and medially into the submandibular nodes.[1]

Surgical Approaches to the Orbit

Access to the orbital contents without osteotomy can proceed from the anterior orbit using either transcutaneous or transconjunctival approaches.

Lid creases form the basis for designing most transcutaneous incisions, with the coronal incision being a notable exception. For any orbital surgery, the cornea should be protected by placement of a corneal shield or tarsorrhaphy suture over eye lubricant. Incision design should be completed before distorting tissue with local anesthetic.

In the upper lid, the periorbital skin is thin and the supratarsal fold provides a highly cosmetic crease in which to hide an incision. For this reason, the upper blepharoplasty approach is commonly used in this area. The incision is made through the skin and orbicularis muscle at the level of the upper lid crease. A plane can be developed between the orbicularis oculi and orbital septum to allow control of entry into the orbit. The incision through the periosteum versus the orbital septum depends on the surgical indication. Alternatively, the incision can be hidden in the hair-bearing skin of the lateral brow with a similar area of exposure, but a less cosmetic result.

To expose the superior orbit more broadly with more robust exposure of the medial and lateral walls or to provide access for orbital osteotomies, the coronal incision is the most versatile and cosmetic. This approach consists of an incision at the vertex of the head and postauricular extensions bilaterally. If significant exposure of the root

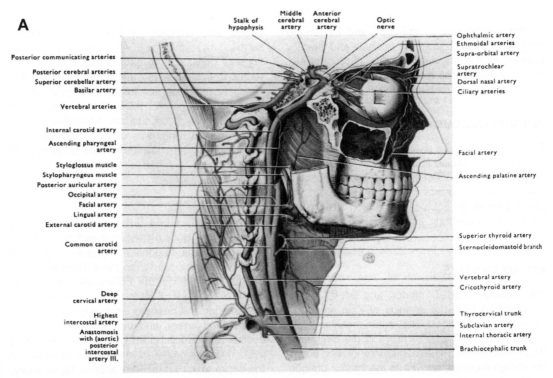

Fig. 8. (A, B) Arterial blood supply of the orbit and its contents. (*Reprinted from* Romanes GJ. Cunningham's textbook of anatomy. 10th edition. Oxford Press; 1962; with permission.)

of the zygoma is anticipated, the inferior extension is moved to the preauricular position. Dissection in the subpericranial plane is prudent inferiorly from the hairline across the orbital rims to protect the facial and supraorbital nerves.

For access to the inferior and lateral orbit, the most often used cutaneous approaches are the subciliary and subtarsal approaches. The subciliary incision is created approximately 2 mm inferior and parallel to the free margin of the lower lid. Dissection to the preseptal plane may proceed through the orbicularis directly or in a stepped manner. Final access to the bony orbit is accomplished by incising the periosteum over the infraorbital rim. The subtarsal approach moves the incision inferiorly to between 6 and 7 mm below the free lid margin while following a lower lid skin crease. Here, the skin is incised and the dissection is stepped through the orbicularis oculi to the septum orbitale and taken down to the infraorbital rim. The periosteum is then incised. Exposure is similar for both approaches, but opinions vary regarding the amount of risk relative to ectropion and cosmetic outcome.

Transconjunctival approaches have gained favor for access to inferior and lateral orbit as well as

B

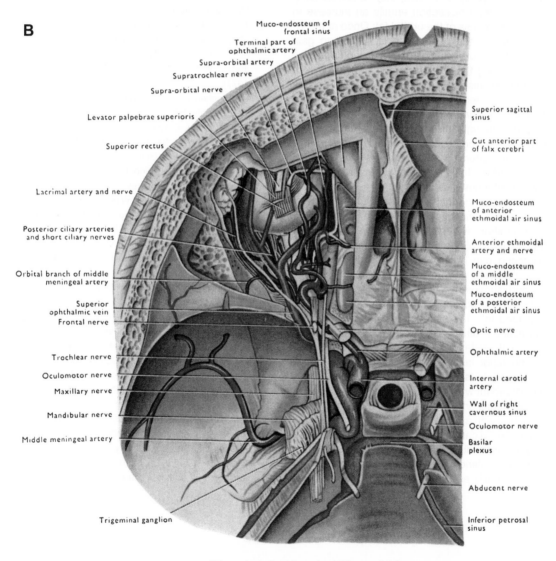

Dissection of orbit and middle cranial fossa.

On the right side the trochlear nerve has been removed, and in the left orbit portions of the structures above the ophthalmic artery have been taken away.

Fig. 8. (continued)

the medial wall, given their cosmetic appeal. The transconjunctival approach often may need to be combined with a lateral canthotomy to obtain comparable access to the transcutaneous approaches. The inferior fornix transconjunctival incision is made through the lower lid conjunctiva after protection of the cornea and injection of local anesthetic. Retraction sutures in the lid margin are helpful adjuncts. This incision is made approximately 2 to 3 mm inferior to the tarsus, which is anterior to the depth of the fornix. This incision should remain lateral to the lower lacrimal punctum. Dissection to the infraorbital rim may proceed either preseptally or postseptally, understanding that postseptal dissection entails an increase in the obtrusiveness of the orbital fat. Once at the infraorbital rim, the periosteum is incised to gain access to the orbital floor. This incision should be located along the anterior inferior rim to prevent unintended disinsertion of the inferior oblique muscle. No attempt is needed to reattach the lower lid retractors or even to suture the conjunctival wound, although this reattachment can be performed in a loose fashion with fine resorbable suture. If a lateral canthotomy is required, resuspension of the lower lid tarsal plate via the lateral canthal attachment is required.

The medial canthal apparatus, lacrimal drainage system, and inferior oblique muscle require consideration with transconjunctival access to the medial orbit. Accordingly, a transcaruncular approach can be used concurrently with or in isolation from the inferior fornix approach to expand surgical access. The incision is placed between the plica semilunaris and caruncle and extended into the superior and inferior fornices. Dissection is directly toward the posterior lacrimal crest just posterior to Horner's muscle. Once at the posterior lacrimal crest, an incision through the periorbita is accomplished for access to the medial orbital wall.

The medial orbital rim and wall may also be approached with a curvilinear incision placed anterior to the medial canthus on the frontal process of the maxilla, extending superiorly to the nasofrontal suture and inferiorly to the inferior rim. This incision can be made as a continuous incision with the inferior lid incision if necessary. The limitation with this approach is the medial canthal attachment at the frontal process of the maxilla. If the canthus is detached for access, meticulous care must be taken to anchor it when closing. The most predictable anchor is transnasal canthoplexy. A middorsal nasal incision may also be used to approach the medial orbital wall, but its limitation is similar to the medial curvilinear incision.[11,12]

REFERENCES

1. Ochs MW, Buckley MJ. Anatomy of the orbit. Oral Maxillofac Surg Clin North Am 1993;5:419–29.
2. Tessier P, Rougier J, Herrouat F, et al. Plastic surgery of the orbit and eyelids: report of the French Society of Ophthalmology. New York: Masson Publishing; 1981 [Wolfe SA, Trans.; original work published 1977].
3. Hollingshead WH. Anatomy for surgeons, vol. 1. Philadelphia: Harper and Row Publishers; 1982.
4. Romanes GJ. Cunningham's textbook of anatomy. 10th edition. London: Oxford University Press; 1964.
5. Rontal E, Rontal M, Guilford FT. Surgical anatomy of the orbit. Ann Otol Rhinol Laryngol 1979;88:382–6.
6. Putterman AM. Cosmetic oculoplastic surgery. 3rd edition. Philadelphia: W.B. Saunders Co; 1999.
7. Robinson TJ, Strac MF. The anatomy of the medial canthal ligament. Br J Plast Surg 1970;1:1–7.
8. Manson PN, Clifford CM, Hill NT, et al. Mechanism of global support and post traumatic enophthalmous 1. The anatomy of the ligament sling and its relationship to intramuscular cone orbital fat. Plast Reconstr Surg 1986;77:193–202.
9. Manson PN, Grivas MA, Rosenbaum A, et al. Studies of enophthalmous: II. The measure of orbital injuries and their treatment by quantitative computed tomography. Plast Reconstr Surg 1986;77:203–14.
10. Abed SF, Shams P, Shen S, et al. Academic study of cranio-orbital foramen and its significant in orbital surgery. Plast Reconstr Surg 2012;129:307e–11e.
11. van der Meulen JC, Gruss JS. Ocular plastic surgery. London: Mosby-Wolfe; 1996.
12. Fattahi T. Blepharoplasty. In: Fonseca RJ, Marciana A, Turvey TA, editors. Oral and maxillofacial surgery. 2nd edition. Philadelphia: Saunders; 2009.

CT & CBCT Imaging
Assessment of the Orbits

David C. Hatcher, DDS, MSc, MRCD(c)[a,b,c,d,*]

KEYWORDS

- Cone beam computed tomography • Orbital fracture • Orbital imaging • Orbital anatomy

KEY POINTS

- The orbits can be visualized quite easily on routine or customized protocols for computed tomography (CT) or cone beam CT (CBCT) scans.
- The complex geometry of the orbits and their midface location make 2-dimensional imaging methods suboptimal for most clinical investigations; detailed orbital investigations are best performed with 3-dimensional imaging methods.
- CT scans are preferred for visualization of the osseous orbital anatomy and fissures while magnetic resonance imaging is preferred for evaluating tumors and inflammation.
- CBCT provides high-resolution anatomic data of the sinonasal spaces, airway, soft tissue surfaces, and bones but does not provide much detail within the soft tissues.

The orbits can be visualized quite easily on routine or customized protocols for computed tomography (CT) or cone beam CT (CBCT) scans. This article discusses CBCT imaging of the orbits, osseous anatomy of the orbits, and CBCT investigation of selected orbital pathosis.

IMAGING

The maxillofacial region and orbits can be imaged with a variety of methods, including panoramic, cephalometry, magnetic resonance imaging (MRI), CT, planer views, and more recently CBCT.[1] The methods include 2-dimensional and 3-dimensional imaging and imaging in supine and upright positions. The complex geometry of the orbits and their midface location make 2-dimensional imaging methods suboptimal for most clinical investigations. Detailed orbital investigations are best performed with 3-dimensional imaging methods. CT scans are preferred for visualization of the osseous orbital anatomy and fissures while MRI is preferred for evaluating tumors and inflammation. A relatively new 3-dimensional imaging technology, CBCT, was introduced into the North American dental and medical markets in May 2001 and thus created a practical, low-cost, and low-dose opportunity for practitioners to visualize the maxillofacial and adjacent anatomy in 3 dimensions.[2] Maturation or evolution of the CBCT systems has trended toward upright imaging, flat panel detectors, graphical (faster) processing, shorter scan times, pulsed dose, flat panel sensors, and smaller voxel sizes. CBCT provides high-resolution anatomic data of the sinonasal spaces, airway, soft tissue surfaces, and bones but does not provide much detail within the soft tissues.

During a CBCT scan, the scanner (radiographic source and a rigidly coupled sensor) rotates, usually 360°, around the head acquiring multiple

Author has nothing to disclose.

[a] Department of Orthodontics, School of Dentistry, University of Pacific, San Francisco, CA, USA; [b] School of Dentistry, University of Southern Nevada, NV, USA; [c] Orofacial Sciences, School of Dentistry, University of California, San Francisco, CA, USA; [d] Private Practice, Diagnostic Digital Imaging, 99 Scripps Drive, # 101, Sacramento, CA 95825, USA
* Diagnostic Digital Imaging, 99 Scripps Drive, # 101, Sacramento, CA 95825.
E-mail address: david@ddicenters.com

Oral Maxillofacial Surg Clin N Am 24 (2012) 537–543
http://dx.doi.org/10.1016/j.coms.2012.07.003
1042-3699/12/$ – see front matter © 2012 Elsevier Inc. All rights reserved.

images (ranging from approximately 150 to 599 separate and unique projection views).[2] Raw image data are collected from the scan and reconstructed into a viewable format. The scan time can range between 5 and 70 seconds depending on machine brand and protocol setting. The radiograph source emits a low milliampere-shaped or divergent beam. The beam size is constrained (circular or rectangular) to match the sensor size but in some cases can be further constrained (collimated) to match the anatomic region of interest. The field of view for a medium field of view scan includes the rostralcaudal area between the cranial base and menton. Following the scan, the resultant image set or (raw) data set is subjected to a reconstruction process that results in the production of a digital volume of anatomic data that can be visualized with specialized software. The smallest subunit of a digital volume is a volume element (voxel). CBCT voxels are generally isotropic (x, y, and z dimensions are equal) and range in size from approximately 0.07 mm to 0.4 mm per side. The average voxel size for an airway study is 0.3 mm^3. Each voxel is assigned a gray scale value that approximates the attenuation value of the represented tissue or space.

DATA VISUALIZATION

The reconstructed volumes are ready for viewing using specialized software. The voxel volume can be retrieved and viewed with various viewing options. Visualization options include multiplanar or orthogonal (coronal, axial, sagittal) viewing angles. The data can be sliced as single voxel row or column at a time. The multiple voxel layers can be combined to create a slab and then visualized. It is possible to produce and visualize oblique and curved slices or slabs. The entire volume can be rendered and visualized from any angle. There are several techniques for visualizing a volume, including shaded surface display and volume rendering. All CBCT units are installed with viewing software, but third-party software is also available for general viewing or specialized applications, such as surgical planning software. Software has been optimized to measure orbital volumes, and the clinical application of this software will be discussed in a subsequent section of the article.

ANATOMIC ACCURACY

The accuracy of CBCT measurement when compared with physical caliper measures has been reported to be 0.00 plus or minus 0.22.[3,4] The precision is also very high. Theoretically the CBCT accuracy should be plus or minus the voxel size. Primary reconstruction of raw scan data results in a digital volume typically has a cylindrical shape (flat panel sensors). This digital volume is composed of isotropic voxels that are stacked in rows and columns. The voxel size for orbital studies ranges from 0.2 mm^3 to 0.4 mm^3. The image quality or ability to detect small features is related to physical characteristics of digital images. The physical characteristics are represented by dynamic range (number of gray levels), volume averaging, modulation transfer function, Nyquist-Shannon sampling theorem, and signal-to-noise ratio.

NYQUIST SAMPLING FREQUENCY

Sampling is the process of converting continuous analog signals, such as anatomy, into discrete digital data by recording data points of the analog signals at regular intervals in space. Quantization is the process of digitizing the amplitude of the continuous analog signals into a set of discrete values. For example, quantization of a black and white picture into a 12-bit (2^{12}) digital image (dynamic range) involves converting the value of each sampled point to an integer value between 0 and 4096, with 0 representing black, 4096 representing white and the values in between representing various shades and intensities of gray. The ultimate goal of sampling is to take enough samples to enable an accurate reconstruction of the original image. The Nyquist-Shannon sampling theorem defines how often each sample should be taken in space for an accurate reconstruction of the original analog signals. Samples are taken in the unit of space in cubic millimeters (defined as a pixel) for a 2-dimensional image, or in a unit of space in cubic millimeters (defined as a voxel) for a 3-dimensional image. The Nyquist-Shannon sampling theorem states that for a continuous, band-limited analog signal to be recovered from a set of sample points, the samples are to be taken at a rate greater than twice the highest frequency of the original analog signal. For example, applying the Nyquist-Shannon sampling theorem in digital image processing to visualize and represent accurately anatomic structures that are at least 0.4 mm, a voxel size of 0.2 mm is required.[5,6] The visual detection of anatomic features can be a function of sampling frequency and contrast variance, which is referred to as the modulation transfer function (MTF). MTF is the contrast at a given spatial frequency relative to the contrast at low frequencies. Spatial frequency can be expressed as line pairs per millimeter and contrast as the ratio of the luminance of white to that of black. The best opportunity to detect fine anatomic detail occurs with a high sampling frequency and high contrast. Low sampling frequency, low contrast, or both reduces the visualization of fine anatomic detail. The contrast ratio decreases with the reduction in signal and the introduction of noise. Spiral CT has higher contrast than CBCT, but it generally has lower spatial frequency, particularly in the longitudinal direction. The maintenance of high contrast and increase in spatial frequency for a spiral CT is associated with a higher dose.[7]

VOLUME AVERAGING

When digitizing the amplitude of a continuous analog signal, the discrete value representing the voxel will be the average of all anatomic structures within the voxel. When the anatomic structures within the voxel are relatively homogenous (that is, the voxel either contains all hard tissue, all soft tissue, or all air), the final average will be representative of the structures. However, when the voxel contains a mixture of soft tissue and air, especially when the original analog signal differs dramatically, the average value of the soft tissue and air will not be representative of either structure. When several voxels in proximity are misrepresented due to the effect of volume averaging, the ambiguous region may result in misinterpretation and may not represent a precise boundary.[8,9]

SIGNAL-TO-NOISE RATIO

Signal is useful information used to build an anatomic image, and it can be corrupted by noise information. The signal is compiled from the multiangular images produced during the image acquisition cycle (150–599 images). Increasing the milliamperes and increasing the number of angular images acquired will increase the signal. There are many sources of noise that can degrade a CBCT image, but the most significant sources are related to patient motion and scatter artifact, particularly scatter artifacts associated with dense objects such as metallic restorations.

ATTENUATION VALUES

Hounsfield units (HU) express the relative attenuation value of various anatomic tissues or spaces. For example, the HU scale transforms the anatomic attenuation coefficient measurements to a scale that is calibrated to give the radiodensity of distilled water (standard pressure and temperature) an HU of zero. The relative HU of other substances are air (-1000 HU), fat (-120 HU), muscle (+ 40 HU) and bone (+ 400 HU). CBCT produces relatively poor contrast between tissues, which has limited its value for the conversion of the tissue attenuation values to HU.[10]

DOSE

The effective dose is expressed as micro/Sieverts (μSv). The effective dose for CBCT machines is not homogeneous with dose variations related to the machine settings (milliamperes, kilovolt [peak] [kV(p)], time), field of view, signal requirements, sensor type, pulse, or continuous exposure. The effective dose for CBCT (87 μSv) is greater than a cephalometric projection (14.2–24.3 μSv) but less than a conventional CT scan (860 μSv).[11,12]

ORBITAL ANATOMY
Osseous Anatomy

The orbit is formed by frontal, maxillary, ethmoid, lacrimal, zygomatic, sphenoid, and palatine bones (**Fig. 1**).

Frontal bone
The frontal bone forms the superior rim and anterior portion of the roof.

Maxillary bone
The maxillary bone (MB) forms the anterior portion of the floor and the inferomedial orbital rim.

Zygomatic bone
The zygomatic bone (ZB) forms inferolateral rim and the anterior portion of the floor and lateral walls.

Lacrimal bone
The lacrimal bone (LB) forms the portion of the medial wall posterior to the maxillary and anterior to the ethmoid bone.

Ethmoid bone
The portion of ethmoid bone (EB) that covers the middle and posterior ethmoid air cells forms the midportion of the medial orbital wall. The ethmoid portion of the orbital can be very thin, fractures easily, and is sometimes referred to as the lamina papyracea.

Palatine bone
The palatine bone (PB) forms a very small portion of the inferomedial wall between the ethmoid, maxillary and sphenoid bones.

Sphenoid bone
The sphenoid bone (SB) forms the posterior portions of the medial and lateral walls. The greater wing of the SB (GWS) is medial and superior to the superior orbital fissure and the lesser wing of SB (LWS) is located lateral and inferior to the superior orbital fissure.

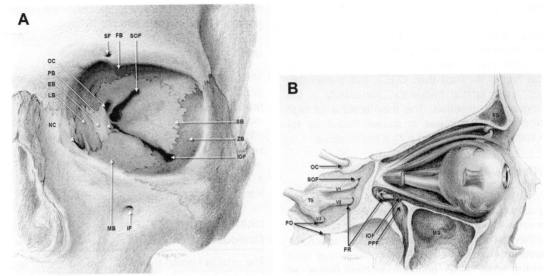

Fig. 1. (*A*) This anatomic illustration shows the osseous anatomy of the left orbit. The 7 bones forming the orbit are: FB; frontal bone; ZB, zygomatic Bone; MB, maxillary bone; LB, lacrimal bone; EB, ethmoid bone; SB, sphenoid bone; PB, palatine bone. The fissures, formina and canals in and adjacent to the orbit are: SOF, superior orbital fissure; IOF, inferior orbital fissure; OC, optic canal; NC, nasolacrimal canal; SF, supraorbital canal and IF, infraorbital canal. Graphics by Robin French. (*B*) This anatomic illustration shows a lateral view of the right orbit and adjacent structures. *Abbreviations:* OC, optic canal; SOF, superior orbital fissure; TG, trigeminal ganglia; V1, cranial nerve V1; V2, cranial nerve V2; V3; cranial nerve V3; FO, foramen ovale; FR, foramen rotundum; IOF, inferior orbital fissure; PPF, pterygopalatine foramen; MS, maxillary sinus; FS, frontal sinus. Graphic by Robin French.

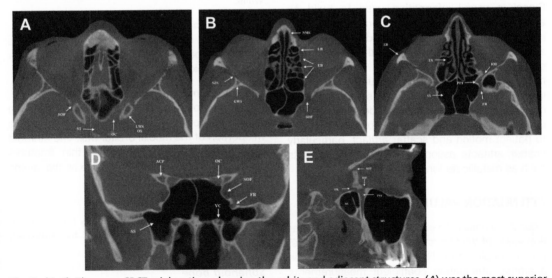

Fig. 2. (*A–C*): These are CBCT axial sections showing the orbits and adjacent structures. (*A*) was the most superior section, and (*C*) was the most inferior section. (*D*) is a coronal section demonstrating the anatomy posterior to the orbits. (*E*) is a sagittal section showing the orbits and adjacent anatomy. *Abbreviations*: SOF, superior orbital fissure; ST, sella turcica; OC, optic canal; LWS OS, lesser wing of sphenoid bone osseous strut; SZS, sphenozygomatic suture; GWS, greater wing of sphenoid bone; EB, ethmoid bone; LB, lacrimal bone; NMS, nasomaxillary suture; ZB, zygomatic bone; ES, ethmoid sinus; SS, sphenoid sinus; PPF, pterygopalatine fissure; FR, foramen rotundum; IOF, inferior orbital fissure; ACP, anterior clinoid process; VC, vidian canal; FS, frontal sinus; MS, maxillary sinus.

FISSURES, FORAMINA, AND CANALS

The major fissures, foramina, and canals within and adjacent to the orbits are the optic canal (OC), superior orbital fissure (SOF), inferior orbital fissure (IOF), foramen rotundum (FR), superior orbital foramen (SF), infraorbital foramen (IF), foramen ovale (FO), and the nasolacrimal canal (NC) (see **Fig. 1**; **Fig. 2**).

Optic Canal

The OC is located in the lesser wing of the SB and contains the cranial nerve 2 and opthalmic artery.

Superior Orbital Fissure

The SOF is located in the SB and separates the greater wing of the sphenoid laterally and the lesser wing of the sphenoid medially. The SOF contains cranial nerves 3, 4, 5 (V1), 6, and superior opthalmic vein.

Inerior Orbital Fissure

The IOF bordered by the ethmoid and maxillary bones on the medial side and the GWS and zygomatic bones medially. The IOF contains cranial nerve 5 (V2), infraorbital artery and vein and inferior ophthalmic veins.

Foramen Rotundum

The FR is located in the SB and caries cranial nerve (V2) from the middle cranial fossa to the superior side of the pterygopalatine fissure and toward the IOF.

Supraorbital Foramen

The SF is located in the frontal bone near the superior orbital rim and contains the supraorbital nerve (V1).

Infraorbital Foramen

The IF is located in the maxillary bone inferior to the infraorbital rim and contains the infraorbital nerve (V2), artery, and vein.

Foramen Ovale

The FO is located in the SB and connects the middle cranial fossa with the infratemporal fossa. The FO contains cranial nerve 5 (V3) and the accessory meningeal artery.

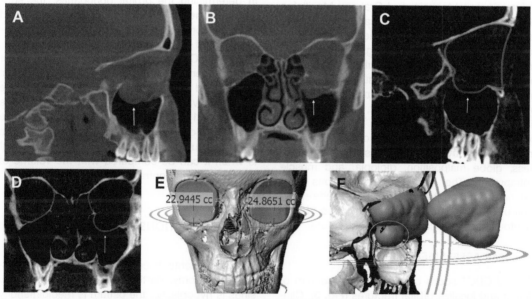

Fig. 3. (*A*) CBCT sagittal section of a 17-year-old girl with a left side orbital floor fracture (blowout fracture). The floor and orbital contents are herniated into the superior region of the left maxillary sinus (*white arrow*). (*B*) Coronal CBCT section of same patient showing orbital floor fracture and inferior displacement of orbital contents (*white arrow*). (*C, D*) CBCT sagittal section of same patient showing segmentation of margins of orbits and herniated portion of the left orbit (*white arrow*) using Stratovan Maxillo software. (*E*) The Stratovan Maxillo software computed the volume of the normal right orbit (22.9445 cc) and the left side with the orbital floor fracture (24.8651 cc). (*F*) An oblique posterior view of the rendered orbital volumes. The yellow oval indicates the herniated portion of the left side orbital contents.

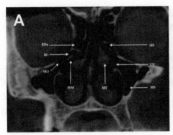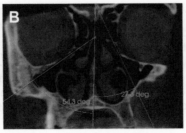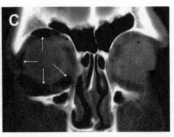

Fig. 4. (A) CBCT coronal view of a patient with a right side hypoplastic sinus. Note the right maxillary ostium was located inferior and medial to the opposite side. *Abbreviations*: Ebu, ethmoid bulla; MI, maxillary infundibulum; MO, maxillary ostium; MM, middle meatus; MT, middle turbinate; MS, maxillary sinus; UP, uncinate process; HS, hiatus similunaris. (B) CBCT coronal view of same patient showing angle formed by the path infundibulum to the midsagittal plane. The angle formed on the side of the hypoplastic sinus is 54° and is twice the angle of the normal sinus side. (C) CT scan coronal view showing orbital air emphysema (*white arrows*) as a sinus endoscopy complication. (*Courtesy of* E. Bradley Strong, MD, Department of Otolaryngology, University of California Davis Medical Center.)

Nasolacrimal Canal

The NC is located in the anteromedial region of the orbit and is bordered by the lacrimal and maxillary bones. The NC contains the lacrimal duct.

ANATOMIC VARIATIONS

The normal orbital volumes are bilaterally symmetric to within 1 cc (Strong EB, Fuller SC, Wiley D. Computer aided analysis of orbital volume: a novel technique. J Oral and Maxillafac Surg 2012. submitted for publication).[13–15] There is a linear relationship between an acquired change in orbital volume and globe position. It has been measured that an acquired enlargement of orbital volume of 1cc can result in 0.62 to 1.6 mm of enopthalmos. Enopthalmos of 2 mm or more can be clinically significant, producing functional or esthetic deformities.[16,17] Significant orbital volume enlargement secondary to orbital fractures can have complications including blindness, globe malposition, diplopia, and muscle entrapment. The fracture complications may extend beyond orbit enlargement to include extrusion of orbital contents, fat atrophy, loss of ligamentous support, scarring, and contracture.

VOLUME ASSESSMENT OF ORBITS

CT and CBCT scans can be used to confirm or detect and localize orbital fractures (**Fig. 3**). Clinical objectives related the assessment of orbital fractures include determination of acute enopthalmos, muscle entrapment, and orbital bone displacement. Surgical intervention is indicated when there is muscle entrapment and/or significant enopthalmos and orbital bone displacement. Enopthalmos and muscle entrapment can be clinically assessed, while the evaluation of orbital bone displacement is an imaging endeavor. Clinical experience in assessing the degree of orbital bone displacement has historically been the state-of-the-art practice, but third-party software (Stratovan Maxillo, Stratovan Corporation, Sacramento, California) has been recently developed to assess orbital volume. The Stratovan Maxillo software employs a semiautomated and novel process to bilaterally measure orbital volumes. In determining the orbital boundaries, the software segments off the osseous margins and uses a proprietary algorithm to create pseudosurface to bind the open spaces in the bony orbit existing from CT volume averaging defects, anterior orbital aperture, optic canal, superior orbital fissure, and inferior orbital fissure. This software has been validated, showing that the average error of 0.1 cc for a single operator and the inter-operator error was less than 0.2 cc. The optimal volume assessment of an involved orbit is when it can be compared with the volume of the un-involved contralateral orbit.

ORBITAL RELATIONSHIP TO OSTIOMEATAL UNITS

The orbital contents can be at risk during a maxillary antrostomy, particularly when the maxillary sinus is hypoplastic; the ostium is medioinferiorly positioned, and the infundibulum has a relatively horizontal angulation. The altered ostiomeatal anatomy associated with a hypoplastic maxillary sinus exposes the medioinferior sinus wall to disruption from a microdebrider during endoscopic surgery (**Fig. 4**). Orbital complications from sinus surgery include aspiration of orbital fat, rectus muscle trauma, scarring and sino-orbital communication.

SUMMARY

CT scans are preferred for visualization of the osseous orbital anatomy and fissures, while MRI is preferred for evaluating tumors and inflammation. A relatively new 3-dimensional imaging technology, CBCT, was introduced into the North American dental and medical markets in May 2001 and thus created a practical, low-cost, and low-dose opportunity for practitioners to visualize the maxillofacial and adjacent anatomy in 3 dimensions.[2]

REFERENCES

1. Hatcher DC. Cone beam computed tomography: craniofacial and airway analysis. Sleep Med Clin 2010;5:59–70.
2. Hatcher DC. Operational principles for cone beam CT. J Am Dent Assoc 2010;141(Suppl 3):3S–6S.
3. Stratemann S, Huang JC, Maki K, et al. Comparison of cone beam computed tomography (CBCT) imaging to physical measures. Dentomaxillofac Radiol 2008;37:1–14.
4. Stratemann S, Huang JC, Maki K, et al. Methods for evaluating the human mandible using cone beam computed tomography (CBCT). Am J Orthod Dentofacial Orthop 2010;137:S58–70.
5. Diniz P, Da Silva E, Netto S. Digital signal processing: system analysis and design. New York: Cambridge University Press; 2002. p. 24.
6. Blackledge J. Digital signal processing: mathematical and computational methods, software development, and applications. Chichester (England): Horwood; 2003. p. 93.
7. Watanabe H, Honda E, Tetsumrua A, et al. A comparative study for spatial resolution and subjective image characteristics of multi-slice CT and a cone-beam CT for dental use. Eur J Radiol 2011;77(3):397–402.
8. Zou Y, Sidky EY, Pan X. Partial volume and aliasing artifacts in helical cone-beam CT. Phys Med Biol 2004;49(11):2365–75.
9. Goodenough D. Tomographic imaging. In: Beutel J, Kundel HL, Van Metter RL, editors. Handbook of medical imaging, Vol. 1. Physics and psychophysics. Bellingham (Washington): SPIE Press; 2000. p. 511–52.
10. Yamashina A, Tanimoto K, Sutthiprapaporn P, et al. The reliability of computed tomography (CT) values and dimensional measurements of the oropharyngeal region using cone beam CT: comparison with multi-detector CT. Dentomaxillofac Radiol 2008; 37(5):245–51.
11. Ludlow JB, Ivanovic M. Compariative dosimetery of dental CBCT devices and 64-slice CT for oral and maxillofacial radiology. Oral Surg Oral Med Oral Pathol Oral Radiol Endod 2008;106(1):106–14.
12. Ludlow JB, Davies-Ludlow LE, White SC. Patient risk related to common dental radiographic examinations: the impact of 2007 Internal Commission on Radiological Protection recommendations regarding dose calculation. J Am Dent Assoc 2008;139:1237–43.
13. Fan X, Li J, Zhu J, et al. Computer-assisted orbital volume measurement in surgical correction of late enophthalmos caused by blowout fracture. Ophthal Plast Reconstr Surg 2003;19:207–11.
14. Whitehouse RW, Batterbury M, Jackson A, et al. Prediction of enopthalmos by computed tomography after 'blow out' orbital fractures. Br J Ophthalmol 1994;78:618–20.
15. Raskin EM, Millman AL, Lubkin V, et al. Prediction of late enophthalmos by volumetric analysis of orbital fractures. Ophthal Plast Reconstr Surg 1998;14: 19–26.
16. Osguthorpe JD. Ortibital wall fractures: evaluation and management. Otolaryngol head Neck Surg 1991;105:702–7.
17. Parsons GS, Mathog RH. Orbital wall and volume relationships. Arch Otolaryngol Head Neck Surg 1988;114:743–7.

Growth and Development of the Orbit

Aaron J. Berger, MD, PhD, David Kahn, MD*

KEYWORDS

• Development • Orbit • Aging

KEY POINTS

- The diagnosis and treatment of patients with orbital/periorbital abnormalities requires knowledge of congenital differences and awareness of the changes that occur as individuals age.
- Embryological development and migration of the eyes determines the formation of the surrounding orbital soft tissue and skeletal elements.
- Congenital anomalies of the orbit result from primary defects in the structural architecture of the bony orbit (eg, facial clefts and craniosynostosis) or as a result of defects in development of the eyeball (eg, anophthalmos) and surrounding soft tissues.
- The orbits complete half of postnatal development by age 2, and adult dimensions of the orbit are attained by age 7.
- The first signs of aging in the face become apparent in the late 20s and early 30s, and involve the skin and soft tissues of the face.
- Changes to the bony architecture have been recognized and described but no longitudinal studies using modern imaging technologies have been performed.

INTRODUCTION

Every surgeon operating on the face, and particularly around the eye, should possess a working knowledge of the critical details related to development of the human orbit and recognized changes that occur during the course of aging. The anatomy of the orbit and periorbital region is complex, and the diagnosis and treatment of patients with orbital/periorbital abnormalities requires expertise in congenital differences and awareness of the changes that occur as individuals age.

RELEVANT ANATOMY
Osseous Anatomy

The bones of the face are considered to hang from the skull, with attachments at the frontozygomatic, frontonasal, and frontoethmoidal sutures, and the sphenoid bone.

Seven bones contribute to the orbit:

1. Orbital process of the frontal bone
2. Lesser wing of the sphenoid bone
3. Orbital plate and frontal process of the maxilla
4. Zygoma
5. Orbital plate of the palatine bone
6. Lacrimal bone
7. Lamina papyracea of the ethmoid bone

Muscular Anatomy

The annulus of Zinn (**Fig. 1**) is a dense fibrous band of connective tissue with firm attachments to the periosteum of the orbital apex and the optic nerve sheath. The 4 rectus muscles of the eye arise from the annulus and insert 5.5 to 8 mm behind the limbus of the globe.[1] The inferior oblique muscle arises just lateral to the nasolacrimal duct ostium in the anterior orbit, whereas the superior oblique muscle arises just superior to the superior rectus

Division of Plastic and Reconstructive Surgery, Stanford Hospital and Clinics, Stanford, CA, USA
* Corresponding author. 770 Welch Road, Suite 400, Palo Alto, CA 94304.
E-mail address: donka1@aol.com

Oral Maxillofacial Surg Clin N Am 24 (2012) 545–555
http://dx.doi.org/10.1016/j.coms.2012.08.001

oralmaxsurgery.theclinics.com

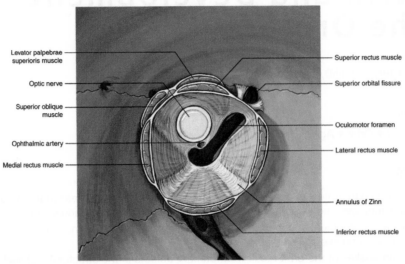

Fig. 1. Annulus of Zinn, anterior surface with origins of the extraocular muscles. (*From* Dutton JJ. Extraocular muscles. In: Dutton JJ, editor. Atlas of clinical and surgical orbital anatomy. 2nd edition. Elsevier; 2011. p. 29–49; with permission.)

muscle. The levator muscle arises from the lesser wing/body of the sphenoid bone.

DEVELOPMENT OF THE ORBIT
Influence of Eye Growth and Migration

Any discussion of orbit development would be incomplete without mention of the importance of the eye and ocular development. The development of the eyes determines the formation of the surrounding orbital soft tissue contents and the bony orbital walls. The growth and migration of the eyes play an important role in the shape and position of the orbits. Growth of the eyes, in particular, provides an expanding force that separates the neural and facial skeletons at the frontomaxillary and frontozygomatic sutures.

The eyeball is derived from surface ectoderm, neural ectoderm, neural crest tissue, and mesoderm. The retina is a direct outgrowth from the forebrain, projecting bilaterally as the optic vesicles. The neuroectodermal optic vesicles induce the overlying surface ectoderm to form the lens placodes. Meningeal ectomesenchyme, of neural crest origin, becomes the sclera, choroid, ciliary bodies, and cornea. Mesoderm invades the structure to form the vitreous body. The extrinsic muscles of the eye are derived from the prechordal somitomeres. Cutaneous ectoderm overlying the cornea form the conjunctiva. Ectodermal folds above and below the cornea become the eyelids.[2]

The eyeballs grow rapidly, and the orbits complete half of their postnatal growth during the first 2 years of life. The adult dimensions of the orbital cavities are usually attained by 7 years of age.[2] Dimensions of the adult orbit include an approximate volume of 30 mL, a lid skin to orbital apex depth of 5 cm, and an overall quadrangular pear shape sweeping toward the medially situated apex.[1] If the globe is absent or microphthalmic (seen in cases of radiation therapy for retinoblastoma), the orbit will fail to reach its normal volume.

FETAL DEVELOPMENT OF THE ORBIT

The scaffolding of the orbital bones is established within the first 2 months of embryogenesis.[3] Migration of neural crest cells over the face follows 2 routes, which meet in the area of the orbit (**Fig. 2**). The frontonasal anlage migrates over the prosencephalon, approaching the orbit from

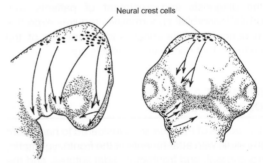

Fig. 2. Neural crest cells arise along the dorsolateral part of the neural tube and migrate ventrally to fill in the upper facial process in 2 waves. The frontonasal anlage migrates over the prosencephalon, whereas the maxillary wave migrates from caudal to cranial. (*From* Johnston MC. A radioautographic study of the migration and fate of cranial neural crest cells in the chick embryo. Anat Rec 1966;156:147; with permission.)

above, whereas the maxillary wave curves around the developing eye from below.[1] The frontonasal process gives rise to the lacrimal and ethmoid bones. The floor and lateral walls of the orbit are components of the maxillary process (**Fig. 3**).

The significance of this migratory pattern plays a role in understanding the pathogenesis of congenital orbital, eyelid, and lacrimal anomalies. For example, failure of fusion between the neural crest waves results in clefting syndromes around the orbit. Additionally, the typical location of dermoid cysts at the frontozygomatic and frontoethmoidal suture line results from sequestration of surface ectoderm in areas of neural crest cell fusion.[1]

The orbital bones ossify and fuse between the sixth and seventh months of gestation. Except for the lesser wing of the sphenoid, which arises from a cartilaginous construct, all of the orbital bones (including the greater wing of the sphenoid) arise from membranous connective tissue.

The eyes gradually converge from an initial 180° relation to each other at 2 months' gestation to a 71° relation at birth. The orbital axis remains somewhat divergent at birth, and postnatal changes in skull growth contribute to the final position of the orbits. In particular, the orbit is nearly hemispheric at birth, and the bony perimeters closely hug the globe (**Fig. 4**).[1]

SINUS FORMATION

The ethmoid sinuses take their shape between the sixth and eighth weeks of gestation, and they are fully developed at birth. However, the remaining paranasal sinuses develop later. The maxillary sinus borders the orbital floor and is fully

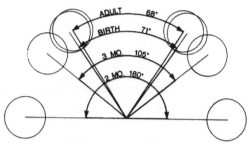

Fig. 4. Convergence of the orbits. Angular separation of the globes at 2 months' gestation, 3 months' gestation, birth, and adulthood. (*From* Fries PD, Katowitz JA. Congenital craniofacial anomalies of ophthalmic importance. Surv Ophthalmol 1990;35: 87; with permission.)

pneumatized at 2 to 4 years of age. The sphenoid and frontal sinuses continue to pneumatize into early adulthood.[1]

EXTRAOCULAR MUSCLE DEVELOPMENT

The 6 extraocular muscles develop from 3 separate mesenchymal areas around 4 weeks' gestation. The associated oculomotor (cranial nerve III) and abducens (cranial nerve VI) nerves grow into the developing muscles around the same time. The muscle cone develops around the optic nerve, and the shared apical tendinous insertions of the 4 rectus muscles become the annulus of Zinn. Just posterior to the superomedial orbital rim, the fibrous trochlea of the superior oblique muscle develops and ultimately becomes cartilaginous.[1]

LACRIMAL SYSTEM DEVELOPMENT

The entire lacrimal drainage apparatus is of ectodermal origin. A solid cord of epithelium forms in the region of the medial lower eyelid in utero. This cord sends projections temporally to form the canaliculi and inferiorly to form the nasolacrimal duct. Canalization of these structures begins at 4 months of gestation and may continue after birth. In fact, the most inferior portion of the nasolacrimal duct is imperforate at birth in 50% to 70% of individuals (**Fig. 5**).[1]

CONGENITAL DEFORMITIES OF THE ORBIT

Congenital anomalies of the orbit can result from primary defects in the structural architecture of the bony orbit or as a result of defects in development of the eyeball and surrounding soft tissues. Because the orbit represents a bridge between the face and the cranium, ocular and adnexal abnormalities are a frequent element of craniofacial anomalies. The major craniofacial anomalies that

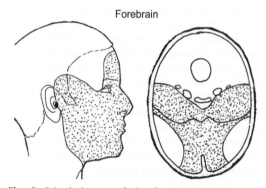

Forebrain

Fig. 3. Stippled area of the face indicate the soft tissues and bones of the skull formed by neural crest cells. (*From* Johnston MC, Bhakdinaronk A, Reid YC. An expanded role of the neural crest in oral and pharyngeal development. In: Bosma JF, editor. The Fourth Symposium on Oral Sensation and Perception. Bethesda (MD): National Institutes of Health; 1973. p. 37–52. HEW Pub No 73–546.)

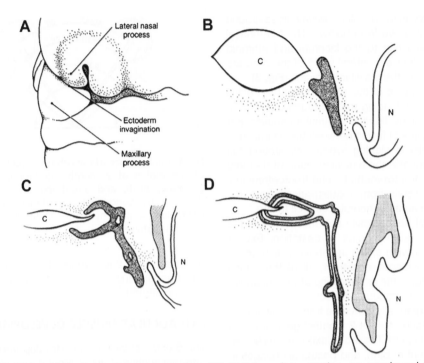

Fig. 5. Embryology of the lacrimal drainage system. (*A*) At 5.5 weeks' gestation, an ectodermal invagination forms between the lateral nasal process and maxillary process, which becomes pinched off from the surface. (*B*) At 6 weeks' gestation, a solid cord of ectoderm is located between the primitive medial canthus and nose. (*C*) At 12 weeks' gestation, proliferation of the cord occurs laterally toward the eyelid and inferiorly toward the inferior turbinate. The isolated cavities shown appear at 3 to 4 months. (*D*) At 7 months, canalization is nearly complete, with only the puncta and valve of Henle remaining imperforate. (*From* Doxanas MT, Anderson RL. Clinical orbital anatomy. Baltimore (MD): Williams & Wilkins; 1984. p. 9; with permission.)

involve the orbits include the craniosynostoses and the clefting syndromes.

Localized Anomalies of the Orbit

Anophthalmia/microphthalmia
Primary localized anomalies of the orbit include microphthalmia/anophthalmia and cystic anomalies. Anophthalmia is rare, and results from failure of optic vesicle development. Microphthalmia results from incomplete invagination of the optic vesicle or closure of the embryonic fissure. Both of these conditions are typically unilateral, and may be found in association with other craniofacial and systemic anomalies, including orbital hypoplasia, facial clefts, basal encephalocele, hemifacial microsomia, mandibulofacial dysostosis, cardiac anomalies, polydactyly, and mental retardation.

Anophthalmia and microphthalmia are often associated with contracture of the conjunctival fornices, phimotic eyelids, and generalized hypoplasia of the periocular soft tissues.[4] Treatment of soft tissue and bone hypoplasia involves the use of conformers and tissue expanders (or serial implantation of progressively larger orbital implants) to stimulate orbit bone development.[5–8]

Cystic anomalies of the orbit
Several congenital cystic structures may develop in or around the orbit, including meningoencephaloceles, mucoceles, dermoid cysts, teratomas, and epithelial cysts.[4] Dermoid cysts are the most common congenital orbital anomalies, and they arise from ectodermal nests that are trapped by fusion of the bony sutures around the orbit. They typically develop around the frontozygomatic suture but can also been found at the frontonasal and frontolacrimal sutures. They usually present during the first decade of life as a well-circumscribed, firm, rubbery subcutaneous mass just below the temporal eyebrow.[4]

Craniosynostosis
Craniosynostosis is defined as premature fusion of bony sutures of the skull. Although several well-recognized syndromes are associated with craniosynostosis, it is more commonly sporadic in appearance. The phenotypic pattern (ie, the abnormal shape of the skull) is the direct result of

the sutures involved. Simple craniosynostosis refers to the premature closure of a single suture, and compound craniosynostosis involves 2 or more sutures.

Early intervention in craniosynostosis is recommended to permit "expansion of the brain" and capitalize on the plasticity (and regenerative potential) of the calvarium in infants. Early intervention typically results in a better cosmetic result, and also has been proposed to lower intracranial pressure and permit normal visual and mental development. The various surgical techniques to correct craniosynostosis are beyond the scope of this review. In general, cranioplasty for craniosynostosis involves reorganization and reshaping of the calvarium, including frontal and facial bone advancement. Additional procedures, including Le Fort III osteotomies and, more recently, internal distraction devices address maxillary hypoplasia and shallow orbits.[4]

Crouzon syndrome

Crouzon syndrome was first described in 1912 as hereditary craniofacial dysostosis.[9] It is characterized by the triad of compound craniosynostosis, midface retrusion, and exorbitism. Prevalence is 16.5 cases per million live births and accounts for 4.8% of all cases of craniosynostosis, making it the most common of the craniosynostosis syndromes. It is seen in many different ethnic groups and has an autosomal dominant inheritance pattern. However, 25% of cases have no family history of the disorder, suggesting that spontaneous mutations may play a prominent role in this disorder. Molecular analyses have shown that mutations in the FGFR2 gene on chromosome 10q25–q26 can cause Crouzon syndrome.[10,11]

Calvarial suture synostosis in Crouzon syndrome varies, and no single head shape is uniquely characteristic of this syndrome. However, most patients with Crouzon syndrome have brachycephaly from coronal suture synostosis. Radiographic evidence of coronal and sagittal suture synostosis is seen in 96% to 98% of patients, and 79% have lambdoidal synostosis.[12]

The orbit and maxillary bones are affected by premature suture fusion. In particular, the midface retrusion and shallow orbits seen in Crouzon syndrome result from hypoplasia of the ethmoid, frontal, maxillary, and sphenoid bones. The exorbitism these patients experience can result in exposure keratopathy, and preventative treatment should begin early.

Apert syndrome

Apert syndrome (acrocephalosyndactyly type I) was described by Apert[13] in 1906. The craniofacial anomalies seen with Apert syndrome are similar to those seen in Crouzon but are usually more severe; the major difference is that Apert syndrome involves varying degrees of syndactyly. Mutations in the FGFR2 gene are also responsible for Apert syndrome. Although the syndrome is inherited in an autosomal dominant fashion, most cases are sporadic.

The craniosynostotic component of Apert syndrome typically involves the coronal sutures, resulting in brachycephaly, although multiple and variable suture involvement has been described. Similar to Crouzon syndrome, the phenotype includes hypoplasia of the midface, hypertelorism, and shallow orbits with exorbitism.

Pfeiffer syndrome

Pfeiffer syndrome was first described in 1964, and includes the combination of craniosynostosis, broad thumbs and toes, and partial syndactyly of the fingers and toes.[14] This syndrome has been associated with mutations in the FGFR2 and FGFR1 genes. These patients usually present with bilateral coronal synostosis, and the ophthalmic manifestations are similar to those seen in Apert and Crouzon syndromes, although usually less severe.[9]

Facial clefting syndromes

Facial clefts result from defects in opposition of junctional structures. Tessier[15] developed an anatomic classification system for this diverse set of congenital facial anomalies in 1976. The Tessier classification system numbers the clefts based on their location in relation to the orbit. Each cleft is numbered from 0 to 14 in a clock-like circle, beginning at 0 in the lower facial midline and running clockwise on the right side of the face (counterclockwise on the left), ending at 14 in the upper facial midline cleft (**Fig. 6**). The Tessier classification is purely descriptive and provides no pathogenetic or etiologic information. The cause of facial clefts is poorly understood, and likely a result of both genetic and environmental influences.

Several syndromes, some with known genetic origin, display periorbital clefts, including Treacher Collins syndrome, oculoauriculovertebral dysplasia, and hemifacial microsomia. Treacher Collins syndrome has been associated with a balanced translocation of chromosome 5, affecting the TCOF1 gene (codes for treacle, a nucleolar trafficking protein).[16,17] The syndrome includes hypoplasia of the mandible and zygoma, antimongoloid palpebral slant, pseudocoloboma (or true notching) at the lateral lower lid, hypoplasia of the lashes over the medial two-thirds of

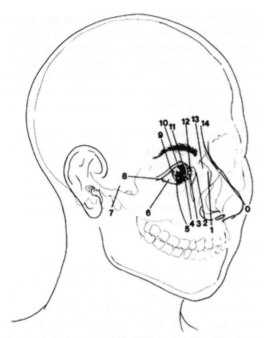

Fig. 6. Facial clefts. Skull with adnexal soft tissue showing Tessier's classification of facial clefts. (*From* Fries J, Katowitz JA. Congenital craniofacial anomalies of ophthalmic importance. Surv Ophthalmol 1990; 35(2):87–119; with permission.)

the lower lid, external and middle ear abnormalities, deafness, macrostomia with malocclusion and abnormal dentition, pretragal fistulae, and inferior extension of the sideburns onto the upper cheek.[18] Oculoauriculovertebral dysplasia, which includes Goldenhar syndrome, presents with unilateral aplasia/hypoplasia of the mandibular ramus, external ear abnormalities, and preauricular fistulae. Ocular anomalies associated with oculoauriculovertebral dysplasia may include corneoscleral dermoids, upper eyelid colobomas, ptosis, nasolacrimal anomalies, horizontal palpebral fissure shortening, and eyelid skin tags.[9] Hemifacial microsomia demonstrates a highly variable phenotype, which may include microphthalmia, and associated small orbital size/volume.[9]

Hypertelorism and hypotelorism
Orbital hypertelorism is defined as an abnormally wide distance between the orbits. It is not a syndrome but rather a physical finding found in a variety of craniofacial anomalies. The normal distance between the orbits is approximately 16 mm at birth, and increases to 25 to 28 mm in adults.[19] Hypotelorism (narrowed interorbital distance) is the result of premature fusion of the metopic suture. This synostosis restricts growth

perpendicular to the midline suture, resulting in trigonocephaly (triangular-shaped cranial vault).

Anatomically, the anterior ethmoid air cells are widened in hypertelorism, with an associated increase in the soft tissue, bone, and cartilage between the medial canthi.[20] Several facial clefts, craniosynostoses, and meningoencephaloceles have been associated with hypertelorism. Surgical correction of the condition involves osteotomies to all 4 walls of the orbits, removal of excess intervening tissues, and a narrowing of the space between the orbits.[4]

Meningoencephalocele
A meningoencephalocele is defined as a herniation of brain and meningeal tissue through defects in the calvarial skeleton. Herniation into the orbit is usually associated with facial clefts that may occur between the sutures of the frontal, ethmoidal, lacrimal, or nasal bones.

Other rare congenital anomalies affecting the orbit
Anencephaly, the absence of the brain, is a severe congenital birth defect that is incompatible with life. The vault of the skull is absent, and the orbits are shallow and tilted upward. Cyclopia/synophthalmos is another rare congenital anomaly characterized by a single eye situated in a single median orbit. This disorder results from a failure of lateralization of the midline facial structures.[4]

Changes occurring within and around the orbit with aging
Aging is a dynamic process that involves gravitational forces, atrophy, changes in skin elasticity, and changes to the bony skeleton. The attributes of a youthful periorbital area include a palpebral fissure that is narrow, a lower lid that is short, contours that are smooth and a cheek that is full.[21–23] The hallmarks of the aging periorbital region can include descent of the brow with resultant lateral hooding, the development of crow's feet, changes in pigmentation and texture, the perception of redundant and lax lid skin (dermatochalasis), and an increasing prominence of the lid–cheek junction and tear trough. The first signs of aging typically become apparent in the late 20s and early 30s, and involve the skin and soft tissues of the face.

Surgical procedures designed to reverse the effects of aging have progressed from "skin tightening" facelifts to interventions focused on facial reshaping and filling areas of atrophy. This progression reflects a greater awareness among cosmetic surgeons of the changes that occur as humans age.

Historically, studies of the aging face have relied on 2-dimensional standard photography and surgeon gestalt. A particular procedure may improve the signs of aging; hence, aging must occur in reverse to what the surgeon had performed. For example, elevating the lid–check junction created a more youthful smooth contoured–appearing eyelid, thus the lid–cheek junction must descend with age.

More recently, 3-dimensional analyses (with CT and MRI) and studies incorporating cephalometric data have been performed to evaluate changes that occur within the aging face.[24–26] However, no longitudinal studies of the aging face have been conducted using modern imaging techniques, and most studies have relied on mother/daughter comparisons or pooling of imaging data from different age groups (ie, cross-sectional studies). Critical analysis of the published literature reveals that, factual/scientific knowledge of changes occurring in the face and periorbital area as a person ages is limited.

Skin and soft tissue changes

With respect to the periorbital region, aging changes are first noted in the skin, including thinning of the skin, changes in pigment and texture, and the appearance of dynamic rhytids at the lateral canthi, known as *crow's feet*. Dermatochalasis (redundant eyelid skin) becomes apparent with increasing laxity to the upper eyelid, and can lead to the appearance of pseudoptosis. Lower lid skin and orbital septum laxity leads to the development of infraorbital festoons or bags.[27]

With respect to the subcutaneous soft tissues, orbicularis muscle laxity and changes in fat position contribute to the signs of aging. What actually occurs is unclear. Some suggest that lower lid fat protrudes, and malar fat descends, resulting in the nasojugal groove becoming more prominent.[27] Others have suggested that the atrophy or descent of the fat underneath the orbicularis muscle (retro-orbicularis and suborbicularis oculi fat) is the cause of the changes in eyelid contour and shape.[28] Camp and colleagues[25] compared 3-dimensional images of matched mother/daughter faces, and showed that there is a consistent pattern of atrophy and regression of soft tissues associated with the medial canthus and nasojugal groove, with the greatest atrophy in the medial canthal region and soft tissues caudal to the lower lid. Additionally, an increase in laxity of the canthal tendons can contribute to the aging appearance of the eye, contributing to the development of increasing scleral show, and possible ectropion.[29]

Lambros[30] compared closely matched photographs of individuals taken over time, attempting to control for differences in the images and then creating animations of these aligned images. He found that descent was not a major component of the changes seen with aging, particularly in the lid–cheek junction. In a similar fashion, the authors and some of their colleagues have observed that the brows seem to descend far less than surgeons elevate them, and that many patients have a false image of how they appeared in youth. Yaremchuk and colleagues,[31] in their article on reversing brow lifts, reviewed some of the literature regarding brow position, which seem to confirm that eyebrows may change shape but do not seem to change position consistently or significantly. More recently, Papageorgiou and colleagues[32] even challenged the concept of volume loss in the brow, noting a trend toward an increase in galeal and brow fat volumes.

In summary, with respect to the effects of aging on the periorbital soft tissues, the jury is still out. Based on the authors' review of the literature, their current working hypothesis is that descent or gravitational changes may play a role, but those effects are probably far less significant than traditionally thought. It seems to the authors that changes in fat distribution result in an unmasking of the differences in soft tissue thickness and texture, exposing the underlying musculoskeletal framework. They believe that some atrophy of the retro-orbicularis oculi and suborbicularis oculi fat pads occurs, and likely thinning of the subdermal fat. Finally, the changes from aging that the body undergoes are likely similar for all patients, and the differences in appearance between individuals probably relates to their own anatomic relationships (eg, vector relationship of the globe to the orbital rim).

Bony changes

In addition to soft tissue changes, including atrophy and descent, skeletal changes play a role in the aging face. Recent data support the concept that the aging process is associated with a loss of projection of the midface skeleton.[23,26,33–35]

Past studies by the senior author (D.K.) analyzing the midface, orbit, and mandible in 120 subjects have shown that bony aging of the orbit and midface is a process primarily of contraction and morphologic change.[35–38] Additionally, Richard and colleagues[33] reviewed CT scans on 100 consecutive patients, comparing a young cohort with an older cohort. They noted statistically significant decreases in glabellar, orbital, maxillary, and pyriform angles. Although previously reported by Pessa and colleagues,[34] they also note a relative rotation of the facial skeleton around the orbit. The frontal bone is observed to move anteriorly and inferiorly, whereas the maxilla moves posteriorly and superiorly. This angular rotation of the bones results in loss of support to the overlying soft tissues (**Figs. 7** and **8**).

Matros and colleagues[39] showed that skeletal implants may be used to achieve a more youthful appearance, including augmentation of the malar

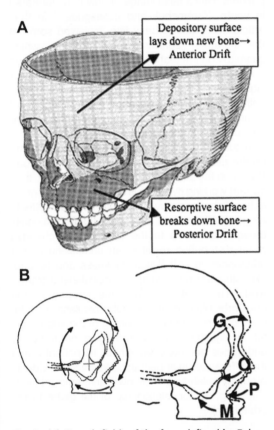

Fig. 7. (A) Growth fields of the face, defined by Enlow, show resorption and deposition within the craniofacial bones. (B) Lambros's algorithm refers to an apparent clockwise rotation of the facial bones when viewing the right side of the face from a lateral direction, which leads to a posterior movement of the inferior maxilla (M) and pyriform (P), and to an anterior movement of the superior orbits (O) and glabella (G). ([A] From Enlow DH. The human face: an account of the postnatal growth and development of the craniofacial skeleton. New York: Harper and Row Publishers; 1968. p. 196; and [B] Pessa JE. An algorithm of facial aging: verification of Lambros's theory by three-dimensional stereolithography, with reference to the pathogenesis of midfacial aging, scleral show, and the lateral suborbital trough deformity. Plast Reconstr Surg 2000;106:479–88 [discussion: 489–90; with permission.)

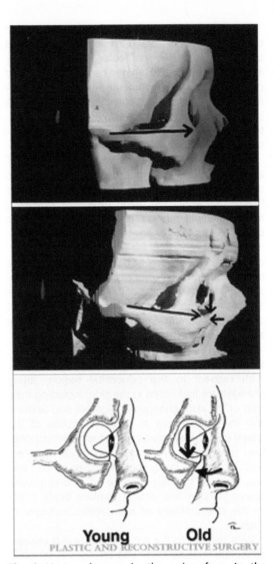

Fig. 8. Vector changes in the aging face. In the youthful face, the vector from the zygomatic arch to the mid-orbit (*long arrow*) is parallel to the horizon (head in cranial base position). As one ages, the vector from the zygomatic arch to the mid-orbit is significantly deflected (*long arrow*). This event is secondary to a vector shift of the orbital rim inferiorly and posteriorly (*short arrows*). The vector of change of the soft tissues of the midface is also inferior and posterior and mimics the vector of change of the orbital rim (*arrows*). This change in orbital rim position has been suggested to be a significant factor in midfacial aging, in addition to pyriform remodeling. (*From* Pessa JE. An algorithm of facial aging: verification of Lambros's theory by three-dimensional stereolithography, with reference to the pathogenesis of midfacial aging, scleral show, and the lateral suborbital trough deformity. Plast Reconstr Surg 2000;106:479–88 [discussion: 489–90]; with permission.)

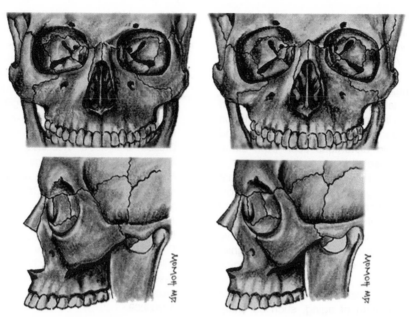

Fig. 9. Summary of age-related changes to the midface skeleton. (*Left*) Features of a youthful skull include a malar eminence, infraorbital rim, and piriform aperture that are positioned anterior and vertical in the sagittal plane. The orbital aperture is small with a horizontally positioned inferior orbital rim. (*Right*) Older patients have a retroclined malar eminence, infraorbital rim, and piriform aperture compared with that of young patients. The orbital aperture area is increased secondary to progressive curve distortion of orbital rim superomedially and inferolaterally. (*From* Matros E, Momoh A, Yaremchuk MJ. The aging midfacial skeleton: implications for rejuvenation and reconstruction using implants. Facial Plast Surg 2009;25:252–9; with permission.)

eminence, infraorbital rim, and pyriform aperture (**Fig. 9**). In particular, as previously shown by Yaremchuk and Kahn,[40] they found that infraorbital implants are the most important for correcting midface deformity (**Fig. 10**).

Analyses by the senior author have identified a series of bony changes in the orbital anatomy that occur with aging. In particular, superomedial and inferolateral rim remodeling play an important role in the aging orbit. Additionally, the orbital aperture is noted to widen and increase in area with aging. These changes have been attributed to recession of the facial bones comprising the orbit, especially the orbital rims.[38] This bony remodeling plays a role in the appearance of the overlying soft tissues. The superomedial rim remodeling likely contributes to the unmasking of medial upper lid fat. The inferolateral rim remodeling may contribute to the formation of crow's feet and lower lid lag.

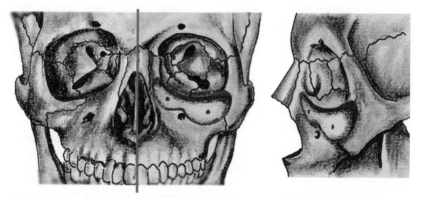

Fig. 10. Infraorbital implants developed to match the skeletally deficient areas of orbits in older patients. These implants increase infraorbital projection in patients with negative vector proportions, and concomitant subperiosteal degloving allows for resuspension of the cheek soft tissues via suturing to the implant. (*From* Matros E, Momoh A, Yaremchuk MJ. The aging midfacial skeleton: implications for rejuvenation and reconstruction using implants. Facial Plast Surg 2009;25:252–9; with permission.)

Aging of the orbit involves a combination of bone remodeling and overlying soft tissue atrophy and repositioning. According to Zimbler and colleagues,[41] "A youthful face…represents a point in time when a particular set of skeletal proportions are ideal for their soft tissue envelope." Therefore, attempts at facial rejuvenation, especially around the orbit, should incorporate volume augmentation for bony loss and soft tissue repositioning and reduction to avoid distortions seen from either approach used in isolation.

Ideally, one would like to offer treatments that reverse the physiologic process of aging.[42] Unfortunately, in 2012, knowledge of how the signs of aging develop is still limited. The authors believe that many of the complications of rejuvenative surgery are from procedures that are designed around a false premise of what occurs in the aging process. As a result, practitioners continue to execute treatment plans that are designed to eliminate the stigmata of aging, such as sharp contour changes and wrinkles, while limiting the risk of complications and unnatural results from overlifting and overresecting.

REFERENCES

1. Bilyk JR, Jacobiec JR. Embryology and anatomy of the orbit and lacrimal system. In: William T, Edward AJ, editors. Duane's Foundations of Clinical Ophthalmology. Volume 1. Philadelphia (PA): Lippincott Williams and Wilkins; 2006.

2. Sperber GH, Gutterman GD, Sperber SM. Craniofacial development. Hamilton (Ontario): BC Decker, Inc; 2001.

3. Ozanics V, Jakobiec FA. Prenatal development of the eye and its adnexa. Ocular anatomy, embryology, and teratology. Philadelphia: Harper and Row; 1982. p. 11–96.

4. Yen MT, Flaharty PM, Anderson RL. Congenital and developmental anomalies of the orbit. In: William T, Edward AJ, editors. Duane's Clinical Ophthalmology. Volume 2. Philadelphia (PA): Lippincott Williams and Wilkins; 2006.

5. Schittkowski MP, Guthoff RF. Injectable self inflating hydrogel pellet expanders for the treatment of orbital volume deficiency in congenital microphthalmos: preliminary results with a new therapeutic approach. Br J Ophthalmol 2006;90:1173–7.

6. Bernardino CR. Congenital anophthalmia: a review of dealing with volume. Middle East Afr J Ophthalmol 2010;17:156–60.

7. Quaranta-Leoni FM. Congenital anophthalmia. Curr Opin Ophthalmol 2011;22:380–4.

8. Dootz GL. The ocularists' management of congenital microphthalmos and anophthalmos. Adv Ophthalmic Plast Reconstr Surg 1992;9:41–56.

9. Forbes BJ. Congenital craniofacial anomalies. Curr Opin Ophthalmol 2010;21:367–74.

10. Preston RA, Post JC, Keats BJ. A gene for Crouzon craniofacial dysostosis maps to the long arm of chromosome 10. Nat Genet 1994;7:149.

11. Reardon W, Winter RM, Rutland P. Mutations in the fibroblast growth factor receptor 2 gene cause Crouzon syndrome. Nat Genet 1994;8:90.

12. Losken HW, Preston RA, Post JC, et al. The gene for Crouzon craniofacial dysostosis maps to chromosome 10q25–q26. Proceedings of the 63rd Annual Meeting of the American Society of Plastic and Reconstructive Surgery. San Diego (CA); 24–30 September 1994.

13. Apert E. De l'acrocephalosyndactylie. Bull Mem Soc Med Hop Paris 1906;243:1310 [in French].

14. Pfeiffer RA. Dominant erbliche Akrocephalosyndaktylie. Z Kinderheilkd 1964;90:301 [in German].

15. Tessier P. Anatomical classification of facial, craniofacial, and latero-facial clefts. J Maxillofac Surg 1976;4:69.

16. Sakai D, Trainor PA. Treacher–Collins syndrome: unmasking the role of Tcof1/treacle. Int J Biochem Cell Biol 2009;41:1229–32.

17. Trainor PA, Dixon J, Dixon MJ. Treacher–Collins syndrome: etiology, pathogenesis and prevention. Eur J Hum Genet 2009;17:275–83.

18. Rogers BO. Berry–Treacher–Collins syndrome: a review of 200 cases. Br J Plast Surg 1964;17:109.

19. Cohen MM, Richieri-Costa A, Guion-Almeida ML, et al. Hypertelorism: interorbital growth, measurements, and pathogenetic considerations. Int J Oral Maxillofac Surg 1995;24:387.

20. Converse JM, Ransohoff J, Mathews ES. Ocular hypertelorism and pseudohypertelorism: Advances in surgical treatment. Plast Reconstr Surg 1970;45:1.

21. Farkas LG, Hreczko TA, Katic MJ. Craniofacial norms in North American Caucasians from birth (one year) to adulthood. Anthropometry of the head and face. New York (NY): Raven Press; 1994.

22. Yaremchuk MJ. Subperiosteal and full-thickness skin rhytidectomy. Plast Reconstr Surg 2001;107:1045–58.

23. Pessa JE, Desvigne LD, Lambros VS, et al. Changes in ocular globe-to-orbital rim position with age: implications for aesthetic blepharoplasty of the lower eyelids. Aesthetic Plast Surg 1999;23:337–42.

24. Gosain AK, Klein MH, Sudhakar PV, et al. Volumetric analysis of soft-tissue changes in the aging midface using high-resolution MRI: implications for facial rejuvenation. Plast Reconstr Surg 2005;115:1143–52.

25. Camp MC, Wong WW, Filip Z, et al. A quantitative analysis of periorbital aging with three-dimensional surface imaging. J Plast Reconstr Aesthet Surg 2011;64:148–54.

26. Pessa JE. An algorithm of facial aging: verification of Lambros's theory by three-dimensional stereolithography, with reference to the pathogenesis of

midfacial aging, scleral show, and the lateral suborbital trough deformity. Plast Reconstr Surg 2000; 106:479–88 [discussion: 489–90].

27. Love LP, Farrior EH. Periocular anatomy and aging. Facial Plast Surg Clin North Am 2010;18:411–7.

28. Rohrich RJ, Arbique GM, Wong C, et al. The anatomy of suborbicularis fat: implications for periorbital rejuvenation. Plast Reconstr Surg 2009;124: 946–51.

29. Erbagci I, Erbagci H, Kizilkan N, et al. The effect of age and gender on the anatomic structure of Caucasian healthy eyelids. Saudi Med J 2005;26: 1535–8.

30. Lambros V. Observations on periorbital and midface aging. Plast Reconstr Surg 2007;120:1367–76 [discussion: 1377].

31. Yaremchuk MJ, O'Sullivan N, Benslimane F. Reversing brow lifts. Aesthet Surg J 2007;27:367–75.

32. Papageorgiou KI, Mancini R, Garneau HC, et al. A three-dimensional construct of the aging eyebrow the illusion of volume loss. Aesthet Surg J 2012;32: 46–57.

33. Richard MJ, Morris C, Deen BF, et al. Analysis of the anatomic changes of the aging facial skeleton using computer-assisted tomography. Ophthal Plast Reconstr Surg 2009;25:382–6.

34. Pessa JE, Zadoo VP, Mutimer KL, et al. Relative maxillary retrusion as a natural consequence of aging: combining skeletal and soft-tissue changes into an integrated model of midfacial aging. Plast Reconstr Surg 1998;102:205–12.

35. Shaw RB Jr, Kahn DM. Aging of the midface bony elements: a three-dimensional computed tomographic study. Plast Reconstr Surg 2007;119: 675–81 [discussion: 682–3].

36. Shaw RB Jr, Katzel EB, Koltz PF, et al. Aging of the mandible and its aesthetic implications. Plast Reconstr Surg 2010;125:332–42.

37. Shaw RB Jr, Katzel EB, Koltz PF, et al. Aging of the facial skeleton: aesthetic implications and rejuvenation strategies. Plast Reconstr Surg 2011;127:374–83.

38. Kahn DM, Shaw RB Jr. Aging of the bony orbit: a three-dimensional computed tomographic study. Aesthet Surg J 2008;28:258–64.

39. Matros E, Momoh A, Yaremchuk MJ. The aging midfacial skeleton: implications for rejuvenation and reconstruction using implants. Facial Plast Surg 2009;25:252–9.

40. Yaremchuk MJ, Kahn DM. Periorbital skeletal augmentation to improve blepharoplasty and midfacial results. Plast Reconstr Surg 2009;124:2151–60.

41. Zimbler MS, Kokoska MS, Thomas JR. Anatomy and pathophysiology of facial aging. Facial Plast Surg Clin North Am 2001;9:179–87, vii.

42. Haddock NT, Saadeh PB, Boutros S, et al. The tear trough and lid/cheek junction: anatomy and implications for surgical correction. Plast Reconstr Surg 2009;123:1332–40 [discussion: 1341–2].

Surgical Ophthalmologic Examination

Joel Powell, DDS, MD, MSc[a],*, Justine Moe, DDS[b],
Martin B. Steed, DDS[b]

KEYWORDS

- Eye • Ocular • Ophthalmology • Trauma • Exam • Fundoscopy • Vision • Pupils

KEY POINTS

- Vital signs of the eye are vision, pupils, and intraocular pressure. They need to be monitored perioperatively.
- The finding of a pointed pupil in the setting of trauma raises a high suspicion for an open globe injury and precludes further manipulation of the globe.
- Traumatic hyphemas need to be followed closely for rebleeding, and orbital reconstruction should be delayed until they are stabilized or resolved.
- The absence of a red reflex and identification of posterior segment blood on fundoscopic examination raise a high suspicion for a posterior segment injury and require immediate ophthalmologic evaluation.
- A relative afferent pupillary defect, detected by the swinging flashlight test, is indicative of a blind or partially blind eye and requires identification of its cause.

INTRODUCTION

Oral and maxillofacial surgeons are frequently called to assess and treat facial injuries, including those of the orbit and nearby structures. Ocular trauma constitutes approximately 3% of all emergency department visits in the United States.[1] Most encounters for eye and adnexal tissue complaints are related to trauma, followed by ocular complaints related to workplace injury.[1–3] From 2 to 2.5 million ocular injuries occur annually in the United States,[4,5] with the incidence of ocular injury in major trauma ranging from 2% to 16%.[4,6–8] More than 90% of midfacial fractures are associated with injury to the eye and/or adnexa, of which nearly one-third are moderate to severe injuries.[8] More than one-half of ocular injuries are treated in the emergency department, but nearly 40% are treated in private physician offices, followed by other outpatient and inpatient facilities.[6]

Although the eyes make up a small proportion of total body surface area, visual impairment carries a disproportionately high level of disability. The maxillofacial surgeon should be able to conduct a thorough and expedient assessment of the eye after blunt or sharp midfacial trauma and perioperatively for the many surgical procedures that involve the orbit and surrounding soft tissues. Recognition of potentially sight-threatening disorders is of the highest priority, and prevention of secondary injury is equally important.[5] Proficiency with the relevant anatomy and ophthalmologic examination is paramount for the oral and maxillofacial surgeon to perform a rapid, appropriate triage and to arrive at potentially critical diagnoses. Failure to recognize an ocular injury before or after

The authors have nothing to disclose.
[a] Private Practice, 18 Acadia Street, Dartmouth, Nova Scotia B2Y 4H3, Canada; [b] Division of Oral and Maxillofacial Surgery, Emory University School of Medicine, 1365 Clifton Road, Suite 2300, B, Atlanta, GA 30322, USA
* Corresponding author.
E-mail address: Dr.Joel.Powell@mac.com

Oral Maxillofacial Surg Clin N Am 24 (2012) 557–572
http://dx.doi.org/10.1016/j.coms.2012.07.001
1042-3699/12/$ – see front matter © 2012 Elsevier Inc. All rights reserved.

surgical intervention could lead to permanently reduced vision or even complete blindness.

OPHTHALMOLOGIC HISTORY AND EXAMINATION

Once the orbital and ocular examination can be obtained, modeling the examination after an ophthalmology note is useful. A sample ophthalmologic or oculoplastic note is represented in **Fig. 1**.[9] Familiarity with the nomenclature, Abbreviations, and examinations of an ophthalmology consult is useful and aids in communication between specialists, including such terms as the Birmingham Eye Trauma Terminology System (**Fig. 2**).[10] Ophthalmologists often refer to and differentiate between anterior segment injuries (cornea, iris, anterior chamber, ciliary body, and lens) and posterior segment injuries (vitreous, choroid, and retina).

The organized history can be accomplished in a few minutes and includes a detailed history of present illness (indicated on trauma note as HPI, past medical history (indicated as PMH), past ocular history (indicated as POH), allergies (indicated as ALL), family history (indicated as FH), and medications (indicated as Meds). Once these are obtained, the physical examination will focus on obtaining measurements of the patient's vision (indicated on trauma note as V), pupils (indicated as P), ocular pressure (indicated as Tap), confrontational fields (indicated as CF), and extraocular muscle (EOM) movements. The examination can then be completed with a slit lamp examination (SLE) and the dilated fundus examination (DFE).[9]

History of Present Illness

Once appropriate, the ocular history needs to assess the nature of the injury/injuries (What happened?) including the mechanism (How did it happen?) and timing (When did it happen?). Any visual symptoms should be elicited, including reduced or altered vision, diplopia (double vision), floaters, pain, discharge, dyschromatopsia (altered color vision), and flashing lights.[11,12] These symptoms should be characterized in terms of location (focal or diffuse, unilateral or bilateral?), degree (mild, moderate, or severe?), duration (brief, intermittent, or persistent?), frequency, and rate of onset (rapid, gradual, or asymptomatic—perhaps only noted when the opposite eye was covered?).[11,12] These findings give clues that will guide the physical examination (**Table 1**).

Birmingham Eye Trauma Terminology System (BETTS) Glossary of Terms

Term	Definition and Explanation
Eyewall	Sclera and Cornea
Closed globe injury	No full thickness wound of the eyewall
Open globe injury	Full thickness wound of the eyewall
Contusion	There is no full thickness wound. *The injury is etither due to direct energy delivery by the object (ex: choroidal rupture) or to the changes in the shape of the globe.*
Lamellar laceration	Partial thickness wound of the eyewall
Rupture	Full thickness wound of the eyewall, caused by a blunt object. *Since the eye is filled with incompressible liquid, the impact results in momentary increase of the IOP. The eyewall yields at its weakest point. The actual wound is produced by an inside out mechanism.*
Laceration	Full thickness wound of the eyewall, caused by a sharp object *The wound occurs at the impact site by an outside-in mechanism.*
Penetrating Injury	Entrance wound *If more than one wound is present, each must have been caused by a different agent.*
Perforating injury	Entrance and exit wounds *Both wounds caused by the same agent.*

Fig. 1. Birmingham Eye Trauma Terminology System (BETTS).[10]

Sample Ophthalmologic Trauma Note

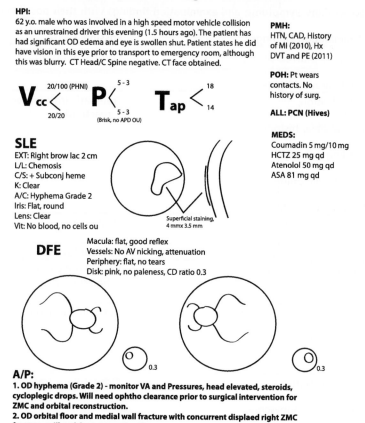

HPI:
62 y.o. male who was involved in a high speed motor vehicle collision as an unrestrained driver this evening (1.5 hours ago). The patient has had significant OD edema and eye is swollen shut. Patient states he did have vision in this eye prior to transport to emergency room, although this was blurry. CT Head/C Spine negative. CT face obtained.

PMH:
HTN, CAD, History of MI (2010), Hx DVT and PE (2011)

POH: Pt wears contacts. No history of surg.

ALL: PCN (Hives)

MEDS:
Coumadin 5 mg/10 mg
HCTZ 25 mg qd
Atenolol 50 mg qd
ASA 81 mg qd

$$V_{cc} < \begin{array}{c} 20/100 \text{ (PHNI)} \\ \\ 20/20 \end{array} \quad P < \begin{array}{c} 5\text{-}3 \\ \\ 5\text{-}3 \\ \text{(Brisk, no APD OU)} \end{array} \quad T_{ap} < \begin{array}{c} 18 \\ \\ 14 \end{array}$$

SLE
EXT: Right brow lac 2 cm
L/L: Chemosis
C/S: + Subconj heme
K: Clear
A/C: Hyphema Grade 2
Iris: Flat, round
Lens: Clear
Vit: No blood, no cells ou

Superficial staining, 4 mm x 3.5 mm

DFE
Macula: flat, good reflex
Vessels: No AV nicking, attenuation
Periphery: flat, no tears
Disk: pink, no paleness, CD ratio 0.3

0.3   0.3

A/P:
1. OD hyphema (Grade 2) - monitor VA and Pressures, head elevated, steroids, cycloplegic drops. Will need ophtho clearance prior to surgical intervention for ZMC and orbital reconstruction.
2. OD orbital floor and medial wall fracture with concurrent displaed right ZMC fracture - will anticipate reconstruction.
3. OD corneal abrasion - will treat with emycin qid

Fig. 2. A sample ophthalmology trauma note. By convention, right eye findings are denoted first or superiorly. *Abbreviations:* A/C, anterior chamber; APD, afferent pupillary defect; ASA, aspirin; AV, atrioventricular; CAD, coronary artery disease; CF, confrontational fields; C/S, conjunctiva and sclera; CT, computed tomography; DVT, deep venous thrombosis; EOMI, EOMs intact; EXT, external; HCTZ, hydrochlorothiazide; HTN, hypertension; Hx, history; K, cornea; L/L, lids and lacrimation; OD, oculus dexter or right eye; OS, oculus sinister or left eye; OU, oculus uterque or both eyes; P, pupils; PCN, penicillin; PE, pulmonary embolism; PHNI, pinhole no improvement; Pt, patient; Tap, pressure; VA, visual acuity; Vcc, vision with glasses; Vit, vitreous; ZMC, zygomaticomaxillary complex.

Past Medical History

Past medical history should focus on general state of health and inquire about conditions that contribute to ocular pathologic conditions in the trauma setting such as sickle cell anemia (trait or disease), diabetes, hypertension, coronary artery disease, connective tissue disorders, thyroid dysfunction, and acquired or congenital coagulopathic conditions including von Willebrand disease and hemophilia A/B.[11–13] Tetanus status should also be documented.

Past Ocular History

Prior ocular history has implications for physical examination and management, and current complaints and findings need to be put in the context of preexisting conditions. The history should include previous ocular trauma, use of corrective lenses, and ocular conditions including corneal scarring, amblyopia, glaucoma, macular degeneration, cataracts, Graves disease, diabetic retinopathy, and optic neuropathy.[4,14,15] Previous ocular surgeries should be documented. Notably, prior radial keratotomy or recent laser in situ keratomileusis can increase the risk for corneal complications of trauma, and incision sites for corneal transplantation, glaucoma surgery, and cataract surgery are more likely to rupture in trauma to the globe (**Table 2**).[5]

Allergies

Obtain information on any historical allergies and the subsequent reaction.

Table 1
Correlation between signs, symptoms, and examination findings with their possible cause

Sign/Symptom/Examination Findings	Possible Cause
Foreign body sensation, blurred vision, sharp pain, photophobia, halo around lights	Corneal abrasion
Pain, tearing, blurred vision, photophobia with consensual photophobia, history of ocular trauma in preceding 2–3 days, traumatic miosis (immediate) developing to traumatic mydriasis, cells and flare on SLE	Traumatic iritis (anterior chamber reaction)
Pain, blurred vision, layering of blood in anterior chamber	Hyphema
Decreased vision, monocular diplopia	Lens subluxation or lens dislocation
Floaters, flashing lights (photopsia), unable to visualize fundus on DFE	Retinal detachment with vitreous hemorrhage
Pain, decreasing vision, proptosis, relative afferent papillary defect, increased IOP, red desaturation, ophthalmoplegia	Retrobulbar hemorrhage
Binocular diplopia, restricted eye movement, periorbital ecchymoses/emphysema, V2 hypoesthesia	Orbital floor fracture
Photophobia, restricted eye movement, nausea and vomiting, bradycardia	Oculocardiac reflex
Severe conjunctival hemorrhage, hyphema, hemorrhagic chemosis, flat anterior chamber, teardrop or pointed pupil, iris herniation	Ruptured globe

Family History

Family history is pertinent in many ocular disorders, including refractive errors, strabismus, amblyopia, glaucoma, or cataracts, retinal detachment, retinal dystrophy, and macular degeneration.[9,11,12]

Table 2
Ocular problem history items

Macular degeneration	Cataracts
Graves disease	Neoplasm
Vitrectomy	Retinal detachment
Hyphema	Floaters
Laser eye surgery	Contact lenses
Flashing lights	Reading glasses

Medications

Several medications can influence the outcome of orbital trauma and orbital surgery.[13] Anticoagulant therapy including aspirin, warfarin, low molecular weight heparin, and clopidogrel can complicate surgery and should be documented.

Physical Examination

Life-threatening injuries should be addressed first as per standard Advanced Trauma Life Suppost protocols. For patients with a history of ocular trauma, the examiner should conduct a systematic physical examination. Extreme care should be taken during the examination to avoid inadvertently applying pressure on the globe, which can cause herniation of intraocular contents in the event of an open globe injury.[16]

The head, scalp, face, and periorbital tissues should be evaluated on gross inspection and palpation. Common findings in orbital adnexal injury are given (**Box 1**). Neurologic examination should include evaluation of infraorbital nerve (V2) sensation and facial nerve (cranial nerve VII) motor function.

Lower medial lid lacerations may suggest injury to the lacrimal drainage system, especially in the presence of pooling of tears at the medial angle of the eye and lacrimation (epiphora).[10,17] Lacerations of the lateral brow or midglabellar regions should alert the surgeon to the possibility of posttraumatic optic neuropathy.[17] Such findings are discussed in more depth later in this article. Fat prolapsed through an eyelid laceration is strongly suggestive of a full-thickness lid injury and underlying globe injury.[16,17] Notably, full-thickness upper lid lacerations are frequently associated with damage to the lower aspect of the globe and inferior corneal limbus as a result of Bell phenomenon, the reflexive upward rotation of the globe with forced closure of the eye, such as might occur in anticipation of a blow.[16,17]

Examination of the conjunctiva and eye itself should then be performed. Lid edema, blepharospasm, and pain may severely limit examination, especially in the posttraumatic setting. Topical anesthetic solution such as proparacaine may be necessary; occasionally, systemic analgesics or even facial nerve block can facilitate lid opening.[5,12] Gentle lid retraction using a Demarres retractor, lid

speculum, or 2 large paper clips bent under at the ends in a U-shape with a hemostat can also facilitate examination.[5]

Common findings in orbital injury are given in **Box 2**. The bulbar conjunctiva is observed under direct vision and palpebral conjunctiva may be observed with gentle lid eversion.[12] Suspected corneal laceration is further evaluated in the SLE and is discussed later. Corneal sensitivity is mediated by the ophthalmic branch of cranial nerve V and may be evaluated by gentle touch with a cotton swab.[12] Contact should elicit a rapid blink in both eyes, called the corneal reflex or blink reflex, via cranial nerve VII. Globe malposition including dystopia and enophthalmos should be noted but may not be evident on initial examination as a result of edema and hemorrhage in the immediate posttrauma setting. If globe rupture is confirmed or highly likely during the examination, a Fox shield

---

Box 1
Orbital adnexal tissue injuries

- Edema
- Ecchymosis
- Contusion
- Hematoma
- Foreign bodies
- Subcutaneous emphysema/crepitus
- Orbital rim step deformities
- Infraorbital nerve hypoesthesia
- Lid laceration
  - Fat prolapse
  - Nasolacrimal apparatus injury/epiphora

Box 2
Common findings in orbital injury

- Globe malpositioning
  - Proptosis/exophthalmos
  - Enophthalmos
- Conjunctiva
  - Erythema
  - Edema/chemosis
    - Pale
    - Hemorrhagic
  - Foreign bodies
  - Conjunctival tears
  - Reduced conjunctival reflex
- Subconjunctival hemorrhage
- Cornea
  - Clouding
  - Laceration
  - Abrasion
- Pupil
  - Pointed
  - Fixed
  - Dilated ("blown")
  - Anisocoria
- Anterior chamber
  - Hyphema
  - Hypopyon

(no patch) should be placed over the eye and an ophthalmologist should be emergently consulted.[5]

Vision, pupils, and pressure

Although there is a plethora of sophisticated testing available for the eyes themselves, this article will focus on those applicable to the maxillofacial trauma surgeon. The initial basic armamentarium typically includes a near card, penlight, and ophthalmoscope (**Fig. 3**). The patient's vision, pupil, and ocular pressure are often referred to as the "vital signs" of the eye.[9] These measurements should be obtained first, before any dilation of the eyes, and are the most important to monitor routinely before and after any surgical interventions. Visual fields, EOMs, forced ductions, SLE, and DFE are less critical from a timing perspective and are best done as part of a secondary survey in an acute trauma or emergency situation. In the early posttraumatic setting, only parts of the eye examination may initially be possible in patients with severe injuries or altered mental status and those who have been administered analgesics, sedatives, or anesthesia.[5]

Vision

Visual acuity is the most important aspect of the ocular examination and is a good place to start because it has significant prognostic importance and can quickly rule out certain conditions.

Visual acuity is best measured with a Snellen eye chart positioned 20 ft from the subject. Each eye is tested separately, and the result is read off the chart based on the smallest line the patient can read or clearly see. The interpretation is straightforward,

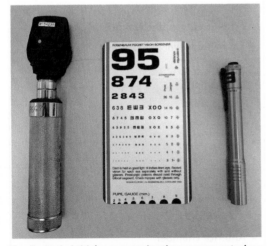

Fig. 3. Basic initial eye examination armamentarium. Includes a direct ophthalmoscope, near card (eg, the Rosenbaum Pocket Vision Screener, Grafco, Atlanta, GA, USA), and a penlight.

in that the recorded number (eg, 20/30) represents the distance the patient is from the chart (20 ft) and the second number is the distance the average person would be to see that same line (30 ft).

In the trauma environment, patients are frequently assessed in examination rooms of limited size, on a gurney, or in an intensive care unit bed and without the availability of the 20-ft charts, making such distance testing impossible or impractical. Therefore, near cards, as shown in **Fig. 3**, are more frequently used and are generally held about 35 cm (14 in) from the eyes. Various cards are available for testing at different distances, and the manufacturer's instructions on the card should always be followed. Near cards, however, do have limitations: although distance vision requires very little accommodation, near vision relies markedly on accommodation. Thus, testing visual acuity at distances less than 20 ft will be less accurate for a patient with uncorrected refractive error such as astigmatism, myopia (nearsightedness), or hyperopia (farsightedness).[18] For example, one must be cautious of older patients who may have presbyopia, an age-related difficulty focusing on near objects in the best of circumstances secondary to age-related changes to the lenses instead of to a traumatic cause.

The only vision assessment that matters is the "best corrected vision." Therefore visual acuity should always be measured with the patient's corrective lenses if possible. If the patient's glasses are not available, refractive error can be corrected with a +2.50 lens taking the place of an older patient's reading glasses or with a "pinhole test," which reduces refractive blur in the ametropic eye (an eye with a refractive or focusing error), thereby allowing measurement of corrected visual acuity (**Fig. 4**).[9,18]

If the patient is illiterate or does not speak the language on the vision chart, other aids for visual acuity are available such as the tumbling E or picture charts.[9] If visual acuity is extremely poor and chart testing fails, the patient is first asked to count fingers (recorded as confrontational fields at farthest distance patient responds correctly); if negative, followed by gross hand movements; if negative, then light perception (recorded as direction of pointed light source); if negative, nil perception of light is recorded.[5,11,12] Using a standard format for recording results for each eye allows rapid and accurate review by colleagues, including ophthalmologists.

It is worth noting that there are free applications available on smart phones, such as Apple's iPhone (Apple Inc, Cupertino, CA, USA) that contain pupil size gauges, rulers, near vision charts, picture

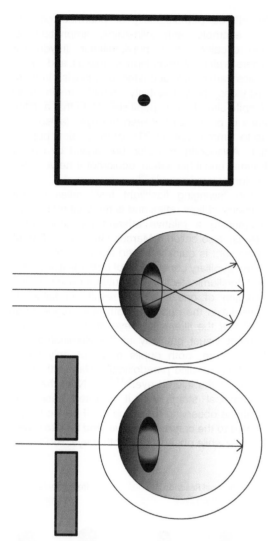

Fig. 4. Pinhole test. A small hole is punched in a paper card. The paper blocks most of the misaligned light rays that cause visual blur and allows the central rays to focus on the retina.

charts, color testing charts, and even sample fundoscopic images. This can eliminate a clinician having to carry these cards, and the potential for them to become damaged or faded and therefore less effective. Eye Handbook, Eye Test, and Eye Chart are a few examples of applications available for the iPhone.

Although the lack of light perception is a very clear finding of severe ophthalmic injury, some other significant ocular injuries including peripheral retinal tears and some penetrating injuries may present with normal central vision and normal visual acuity testing. Furthermore, in the posttraumatic setting, blood, debris, contaminated tear films, and even periorbital edema

can affect accuracy by falsely reducing the recorded visual acuity.

Another valuable test in the verbal, cooperative patient is red color saturation, which is the most sensitive and best overall measure of optic nerve function.[17] With a red object held in front of the patient, each eye is evaluated separately and the patient is asked whether the object seems to have the same color (hue) and brightness (intensity) in each eye. Following damage to the optic nerve, for example in cases of optic neuritis or increased intraocular pressure (IOP), the red object will appear more dull, brown, or grayish to the affected eye compared with the contralateral eye.[17] Similarly, the white light intensity test, although less sensitive, is another test of optic nerve function in which a bright white light is shone into both eyes separately and the patient is asked to comment on the relative brightness of the light in each eye.[17]

Pupils

Examination of the pupils constitutes the second ocular vital sign and may be the only possible measure of optic function in the nonverbal or uncooperative patient. Although not strictly part of the pupillary examination, a quick and easy item to evaluate at this stage is the red reflex of each eye. It is the phenomenon commonly noted in flash photography whereby a red-orange reflection of light is seen in the center of the pupil (the infamous "red eye"). It comes from light reflected off the choroid layer, producing an aerial image of the blood-filled choroid, which is superimposed on the pupil.[18] Best done in a subdued-light environment, it can be checked with a regular flashlight and will always be done at the time of DFE; the technique is described later. Anything interfering with light transmission to or from the back of the eye will produce an abnormal red reflex, and will give either a whitish color from light being reflected back out prematurely or a black color as a result of interference with light transmission or reflection.

An abnormal white reflex can be caused by a swollen cornea (possible sign of glaucoma), cataract, tumor, retinal infection, or retinal detachment. A black reflex can be caused by a cataract, scar, or bleeding inside the eye. A white or black reflex is abnormal and warrants ophthalmology consultation. Note that there can be a slight difference in the red reflex quality between the 2 eyes as a result of an asymmetry in corrective lenses (eg, one eye normal and the other very nearsighted).

Returning to the formal pupillary examination, the pupils should be round and symmetric. An asymmetric pupil, or "corectopia," may indicate an open globe injury, especially if teardrop-shaped, with the point of the teardrop frequently pointing to the site of the penetration (**Fig. 5**).[14] In these cases, the clinician should be very careful not to apply any pressure to the globe during further examination. Note that an abnormally shaped pupil can be preexisting, such as a congenital coloboma of the iris, but this should be easily confirmed by the patient history (see **Fig. 5**).

Reactivity to bright light may be assessed with a penlight or direct ophthalmoscope, the brighter light source of the latter allowing for easier examination and more accurate findings. Baseline pupillary size in millimeters should be recorded for each eye, and constriction to light should be noted with both a written size of the constricted pupil and the relative speed of constriction (trace, sluggish, or brisk).

Normal pupillary constriction to light, or an intact "direct light reflex," depends on passage of light through the eye, retinal and optic nerve function in the afferent limb, and oculomotor nerve function in the efferent limb. Pupillary size is mediated by sympathetic and parasympathetic input that may be altered pathologically or pharmacologically. For example, anticholinergics, amphetamines, and cocaine cause pupillodilation (mydriasis), whereas alcohol, neuroleptics, opioids, and cholinergics cause pupilloconstriction (miosis). In these instances, pupil reactivity should remain intact despite alterations in pupil size. Note that a difference in pupil size between the eyes (anisocoria) up to 1 mm occurs in 20% of the healthy population. Anisocoria may also be caused by uveitis, trauma, uncal herniation, oculomotor nerve palsy, or Horner syndrome.[14,19]

The "swinging flashlight test" relies on the consensual light reflex and is the best method for diagnosing a relative afferent papillary defect (RAPD), also called a Marcus-Gunn pupil (**Fig. 6**). While light is quickly moved from one eye to the other, pupillary constriction of both the illuminated and nonilluminated eyes should be observed. Illumination of one eye that results in failure to constrict in the pupils of both eyes suggests an RAPD of the illuminated eye or a defect of the afferent visual pathway of the illuminated eye. Furthermore, both pupils may not only fail to constrict but also paradoxically dilate with illumination of the injured eye.[5,11,12,18] Note that from a practical standpoint, it is often easiest to continue observing the same pupil as the light is moved to the contralateral eye, and then to repeat the test while observing the other eye. RAPDs are

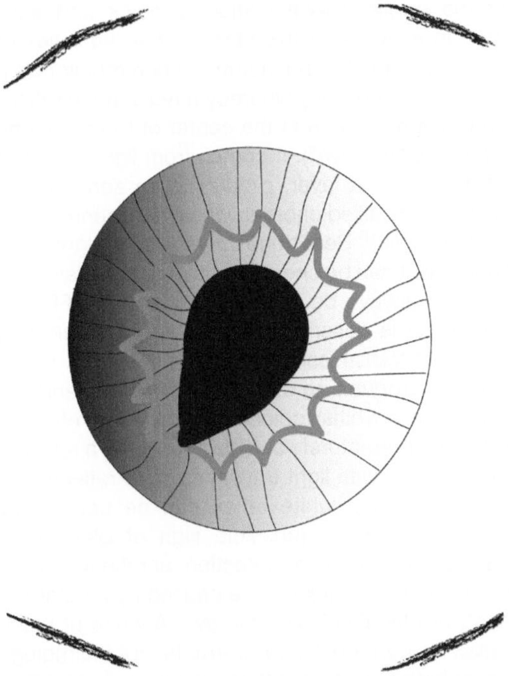

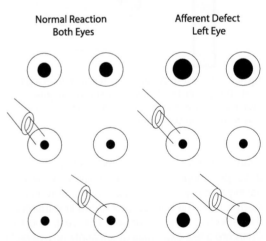

Fig. 5. Peaked pupil. A peaked pupil is indicative of a full-thickness wound of the eye wall or "open globe." The peak points to the location of the wound that has violated both the sclera and cornea. Once an open globe is identified, the eye should not be manipulated or palpated but simply shielded, and an urgent ophthalmology consult obtained.

Fig. 6. Swinging light test. Used to detect afferent papillary defect. When a light is shined back and forth between 2 normal eyes, the pupils constrict, then dilate slightly as the beam passes over the nose, and then constrict again when it reaches the other eye. If one eye is partially blind and light is shined in the uninjured eye, there is constriction in both eyes. When the light is shined in the injured eye, both eyes seem to dilate a little. This phenomenon is called a Marcus Gunn pupil.

graded on a scale of increasing severity of 1 to 4, but the most important aspect is to recognize it.[18]

The final part of the pupil examination in the responsive patient is synkinesis, or pupillary constriction during near vision, which is often erroneously referred to as pupillary accommodation.[17] Note that accommodation for near vision and the concomitant pupillary response constitute a complex process. It is consists of ocular convergence, lens thickening to allow convergence of light rays entering the eye, and pupillary constriction to try to achieve a pinhole type of effect to reduce blurring from the periphery of the cornea, thus allowing proper focusing on near objects. This test has limited value in evaluating ocular trauma and is more appropriately part of a complex neuro-ophthalmologic evaluation.

The standard format to record these findings should be used (**Fig. 2**). The notations "PERRL" (Pupils Equal, Round and Reactive to Light) or "PERRLA" (which includes accommodation) are poorly descriptive and should be avoided.[17]

IOP

IOP is a measure of the fluid pressure within the closed compartment of the globe and is determined by the balance of aqueous humor production and drainage.[11] Normal IOP is between 10 and 21 mm Hg (mean 15 mm Hg) but can fluctuate by 3 to 6 mm Hg or more during the day. Gentle digital palpation of the closed upper lid is a crude assessment of IOP; although slight increases in IOP cannot be detected, a "rock-hard" eye should raise concern for marked increases in IOP.[12] It is most accurately determined through applanation tonometry, in which the amount of force required to flatten the cornea by a predetermined amount reflects the IOP.[11] The Goldman Applanation Tonometer (Haag Streit, USA and Reliance Medical Products, Mason, Ohio), which is used during an SLE, is preferred by ophthalmologists.[11] However, its use is not always possible or practical, particularly in a postoperative situation.

An acceptable alternative is the Tono-Pen (Medtronic Ophthalmics, Jacksonville, FL, USA) (**Fig. 7**), a handheld, portable applanation tonometry device

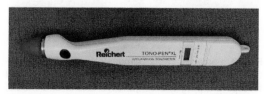

Fig. 7. The handheld Tono-Pen (Medtronic Ophthalmics, Jacksonville, FL, USA) is an acceptable applanation tonometry device, particularly useful postoperatively.

that is easy to use and provides fairly accurate measurements of IOP, although it requires daily calibration.[8,11] Always read and follow the manufacturer's instructions for use of such a device. Topical anesthetic must be applied to the eye before its use. Note that prior application of dilating drops (mydriatics) can falsely elevate readings. If an open globe injury is strongly suspected or confirmed, IOP measurement should be conducted only by an ophthalmologist.[18]

Low IOP may result from ruptured globe or retinal detachment.[12,18] Elevated IOP can be caused by glaucoma, hyphema, or orbital compartment syndrome, such as from retrobulbar hemorrhage.[12,18] IOP greater than 30 mm Hg requires urgent ophthalmologic consultation.[18] In the posttraumatic setting, IOP greater than 40 mm Hg is suggestive of orbital compartment syndrome and is a clear indication to perform a lateral canthotomy.[20]

Motility and Diplopia (EOM)

Double vision, called *diplopia*, can involve one eye (monocular) or both (binocular) and is easily assessed bedside. Most important, ask the patient if he or she is experiencing any diplopia, because objective tests have limitations and do not always correlate perfectly with patient symptoms.[21] To test for dipoplia in primary gaze position, hold a finger or object approximately 3 ft in front of the patient, who should be comfortably looking straight ahead, and ask if he or she sees one image.[17] Diplopia can be horizontal, vertical, or torsional and can be checked by orienting the object horizontally for testing vertical diplopia, and so forth. The presence of esotropia (inward deviation of an eye) or exotropia (outward deviation) should raise suspicion for binocular diplopia.[5,12]

A carefully performed and documented ocular motility assessment is critical in all patients complaining of binocular diplopia or who have a suspected orbital wall or floor fracture. EOMs are most easily assessed by having the patient follow an object to move the eyes to 6 positions of gaze using the standard "H" pattern (**Fig. 8**).[5,11,12] Alternatively, one may have the patient fix his or her gaze on a fixed object straight ahead, and the examiner may instruct and guide the patient to move the head through these motions. Although these tests do not individually isolate extraocular muscles, they test all "duction" and "version" movements (adduction, abduction, elevation, depression, inversion, eversion), and impaired motility in any of these positions of gaze is sufficient to identify a deficit in a specific extraocular muscle or muscles.[11] EOMs should be evaluated

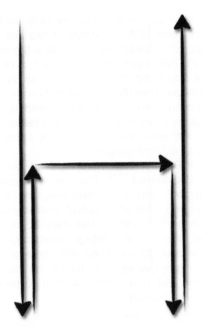

Fig. 8. EOM assessment. EOMs are most easily assessed in the 6 positions of gaze using the standard "H" pattern (upper right, lower right, right, left, lower left, upper left).

in terms of speed, smoothness, range, and symmetry, and any unsteadiness of fixation (nystagmus) should be recorded.[5] The patient should be asked to report diplopia during this test. In addition, the sclera and conjunctiva may simultaneously be grossly inspected for traumatic lesions. The authors find the use of one hand to retract the upper eyelids during these movements effective in improving visualization during the examination, particularly during downward gaze.

Note that diplopia in the extremes of the visual fields is normal and that vision between the primary and inferior gazes is the most functionally important, with diplopia in this range being the most disturbing for patients. Defects in motility, diplopia, and the test used to determine it should be recorded (eg, the "H") in plain descriptive language. More sophisticated tests used to quantify diplopia including the prism cover test and Goldmann diplopia field test may best be left to the ophthalmologists, because they are not critical for the maxillofacial examination in the posttraumatic setting and immediate perioperative period.[22] However, these tests may be very useful in quantitatively monitoring the long-term resolution of diplopia postoperatively.

If an abnormality in extraocular motility is detected, particularly on superior gaze, a forced duction test is indicated to differentiate true restriction and muscle incarceration from other disturbances of motility, including cranial nerve palsy, direct

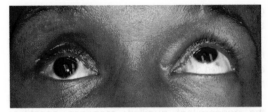

Fig. 9. Limited ocular mobility of the right eye on superior gaze.

muscle trauma, hemorrhage, edema, orbital foreign body, and infection (**Fig. 9**).[5] If the patient requires urgent or emergent surgery for other injuries, this test may be completed under general anesthesia at the time of operation. Otherwise, forced duction should be completed during the initial evaluation with the use of topical anesthetic solution. A 0.3- or 0.5-mm fine-toothed forcep is used to grasp the conjunctiva below the inferior limbus and an attempt is made to pull the eye in the direction of the movement deficit.[5,23] Alternatively, the use of 2 forceps to grasp the conjunctiva on opposite sides of the eye allows for excellent control of the ocular movement and reduces the risk of inadvertently slipping and causing an iatrogenic corneal abrasion.[5] In this case, an assistant to provide lid retraction may be necessary (**Fig. 10**).

Note that although the method of grasping the actual extraocular muscle (most commonly the inferior rectus) to complete the forced duction test is often described, this technique is not only unnecessary but is more difficult to perform, is painful for the awake patient, and can potentially injure the muscle or surrounding tissues, because "blind" grasping is usually required, often because of concurrent chemosis.

A "positive forced duction" by convention refers to an abnormal resistance to movement and may

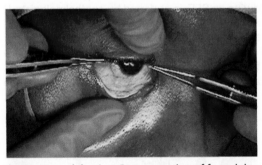

Fig. 10. Forced duction. Demonstration of forced duction superiorly under topical anesthetic using small forceps grasping the conjunctiva lateral and medial to the cornea. The eye should be able to easily and smoothly be rotated with minimal discomfort if unimpeded.

imply muscle restriction, which occurs commonly following entrapment of soft tissues in orbital bony fractures.[5]

Orbital edema may also cause a positive forced duction test; a short interval of observation can help differentiate edema from true muscle restriction.[5] Furthermore, most cases of posttraumatic diplopia result from temporary muscular dysfunction secondary to edema, and in the absence of entrapment or other indications for surgical intervention, such diplopia needs only to be followed over time, because most cases resolve within 7 to 10 days.[24]

True entrapment implies a degree of existing and active soft tissue damage. The likelihood of ongoing tissue damage that could result in permanent scarring with resultant diplopia and its serious functional consequences is reason for prompt surgical intervention.[25,26] In addition, entrapment diagnosed clinically and radiographically in the presence of diplopia and unresolved oculocardiac reflex consisting of bradycardia, heart block, nausea, and syncope is an indication for urgent surgical repair.[11,18]

Visual Field Testing (Confrontational Fields)

The central visual field test measures gross central retinal or macular function in the cooperative patient. Both eyes are evaluated separately, with the patient facing at the clinician from a distance of 2 ft. Without moving his or her eyes, the patient should be able to see all features of the clinician's face without any darkness or blurriness, including the ears and chin.[17]

The peripheral visual field is then assessed using confrontation testing. With the patient seated opposite to the clinician at a distance of 2 to 3 ft, both focus on the other's opposite eye (eg, the patient's right eye focuses on the clinician's left eye), and their contralateral eyes are covered. The clinician moves a finger from the periphery toward midline, keeping it equidistant between the 2 individuals. The finger should be visible to both the patient and clinician at roughly the same time. The examination is repeated in all 4 quadrants (superior, inferior, temporal and nasal) and for both eyes.[5,11,12] More sophisticated visual field testing is available but is generally reserved for the complex neurologic evaluation.

SLE

The SLE (**Fig. 11**) is a technique for which, like many other aspects of the examination, the surgeon requires time and practice to become proficient. A binocular microscope is used that allows the surgeon a 3-dimensional view of the eye. With this tool, the eye is examined with

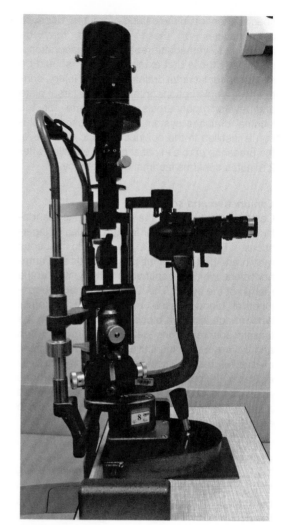

Fig. 11. Slit lamp.

a beam or "slit" of light whose height and width can be adjusted.[9] It is used in the acute trauma setting for evaluation of the anterior segment of the eye and can facilitate foreign body removal in the emergency department setting. An organized examination will include the following and be represented in the trauma note (see **Fig. 2**) under "SLE."

External examination

The external examination evaluates both eyes, identifying features such as periorbital edema, ecchymoses, lacerations, and foreign bodies. The patient's cranial nerve V2 and VII functions should be assessed.

Lids and lacrimation

All elements of the tear-producing and -collecting system are subject to lacerations and require special attention in the setting of trauma, because discontinuities of these structures may be amenable to immediate repair. Eyelid lacerations, particularly those that extend medially, should be evaluated for lacrimal drainage system injury, canthal tendon disruption, or injury to the tarsal plate and levator aponeurosis. To evaluate for the lacrimal drainage system, 10% fluorescein solution is instilled in the conjunctival sac of the eye; the presence of dye in nasal mucus expelled after 2 minutes confirms lacrimal duct patency.[12]

Conjunctiva and sclera

Careful examination of the conjunctiva is mandatory to rule out intraocular foreign bodies or lacerations. The conjunctiva is a thin mucous membrane that covers the posterior lids and anterior sclera, which is continuous with the skin at the margin of the eyelid. The rupture of small subconjunctival blood vessels causes subconjunctival hemorrhage in which blood is extravasated in the loosely adherent zone between the conjunctiva and sclera. Subconjunctival hemorrhage should always be distinguished from chemosis, which is edema of the conjunctiva. Although a hemorrhage appears flat and smooth, chemosis presents as a raised area with erythema and edema. Both are often found simultaneously.

Cornea

The cornea and sclera are often referred to as the "anterior segment" of the eye. Together they form the anterior structural wall of the eye. The cornea is the clear window through which light must travel to eventually reach the retina. A corneal laceration is a partial- or full-thickness injury to the cornea. A partial-thickness injury does not violate the globe of the eye (abrasion). A full-thickness injury penetrates completely through the cornea, causing a ruptured globe.[10] Globe rupture occurs when the integrity of the outer membranes of the eye is disrupted by blunt or penetrating trauma. Any full-thickness injury to the cornea, sclera, or both is considered an open globe injury and is approached in the same fashion in the acute setting. Globe rupture represents a major ophthalmologic emergency and always requires surgical intervention. Fluorescein staining is used to identify corneal abrasions and will outline the epithelial defect. Examining the affected area with a cobalt blue filter or light then allows one to carry out the Seidel test for a possible aqueous humor leak. Under white light, if the fluorescein is diluted by extravasated aqueous humor, it appears as a green (dilute) stream within the dark orange (concentrated) dye. Under the blue light, the leak is a swirling stream of green within a background of green.)[12]

Anterior chamber

The anterior chamber is best assessed with an SLE but can be approximated with a penlight. Lit tangentially from the temporal side, the depth of the anterior chamber can be approximated. The presence of red or white blood cells may also be seen (hyphema and hypopyon, respectively). Hyphema should be monitored carefully and is reason for delay of nonemergent surgery and prompt ophthalmology consultation, whereas hypopyon indicates inflammation of the uvea or iris and is less likely to be secondary to trauma unless secondary infection has occurred. Acute glaucoma may also follow trauma through disruption of outflow of aqueous humor, secondary to red blood cells (hyphema), formation of a trabecular meshwork scar, or lens dislocation.[12]

Iris

The amount of light entering the eye is controlled by the iris, the colored portion of the eye, which can be thought of as the aperture of a camera. Rupture of the iris at its root (iridodialysis) can occur following blunt trauma or penetrating injury to the globe. With larger iridodialises, patients may experience a double pupil effect, monocular diplopia, glare, and photophobia. This is commonly associated with hyphema and an irregular pupil. Damage of the trabecular meshwork and peripheral anterior synechiae may lead to IOP elevation.

Lens

Subluxation of the lens may occur due to disruption of the lens zonule fibers. In such instances, the lens margin can be seen, visual acuity can be reduced, and monocular diplopia may be present.

Vitreous

Looking behind the lens, one can see the dark vitreous cavity that makes up the greatest volume of the eye. The vitreous is located between the lens and the retina. It has an average volume of 24 mL and is composed of 98% water, collagen, and glycosaminoglycans such as hyaluronic acid.[16] Floating blood cells in the vitreous humor is suspicious of a retinal hemorrhage or detachment.

DFE

Fundoscopy is probably the most difficult technical skill to acquire, especially in the setting of trauma. The purpose is to examine the posterior segment of the eye including the retina. Normal fundus anatomy is shown in **Fig. 12.**

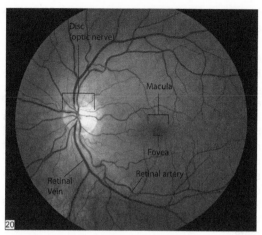

Fig. 12. Normal fundus.

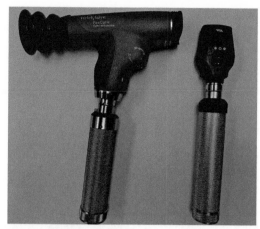

Fig. 13. PanOptic (Welch Allen, Skaneateles Falls, NY, USA) direct ophthalmoscope and traditional direct ophthalmoscope.

The first key to making fundoscopy easier is pupillary dilation. This is accomplished with 1 or 2 drops of a dilating agent such as tropicamide 0.5% or 1% (may last several hours) or phenylephrine hydrochloride 2.5% (shorter acting) and allowing at least 15 minutes to pass for adequate dilation. Contraindications to dilating drops include known or suspected narrow angle glaucoma, known hypersensitivity, or whenever pupillary response is necessary for neurologic monitoring such as in coma or head injuries. In all other situations, pupillary dilation is safe to allow superior visualization.

Different instruments are available for fundoscopy. The indirect ophthalmoscope is a large lens held by the examiner at arm's length with coaxial lighting and allows much larger, superior views of the retina. Two types of direct ophthalmoscopes are available: the traditional flashlight-sized ophthalmoscope commonly found in examination rooms and the panoptic ophthalmoscope, which is much easier to use but less frequently available (**Fig. 13**). The standard, direct ophthalmoscope is by far the most common instrument available in the trauma setting.

With the standard direct ophthalmoscope, the light is set to the largest white, round shape and the focus wheel is positioned on "0." The examiner's glasses, if worn, should be removed. Negative numbers (red) on the focus wheel will correct for nearsightedness and positive for farsightedness, but it may not correlate exactly with the user's prescription. Therefore, the best method is to adjust the focus once the retina is in view to make it clear and crisp.

Ideally, the clinician begins in front of an upright patient, if possible, in a dimly lit environment to reduce glare and pupillary constriction. To examine the patient's right eye, the clinician should be positioned on the patient's right side, with the ophthalmoscope held by the right hand to the right eye (**Fig. 14**A). A similar examination is repeated for the patient's left eye, holding the ophthalmoscope in the left hand to the clinician's left eye. Standing for this examination facilitates visualization nasally, temporally, superiorly, and inferiorly on the retina.

To visualize the fundus efficiently, the ophthalmoscope is first held about 12 in in front of the patient and at about a 15° angle temporally from the patient's midline (see **Fig. 14**B). The free hand is used to help hold the patient's upper eyelid open if necessary, or at least to provide a stable rest and tactile target to prevent touching the patient's eye with the ophthalmoscope as it is brought closer. The patient is told to focus on a distant object in the room and to continue looking at that object. The red reflex should be located immediately, and then "followed in" as the ophthalmoscope is brought nearer to the patient, within a couple of inches or even closer, until the retina is visualized. This 15° angle approach generally allows for rapid location of the optic disc, which is the first area to be examined. If the disc is not immediately located, then the vessels should be traced back to the disc, because the branches of a tree may be followed back to its trunk. Note that the field of view in a direct ophthalmoscope is relatively small, and therefore the angle of examination must be changed to "explore" and visualize different areas of the fundus.

Following examination of the optic disc, about 2 optic disc widths temporally is the slightly darker/

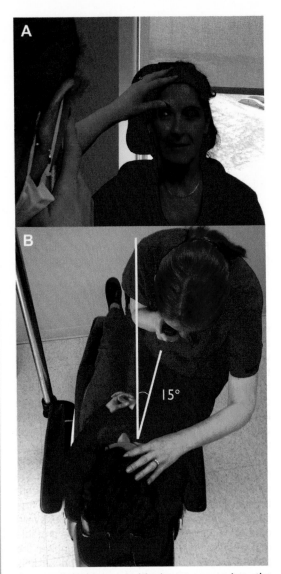

Fig. 14. (*A*)–Proper positioning to examine the patient's right eye showing patient looking straight ahead, round white light, left hand by patient's brow, and the red reflex visualized. (*B*)–Begin with a 15° lateral/temporal angle from patient's direction of view, which allows almost immediate visualization of the optic disc once the fundus is in view.

pigmented macula and fovea within it. Examination time of this area should be minimized, because the macula and fovea are sensitive to the light and it will be uncomfortable for the patient. The upper nasal, upper temporal, lower temporal, and lower nasal quadrants should then be evaluated for the blood vessels and any evidence of hemorrhage, infarction, or retinal detachment. Large white areas, red areas, out-

of-focus areas, or pale undulating folds are abnormal and warrant ophthalmology evaluation.

Posterior segment injuries

Blood in the posterior segment, retinal detachment, retinal hemorrhages, a swollen optic disc, and papilledema are examples of abnormal findings (**Fig. 15**). The presence of a marked vitreous hemorrhage is suspected if there is an abnormal red reflex and is associated with poor visual prognosis in ocular trauma involving the posterior segment (vitreous/choroid/retina). Traumatic vitreous hemorrhage mandates emergent ophthalmologic consultation, because 11% to 44% of vitreous hemorrhages are associated with retinal tears.[16]

Retinal detachments

Severe ocular trauma may result in retinal detachments. The patient may complain of a distinct peripheral visual field cut ("curtain coming down"). On presentation, retinal detachment is usually divided into "macula on," when the fovea is still attached, and "macula off," where the retina is detached centrally.[16] People with macula-on retinal detachments typically have good initial visual acuity and a better prognosis with successful surgery. Rapidly progressive cases are therefore treated as a matter of urgency. Patients may require air injection (pneumatic retinopexy), scleral buckle, vitrectomy, or all 3.

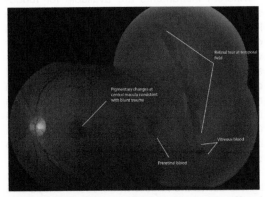

Fig. 15. Fundus photograph of a patient who suffered blunt trauma to the left eye. It shows a series of retinal tears in the temporal periphery of the left eye. Note the shallow subretinal fluid around the largest tear. The presence of fluid is indicated by the glassy loss of details in the underlying choroid. There is also vitreous blood present in front of the largest tear (out of the focal plane) and preretinal blood between the tears and the macula. The central macula shows pigmentary alterations consistent with blunt trauma. (*Courtesy of* Dr G. Baker Hubbard III, MD, Emory University Eye Center, Atlanta, GA.)

Traumatic optic neuropathy

Traumatic optic neuropathy refers to an acute injury of the optic nerve secondary to trauma. Initial fundoscopic examination often reveals a normal optic disc, because the location of injury is usually located within the posterior orbit or optic canal. The disc eventually changes 3 to 4 weeks after the event, becoming markedly pale. The optic nerve axons may be damaged either directly or indirectly and the visual loss may be partial or complete. An indirect injury to the optic nerve typically occurs from the transmission of forces to the optic canal from blunt head trauma. This is in contrast to direct traumatic optic neuropathy, which results from an anatomic disruption of the optic nerve fibers from penetrating orbital trauma, bone fragments within the optic canal, or nerve sheath hematomas.

SUMMARY

Trauma to the eye is not an uncommon occurrence in maxillofacial trauma, and it may occur as a direct result of the original injury, may be secondary to surgical or medical interventions, or may even be iatrogenic as a result of an improper physical examination. *Primum non-nocere* is a well-known phrase in medical and dental training that means, "First, do no harm." It therefore behooves the oral and maxillofacial surgeon to be familiar with the relevant anatomy, to be able to take a pertinent history, and to be proficient in the standardized and physical examination of the eyes, adnexal structures, and optic system. This article has reviewed the proper basic examination techniques and highlighted more advanced techniques, including the SLE and DFE, which greatly augment the gross physical examination. The role of the oral and maxillofacial surgeon is not to diagnose or manage complex ocular injuries. However, familiarity and recognition of *normal* findings will guide the clinician to recognize *abnormalities* via a thorough but directed perioperative ophthalmologic examination, thereby allowing appropriate consultation and communication with an ophthalmologist if necessary.

REFERENCES

1. Nash EA, Margo CE. Patterns of emergency department visits for disorders of the eye and ocular adnexa. Arch Ophthalmol 1998;116:1222–6.
2. Nawar EW, Niska RW, Xu J. National hospital ambulatory medical care survey: 2005 emergency department summary. Adv Data 2007;386:1–32.
3. McGwin G Jr, Hall TA, Xie A, et al. Trends in eye injury in the United States, 1992-2001. Invest Ophthalmol Vis Sci 2006;47:521–7.
4. McGwin G Jr, Xie A, Owsley C. Rate of eye injury in the United States. Arch Ophthalmol 2005;123:970–6.
5. Feliciano DV, Mattox KL, Morre EE. Trauma. 6th edition. New York: The McGraw-Hill Companies; 2007.
6. Guly CM, Guly HR, Bouamra O, et al. Ocular injuries in patients with major trauma. Emerg Med J 2006;23: 915–7.
7. Poon A, McCluskey PJ, Hill DA. Eye injuries in patients with major trauma. J Trauma 1999;46:494–9.
8. al-Qurainy IA, Stassen LF, Dutton GN, et al. The characteristics of midfacial fractures and the association with ocular injury: a prospective study. Br J Oral Maxillofac Surg 1991;29:291–301.
9. Root T. OphthoBook. 1st edition. Charleston (SC): CreateSpace Independent Publishing Platform; 2009.
10. Kuhn F, Morris R, Witherspoon CD, et al. The Birmingham Eye Trauma Terminology system (BETT). J Fr Ophtalmol 2004;27:206–10.
11. Riordan-Eva P, Cunningham E. Vaughan & Ashbury's general ophthalmology. 18th edition. New York: The McGraw-Hill Companies; 2011.
12. Lang GK. Ophthalmology: a pocket textbook atlas. 2nd edition. New York: Thieme New York; 2000.
13. Jamal BT, Diecidue RJ, Taub D, et al. Orbital hemorrhage and compressive optic neuropathy in patients with midfacial fractures receiving low-molecular weight heparin therapy. J Oral Maxillofac Surg 2009;67:1416–9.
14. Robinett D, Kahn J. The physical examination of the eye. Emerg Med Clin North Am 2008;26:1–16.
15. Spraul CW, Grossniklaus HE. Vitreous hemorrhage. Surv Ophthalmol 1997;42:3–39.
16. Bord SP, Linden J. Trauma to the globe and orbit. Emerg Med Clin North Am 2008;26:97–123.
17. Soparkar CN, Patrinely JR. The eye examination in facial trauma for the plastic surgeon. Plast Reconstr Surg 2007;120(7 Suppl 2):49s–56s.
18. Yanoff MY, Duer JS. Ophthalmology. 3rd edition. St. Louis (MO): Mosby; 2008.
19. Adams RD, Victor M, Ropper AH. Adams and Victor's principles of neurology. 7th edition. New York: McGraw-Hill; 2001.
20. Crumpton KL, Shockley LW. Ocular trauma: a quick, illustrated guide to treatment, triage, and medicolegal implications. Emerg Med Rep 1997; 18:223–34.
21. Adams WE, Hatt SR, Leske DA, et al. Comparison of a diplopia questionnaire to the goldmann diplopia field. J AAPOS 2008;12(3):247–51.
22. Holmes JM, Leske DA, Kupersmith MJ. New methods for quantifying diplopia. Ophthalmology 2005;112:2035–9.
23. Kunimoto DY, Kunal DK, Makar MS, et al. The wills eye manual: office and emergency room diagnosis

and treatment of eye disease. 4th edition. Philadelphia: Lippincott Williams & Wilkins; 2004.

24. Miloro M, Ghali GE, Larsen P, et al. Peterson's principles of oral and maxillofacial surgery. 2nd edition. Hamilton (Ontario): BC Decker; 2004.

25. Harris GJ. Orbital blowout fractures: surgical timing and technique. Eye 2006;20:1207–12.

26. Egbert JE, May K, Kersten RC, et al. Pediatric orbital floor fracture: direct extraocular muscle involvement. Ophthalmology 2000;107(10):1875–9.

Traditional and Contemporary Surgical Approaches to the Orbit

Michael R. Markiewicz, DDS, MPH, MD[a],
R. Bryan Bell, DDS, MD[a,b,c],*

KEYWORDS

- Frameless stereotaxy • Orbit • Orbital fractures • Orbital neoplasms • Maxillofacial surgery
- Neuronavigation • Plastic • Wounds and injuries

KEY POINTS

- The surgeon should generally use the approach with which they are most comfortable, which provides for optimal cosmesis, and that results in the least morbidity.
- The authors' preferred approach for most isolated orbital floor fractures is a transconjunctival approach performed at the conjunctival fornix. A lateral canthotomy is not advised.
- An isolated transconjunctival fornix approach combined with upper lid blepharoplasty typically provides adequate access to the orbit for most applications.
- An alternative to a lower lid/transconjunctival approach for isolated orbital floor fractures is endoscopic-assisted transantral repair.

INTRODUCTION

A variety of surgical approaches to the orbit exist, and all carry advantages and disadvantages. In general, the surgical approach used should provide adequate access to the region of interest, should be well concealed, and result in few complications. Contemporary incisions may provide 360-degree access to the external orbital frame and internal orbit and should be imperceptible if performed skillfully. In fact, a single lower lid incision, occasionally combined with an upper eyelid "blepharoplasty" approach alone will provide wide access to the lateral, inferior, and medial orbital walls; result in few complications; and is all that is needed in most operations of the orbit.

Various extensions of lower eyelid approaches, such as the transcaruncular incision or the lateral canthotomy, are useful as well. Occasionally, a coronal incision is required to provide wider access to the orbital roof, frontal-orbital region, or naso-orbital ethmoid complex, and will facilitate circumferential exposure. Direct approaches to the orbit, such as the Lynch, glabellar, medial crease, and superolateral (Wright)[1] incisions result in visible scarring and should be abandoned except in a few instances. This article will focus on common contemporary approaches to the orbit and provides an evidence-based guide to incision selection and design. The anatomy of the orbit is discussed in detail in elsewhere in this issue, therefore only essential points are reviewed.

Funding support: None.

Financial disclosures: The authors have no financial disclosures to declare.

[a] Department of Oral and Maxillofacial Surgery, Oregon Health and Science University, 611 Southwest Campus Drive, SDOMS, Portland, OR 97239, USA; [b] Oral, Head and Neck Cancer Program, Providence Cancer Center, Portland, OR, USA; [c] Trauma Service/Oral and Maxillofacial Surgery Service, Legacy Emanuel Medical Center, Portland, OR, USA

* Corresponding author. 1849 Northwest Kearney, Suite 300, Portland, OR 97209.

E-mail address: bellb@hnsa1.com

Oral Maxillofacial Surg Clin N Am 24 (2012) 573–607

http://dx.doi.org/10.1016/j.coms.2012.08.004

Transcutaneous Approaches

Transcutaneous approaches to the orbit are designed in either the lower (**Fig. 1**) or upper eyelid (**Fig. 2**) to provide access to the orbital rim/floor or upper orbit respectively. Transcutaneous lower eyelid incisions have been described as being placed in a "subciliary" position, as a "subtarsal" or "midlid" approach, or as an "infraorbital" incision (**Fig. 3**). The latter approach leaves a prominent depressed scar and should be avoided. The decision to perform a subciliary or subtarsal incision is based partially on the treating surgeon's training and experience, but data exist that favor the subtarsal approach owing to a lower reported rate of ectropion.[2] In addition to these two lower lid incisions, two basic transcutaneous approaches to the superior orbit, the supraorbital eyebrow and upper eyelid (blepharoplasty) incisions, have been described and remain widely used. The "lateral brow" approach, like the infraorbital approach, results in prominent scarring and should be avoided. The coronal approach and orbital exenteration, direct cutaneous approaches to the orbit, are also discussed. Technique and outcomes between each approach are reviewed. Inference from outcomes data should be tempered by the fact that many reports describe variations of these techniques, making the generalizability of the results difficult.

Access to the inferior, medial, and lateral orbit
Subciliary approach The subciliary, also known as the blepharoplasty or infraciliary incision, was introduced in 1944 by Converse and coleagues.[3] It involves an incision made 2 mm just below the lash line over the tarsal plate. Its major advantage is that it results in little to no perceivable scar and allows for easy extension laterally for exposure of the lateral orbital rim. Once the incision is made, there are 3 pathways available to the underlying orbit—the "skin flap" dissection, the "skin-muscle flap" dissection, and the "stepped skin muscle flap (Converse)" dissection (**Fig. 4**).[4] The "skin-only"

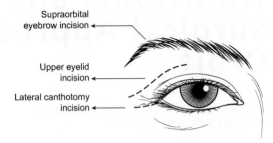

Fig. 2. Approaches to the upper orbit include the supraorbital eyebrow (lateral brow), upper eyelid (blepharoplasty), and lateral canthotomy incisions.

technique is performed by dissecting the thin eyelid skin from incision inferiorly to the orbital rim where the orbicularis oculi and periosteum are incised. This method, however, has been associated with a high rate of complications, such as ectropion, skin necrosis, and ecchymosis and is no longer advocated.[5] The senior author (R.B.B) no longer advocates this approach in the trauma setting, where edema and tissue injury contribute to unfavorable esthetic and functional outcomes. The "nonstepped skin-muscle flap" involves an incision through skin and pretarsal orbicularis oculi until the tarsal plate is encountered. The orbital rim is then approached in a preseptal plane and a periosteal incision is then made just below the orbital septum. The "stepped skin-muscle flap" dissection involves dividing the orbicularis oris muscle 2 to 3 mm below the skin incision, leaving a strip of pretarsal orbicularis oculi to support the lower eyelid. Then, after following a preseptal plane to the orbital rim, an incision is made through periosteum to the orbital bone. The "stepped" technique preserves the pretarsal orbicularis oculi fibers and limits scarring at the eyelid margin while maintaining normal eyelid position. In addition, it limits skin or septal perforations associated with the "skin-only," and "nonstepped skin-muscle" techniques. The "stepped skin-muscle flap" technique is described in the following section as the preferred subciliary technique.

Technique A scleral shield or tarsorrhaphy suture should be placed to protect the globe. For the tarsorrhaphy suture, a 5-0 nylon suture is placed either intermarginally,[6] or as a horizontal mattress.[7] Intermarginal placement involves placing a suture in and out of the tarsal plate in one pass through the tarsal meibomian openings, whereas horizontal mattress placement involves placement of the suture through the skin and tarsi of the upper and lower eyelids bisecting the palpebral fissure. For each technique, the suture should enter the eyelid at the grayline. The incision should be marked approximately 2 mm below the eyelashes along

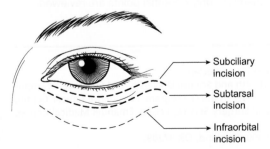

Fig. 1. Approaches to the lower orbit include the subciliary, subtarsal (midlid), and infraorbital incisions.

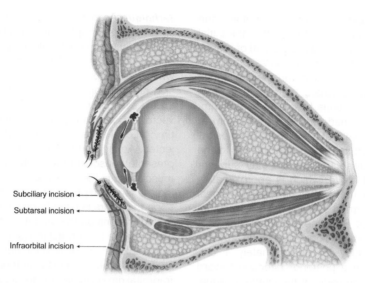

Fig. 3. Transcutaneous approaches to the infraorbital rim and orbital floor include the subciliary, subtarsal, and infraorbital incisions.

the entire length of the eyelid. It may be extended laterally or inferolaterally within a natural skin crease up to 2 cm past the lateral canthus, as the anterior temporal branch of the facial nerve crosses the zygomatic arch approximately 3 cm lateral to the lateral canthus.[8] Local anesthesia is administered after marking the incision. If edema of the eyelid prevents visualization of a natural crease, an injection of hyaluronidase mixed with local anesthetic may be useful.[9] The initial incision should be through skin only down to orbicularis oris. Using the

tarsorrhaphy suture to retract the lower eyelid superiorly, subcutaneous dissection just superior to the pretarsal orbicularis oris toward to the inferior orbital rim is then performed with a pointed scissors or scalpel blade to a depth of 4 to 6 mm. Using a blunted tip scissors, the orbicularis oculi muscle is then dissected in the horizontal direction of its fibers down to the periosteum of the lateral orbital rim. Staying supraperiosteal at the orbital rim makes sure that a supraseptal plane is maintained. After adequate development of a pocket between

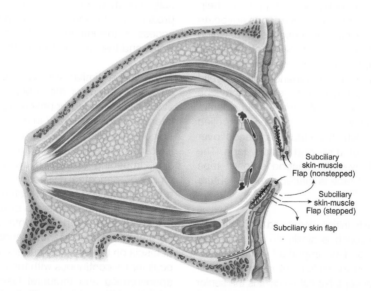

Fig. 4. Following a subciliary incision a skin-muscle (nonstepped), skin-muscle (stepped), or skin-only flap may be developed.

orbicularis oris and the septum orbitale, the muscle is incised inferior to the level of the initial skin incision, making sure to leave a cuff of pretarsal orbicularis oris attached to the tarsal plate. The remaining inferiorly based skin-muscle flap is then retracted inferiorly to where the orbital septum terminates and transitions to orbital periosteum. An incision is then made through periosteum at the zygoma and maxilla at a level 3 to 4 mm below or lateral to the orbital rim to stay inferior to the orbital septum. Dissection should stay superior to the infraorbital nerve, which is approximately 7 mm inferior to the orbital rim. Subperiosteal dissection is performed over the maxilla, zygoma, and inside the orbit. Because the infraorbital rim is superior to the orbital floor, dissection actually takes place inferiorly for approximately 1 cm, then horizontally in a posterior direction toward the orbital apex. The origin of the inferior oblique, which arises from the medial orbital floor just lateral to the origin of the nasolacrimal duct and just posterior to the orbital rim, is stripped during this dissection. The inferior orbital fissure will also be encountered and its contents may be bluntly retracted superiorly along with the rest of the orbital contents to provide access to the orbital floor, medial and lateral orbital walls, and anterior maxilla.

Only periosteal and skin closures are needed. A running 6-0 fast gut stitch may be placed for skin closure. The major disadvantage of the subciliary incision is that it is associated with vertical shortening of the lower eye lid owing to septal and skin scarring.[2] In the authors' experience, this lid retraction commonly results in increased scleral show and, less commonly, in ectropion. To help counteract this process, some surgeons advocate the use of a lower eyelid suspensory suture, which may be placed through the grayline of the lower eyelid in an intermarginal manor and taped to the forehead to maintain superior lower eyelid support ("Frost stitch"). This suture may be removed after resolution of lower eyelid edema. To secure this suture, a layer of tape is applied to the forehead skin, the suture is placed over the tape followed by a second layer of tape. The suture is folded over the second strip of tape and a third strip of tape is placed over the suture and other 2 strips.[10]

Subtarsal approach Initially described by Converse,[2] the subtarsal approach is similar to the subciliary approach, with a few important differences.[11] Because it has been shown to result in fewer complications and has acceptable esthetics, it is the senior author's (R.B.B.) preferred transcutaneous approach to the lower orbit.

Technique As in the subciliary technique, a scleral shield or tarsorrhaphy suture is placed. Marking of the skin incision should take place along the lower border of the tarsal plate in the subtarsal fold, or when edema precludes the presence of normal skin creases, approximately 5 to 7 mm from the lower eyelid margin following an inferolateral vector to a point just past the lateral orbital rim.[2,4] Local anesthetic with vasoconstrictor is injected. An incision is then made through skin and preseptal muscle to the orbital septum. The skin-muscle flap is then elevated superiorly by retracting the tarsorrhaphy suture superiorly and a blunt tipped scissors is used to dissect and spread the orbicularis oris off the orbital septum in an inferior vector to the infraorbital rim (see **Fig. 3**). A double skin hook will assist with inferior retraction of the lower eyelid skin. Once the anterior edge of the infraorbital rim is visualized, an incision through periosteum is made. The orbit, maxilla, and zygoma are then dissected similarly to as described in the subciliary approach (**Fig. 5**). As in the subciliary approach, only periosteal and skin closure is needed. As an alternative to the lower eyelid suspensory suture, a suture may be placed through the lateral canthal tendon and lateral aspect of pretarsal orbicularis oris, providing temporary support to the lower lid during initial healing phases.[12] It may be removed once edema resolves.

Extended lower eyelid approach The extended lower eyelid approach provides additional access to the lateral orbital rim to a point 10 to 12 mm superior to the zygomaticofrontal suture, potentially negating the need for upper eyelid approaches.[13] In addition, this approach provides access to the inferior and lateral orbital rim and walls, and the greater wing of the sphenoid.[13]

Technique A similar approach is taken as previously described for the subciliary incision; however, it is extended approximately 1.0 to 1.5 cm laterally or inferolaterally in a natural skin crease. As noted by Ellis and Zide,[10] the subtarsal incision is placed more inferiorly than the subciliary incision, impeding dissection up the lateral orbital rim. Supraperiosteal dissection of the entire lateral orbital rim staying below the lateral canthal tendon is performed with a scissors or a no. 15 blade to just above the zygomaticofrontal suture. The anterior limb of the lateral canthal tendon is a thickening of fascia on the posterior surface of the orbicularis oculi that is continuous with the fascia of the galea aponeurotica and temporal fascia lateral to the orbital rim. The thicker, posterior limb of the lateral canthal tendon is more difficult to separate from

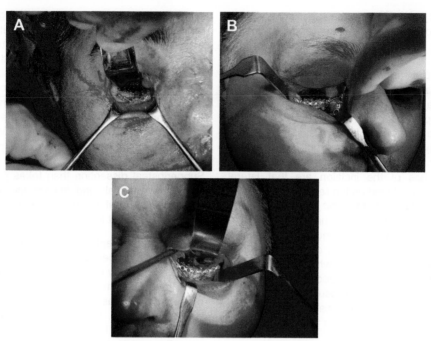

Fig. 5. Subtarsal approach used to access a fracture of the infraorbital rim and floor (*A*). Bilateral (*B, C*) subtarsal approaches used in a patient suffering Le Fort III and orbital rim/floor fractures.

the lateral horn of the levator palpebrae superiors and Lockwood suspensory ligament. The orbicularis oris and anterior limb of the lateral canthal tendon are retracted superiorly and with superior traction on tarsorrhaphy suture, a periosteal incision from just superior to the zygomaticofrontal suture is made downward, connecting to the infraorbital incision. A subperiosteal dissection then takes place stripping the orbital floor, orbital wall, posterior limb of the lateral canthal tendon, Lockwood suspensory ligament, and lateral cheek ligament from Whitnall tubercle of the zygoma.[13] As in the subciliary and subtarsal approaches, only periosteal and skin closure is needed. Lateral canthopexy, however, is not required for lateral canthal tendon repositioning.[10]

Infraorbital (orbital rim) approach Relative indications for an infraorbital approach include conjunctival or orbital pathology, a hypertrophic orbicularis oris muscle, preexisting laceration of the infraorbital rim, persistent globe edema, presence of globe prosthesis, or an unstable globe or corneal injury.[12,14] The advantages of the infraorbital approach are that it is not technically difficult, it is a direct approach to the infraorbital rim, and it does not lead to postoperative lid dysfunction as often as the subciliary and subtarsal approaches. In addition, the medial half of the infraorbital incision may be used for a dacryocystorhinostomy approach owing to its proximity to the lacrimal

gland. Given the unsightly scar associated with the infraorbital incision and other available less morbid approaches to the orbit, however, it should be rarely used. For completeness, it will be reviewed.[11]

Technique The incision is marked in at the level of the infraorbital rim margin in a minor skin crease that is present at the transition of the thin eyelid and thick cheek skin (see **Fig. 1**).[14] This skin crease represents the transition between the orbital and palpebral portions of orbicularis oris and the transition from orbital septum to facial periosteum. Preferably the incision is just within the periorbital skin, because incisions in the thicker skin of the cheek result in a more unsightly scar (see **Fig. 1**). A scleral shield or tarsorrhaphy suture should be placed for protection of the globe. Local anesthesia with vasoconstrictor is injected.

An incision is then made through skin, and then preorbital orbicularis oculi muscle (see **Fig. 3**). Dissection should take placed down to the preorbital periosteum. The periosteum begins to blend with orbital septum 1 to 2 mm inferior to the infraorbital rim and the periosteal incision should be placed just below this transition point. The orbit, maxilla, and zygoma are then dissected in a subperiosteal manor similar to as described in the previous subciliary and subtarsal approaches. To avoid a depressed scar, stepping of the incision may be performed; however, an unsightly scar will usually still persist.[14] As in the subciliary and sub-tarsal approaches, only periosteal and skin closure is needed.

Access to the superior orbit

Supraorbital eyebrow (lateral brow) approach The supraorbital approach offers direct access to the lateral supraorbital rim and frontozygomatic suture. The advantage of the incision is that there are no major neurovascular structures within its vicinity, which makes dissection straightforward. Disadvantages of the incision are that lateral extension is precluded as the resting skin tension lines (RSTLs) lateral to the orbit run perpendicular to the incision resulting in an unsightly scar, and that in women who have undergone previous cosmetic eyebrow removal, a camouflage effect of the brow is restricted. Even when well executed, the incision results in limited access to the supra-orbital rim, and esthetically results in an unsightly scar.[1,10] It is no longer advocated as a first-line approach to the lateral orbit for this reason.

Technique A corneal shield tarsorrhaphy suture should be placed. The upper eyebrow should not be shaved. Local anesthetic with vasoconstrictor is injected into the area of the proposed incision. With bi-digital tension placed superior and inferior to the brow, an incision is made in trichophillic fashion (parallel to the hair shafts of the eyebrow

to the depth of the periosteum) (see **Fig. 1**). Ante-romedial extension of the incision within the brow may improve access; however, inferolateral exten-sion should be avoided, as this would cross the RSTLs (crow's feet) at a 90° angel, resulting in an unsightly scar. Direct inferior extension in "skin only" may take place; however, should stay 6 mm above the lateral canthus to prevent injury to the frontal branch of cranial nerve VII. Follow-ing supraperiosteal undermining, the periosteum overlying the zygomaticofrontal suture is incised. Subperiosteal dissection then takes place along the lateral, medial, and inferior aspects of the superolateral orbital rim. Periosteum and skin closure are all that is needed.

Upper eyelid (blepharoplasty, supratarsal fold) approach The upper eyelid approach is associated with less morbidity than the supraorbital approach to neurovascular strictures located in the periphery of the orbit, such as the frontal branch of the facial nerve (see **Fig. 2**). In contrast to the supraorbital eyebrow incision, however, the upper eyelid inci-sion offers access to virtually the entire supraorbital rim and superior orbit (**Figs. 6** and **7**). Unlike the lower eyelid, where the orbital septum inserts onto the tarsal plate, after its origin at facial perios-teum, in the upper eyelid it inserts and blends with the levator aponeurosis, which is located approxi-mately 10 to 15 mm above the upper eyelid margin.

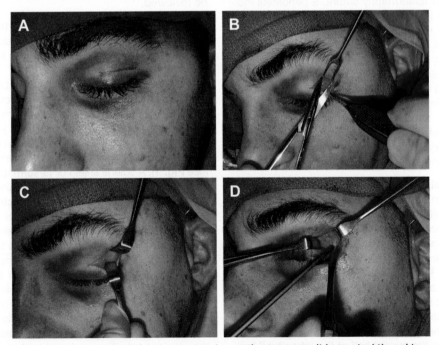

Fig. 6. After skin incision approximately 10 mm superior to the upper eyelid margin (*A*), a skin-muscle flap is developed (*B*). Incision is made through the periosteum (*C*) with further subperiosteal elevation in all directions to access the zygomaticofrontal suture (*D*).

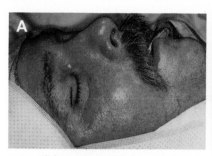
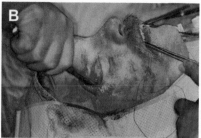

Fig. 7. An upper eyelid approach (A) is used for access to the zygomatic arch for reduction with Dingman elevator (B).

The levator palpebrae superioris originates from the lesser wing of the sphenoid just above the optic foreman. It becomes aponeurotic as it passes superiorly and anteriorly to the equator of the globe. Deep to the orbital septum-Levator aponeurosis complex, lies the Müller muscle–tarsal complex. The sympathetically innervated Müller muscle originates from the inner surface of the levator aponeurosis and inserts onto the superficial surface of the upper tarsal plate.

Technique After placement of a corneal shield or a tarsorrhaphy suture, an incision is marked in the supratarsal fold parallel to the superior palpebral sulcus, a naturally occurring skin line located approximately 10 to 14 mm superior to the upper eyelid margin.[15] If no crease is available because of trauma, congenital anomaly, or involution of levator palpebrae superioris, an incision may easily be marked by comparing with the contralateral side (see **Fig. 6**A). For additional access to the lateral orbit, the incision may be extended into the crow's feet of the lateral orbital skin staying 6 mm superior to the lateral canthus to avoid the frontal branch of the facial nerve. Following injection of local anesthesia with vasoconstrictor, a 1-cm to 2-cm incision is made is made through skin and orbicularis oculi. Alternatively, a skin incision followed by scissors dissection through the orbicularis oris may offer an easier approach (see **Fig. 6**B). A skin-muscle flap is then developed superiorly, medially, and laterally, staying deep to orbicularis oris and superficial to the orbital septum/levator aponeurosis complex. This continues to the supraorbital rim.[16,17] It is important to elevate skin and muscle together to maintain viability to the overlying skin.[10] While retracting the skin-muscle flap superiorly, a periosteal incision is made over the desired area of the superolateral orbital rim with careful attention to maintain bony contact with the periosteal elevator (see **Fig. 6**C). Subperiosteal dissection is then performed in all directions for excellent access to the zygomaticofrontal suture (see **Fig. 6**D). A skin-only flap staying superior to

orbicularis oris may reduce levator palpebrae superioris injury and postoperative ptosis; however, it is associated with an increased risk of bleeding and hematoma, which may lead to detrimental skin necrosis. In addition, the skin-only flap is technically challenging, owing to the skin's close adherence to the thin orbicularis oris muscle of the upper eyelid and risk of a button-hole defect. Unlike inferior orbital transcutaneous approaches, the wound should be closed in 3 layers: periosteum (3-0 polyglactin suture), orbicularis oris (4-0 chromic gut), and skin (running 6-0 fast gut). Failure to close orbicularis muscle may lead to a depression along the orbital rim.

Coronal approach Originally described by Tessier for an approach to the orbits, the coronal incision is an excellent approach for accessing the upper and middle thirds of the face, and the zygomatic arches.[18,19] The major risks of this approach include injury to the temporal and zygomatic branches of the facial nerve, temporal hollowing, scalp hematoma, parietal scalp pain, parasthesia or anesthesia, infection, and nasal orbital hypertrophy.[20] Injury to the temporal branch of the facial nerve can be severely debilitating with patients exhibiting loss of ipsilateral forehead wrinkles, brow ptosis, inability to raise the brow, and visual defects.

Anatomy
The most superficial layer of the scalp is the skin, which is surgically inseparable from the underlying subcutaneous tissue (**Fig. 8**). Under the subcutaneous layer is the musculoaponeurotic layer (galea). These 2 layers are also difficult to separate; therefore, when the galeal aponeurosis and frontalis/occipitalis muscles move, so does the overlying skin.

The musculoaponeurotic layer consists of the paired frontalis and occipitalis muscles, the auricular muscles, and the aponeurosis, which is present between frontalis and occipitalis (occipitofrontalis or epicranius) muscles. The galea, which

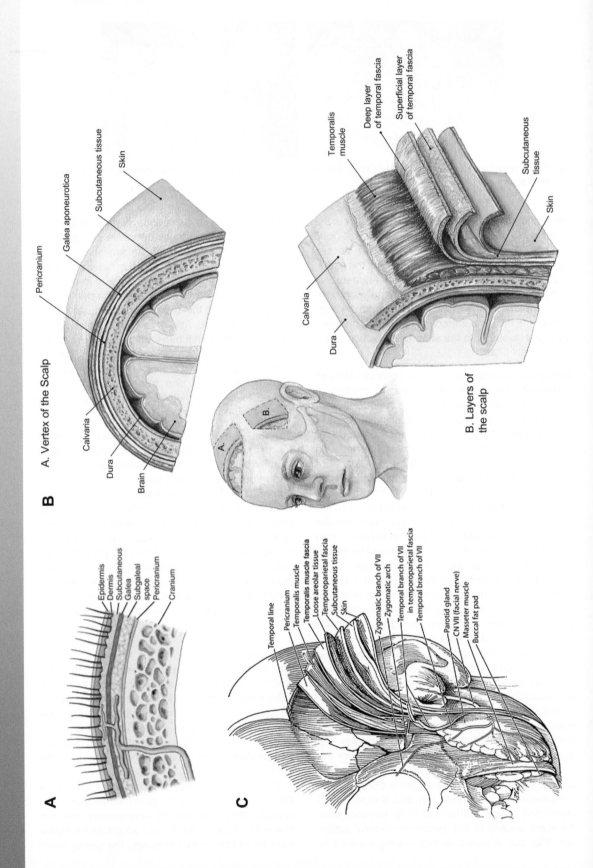

B

A. Vertex of the Scalp

Pericranium

Galea aponeurotica

Subcutaneous tissue

Skin

Calvaria

Dura

Brain

Temporalis muscle

Deep layer of temporal fascia

Superficial layer of temporal fascia

Subcutaneous tissue

Skin

Calvaria

Dura

B. Layers of the scalp

A

Epidermis
Dermis
Subcutaneous
Galea
Subgaleal space
Pericranium
Cranium

C

Temporal line

Pericranium

Temporalis muscle

Temporalis muscle fascia

Loose areolar tissue

Temporoparietal fascia

Subcutaneous tissue

Skin

Zygomatic branch of VII

Zygomatic arch

Temporal branch of VII in temporoparietal fascia

Temporal branch of VII

Parotid gland

CN VII (facial nerve)

Masseter muscle

Buccal fat pad

is a glistening sheet of fibrous tissue approximately 0.5-mm thick, actually only refers to the aponeurosis. Its lateral extension into the temporoparietal region is the temporoparietal fascia (superficial temporal fascia), which is continuous with the superficial musculoaponeurotic system (SMAS) of the face and the superficial cervical fascia (encasing the platysma) of the neck. The superficial temporal vessels travel just superior to the temporoparietal fascia, whereas the temporal branch of the facial nerve travels just deep to this layer. The paired frontalis muscles originate from the galeal aponeurosis and insert on the dermis at the level of the eyebrows. The paired occipitalis muscles originate from lateral two-thirds of the superior nuchal line and external occipital protuberance and insert onto the galeal aponeurosis overlying the occipital bone. An extension of the galeal aponeurosis splits the 2 quadrilateral frontalis muscles at the midline of the forehead.

Inferior to the galea is the loose areolar layer, or the subaponeurotic plane. This layer readily separates from the overlying galea and is the fascial plane the readily separates in trauma. The subgaleal fascia continues anteriorly deep to the orbicularis oris muscles and laterally attaches to the frontal process of the zygomatic arch, and travels on the superior surface of the zygomatic arch, above the external auditory meatus, and the mastoid processes, eventually attaching again to the periosteum at the superior nuchal line. This layer allows for free movement of the overlying skin and musculoaponeurotic layer without disturbing the underlying most inferior layer: the pericranium, which is the periosteal of the skull. The pericranium is more firmly attached at the cranial sutures, but can be elevated as a separate layer.

In the temporoparietal region, beneath the temporoparietal fascia, lies the extension of the subgaleal fascia, which can be dissected as a separate layer in this area but is usually just used as a continuance of the subgaleal plane in the coronal approach. Beneath subgaleal fascia in the temporoparietal region lies the temporalis fascia (deep temporal fascia), which arises superiorly from the superior temporal line where it fuses with pericranium. The temporalis fascia is continuous with the pericranium above the superior temporal lines, the parotidomasseteric fascia below the level of the zygomatic arch, and the cervical fascia incasing the muscles of the neck. At the level of the superior orbital rim, the temporalis fascia divides into a superficial layer, which attaches to the lateral border of the zygomatic arch, and a deep layer, which attaches to the medial border of the zygomatic arch. The middle temporal artery, a branch of the superficial temporal artery, is the primary blood supply to the temporalis fascia. Intervening between the superficial and deep layers is the superficial temporal fat pad. The blood supply to the temporal fat pad is the middle temporal artery, a branch of the superficial temporal artery. Deep to the deep temporalis fascia is the buccal fat pad. The temporalis muscle arises from the deep layers of the temporalis fascia at the temporal fossa, passing medial to the zygomatic arch and inserting onto the coronoid process of the mandible. The blood supply to the temporalis muscle is primarily from the anterior and posterior deep temporal arteries (branches of internal maxillary artery), and secondarily from the superficial temporal artery.

The temporal branch (frontal branch) of the facial nerve exits the parotid gland just inferior to the zygomatic arch.[21,22] In general, the course of the temporal branch of the facial nerve is from a point 0.5 cm below the tragus to a point 1.5 cm above the lateral eyebrow,[22] and it crosses the zygomatic arch between a distance of 0.8 to 3.5 cm anterior to the anterior concavity of the external

---

Fig. 8. (A) The layers of the scalp are the skin (epidermis and then dermis), subcutaneous layer, musculoaponeurotic layer (Galea), loose areolar connective tissue (subgaleal layer), and the pericranium. (B) The layer of the scalp change below the superior temporal lines where the plane below the superficial temporal fascia (temporoparietal fascia) is continuous with the subgaleal layer above the superior temporal lines (C). The temporal branch (frontal branch) of the facial nerve travels just below the temporoparietal fascia. The temporal branch can be found from a point 0.5 cm below the tragus to a point 1.5 cm above the lateral eyebrow while crossing the zygomatic arch between a distance of 0.8 and 3.5 cm anterior to the anterior concavity of the external auditory canal at an average distance of 2 cm anterior to the anterior concavity of the external auditory canal. It crosses the zygomatic arch passing between the under surface of the temporoparietal fascia and the fusion of the zygomatic arch, the superficial layer of temporalis fascia, and subgaleal fascia. As it continues along the undersurface of the temporoparietal fascia, it inserts onto the frontalis muscle at a point approximately 2 cm above the supraorbital rims; however, not before giving off branches to the superior portion of orbicularis oculi, anterior auricular, the corrugator, and the procerus muscle. ([A] *Adapted from* Wells M. Scalp reconstruction. In: Mathes SJ, editor. Plastic surgery. Philadelphia: Saunders; 2006. p. 607–10; with permission. [B] *From* Ducic Y. Reconstruction of the scalp. Facial Plast Surg Clin North Am 2009;17(2):177–87; with permission. [C] *From* Strong EB. Frontal sinus fractures. Operative Techniques in Otolaryngology 2008;19:151–60; with permission.)

auditory canal at an average distance of 2.0 cm anterior to the anterior concavity of the external auditory canal. As the nerve crosses the zygomatic arch, it passes between the under surface of the temporoparietal fascia and the fusion of the zygomatic arch, the superficial layer of temporalis fascia, and subgaleal fascia. Continuing along the undersurface of the temporoparietal fascia, it inserts onto the frontalis muscle no more than 2 cm above the supraorbital rims; however, not before giving off branches to the superior portion of orbicularis oculi, anterior auricular, the corrugator, and the procerus muscles.[23]

Depending on the procedure, the coronal approach may be performed by a subperiosteal dissection in which the periosteum is freed from the superior temporal lines. Proceeding anteriorly, the temporalis muscles are left intact; however, a subgaleal approach may be taken in a plane that is readily separable. The deeper pericranium may be used as a pedicled vascularized flap.

Technique Although shaving the area of incision is an option, leaving the patient's hair in place may be beneficial in assessing the direction of the hair shafts and their growth, minimizing damage to hair follicles. It is not necessary to shave the patient. Before sterile preparation, a comb should be used to part the hair at the proposed incision line, nonpetroleum jelly is applied, and the excess hair is controlled with elastics. The entire head is prepared and draped so that even the occiput is accessible.

When designing an incision, hairline recession at the widow's peak and lateral temporal valleys should be taken into consideration. In men who are balding, the incision should be placed transversely between preauricular areas, several centimeters behind the hairline.[10] The incision may be straight, sinusoidal, or sawtooth (zigzag, stealth) or in a geometric broken-line pattern.[24,25] Other modifications have been described; however, a sinusoidal or sawtooth pattern is better concealed than straight-line incisions.[26] Incisions may also be placed postauricularly if it is not planned to expose zygomatic arches.[27] In women, and men without potential for balding, incisions may be placed anteriorly at the vertex remaining 4 to 5 cm behind the hairline. The incision should be placed behind the hairline in children because it will migrate with growth. Hemicoronal incisions should curve and end toward the hairline at their most anterior aspect to allow for maximal exposure. The most inferior extent of the incision should also be considered. For exposure of the zygomatic arch, the incision may be extended as far as the helix of the ear; however, when exposure to the

temporomandibular joint or infraorbital rims are needed, the incision may be extended as far as the ear lobe.

The initial incision should be made between superior temporal lines down to the loose areolar connective tissue of the subgaleal plane. The initial incision is made only to the superior temporal lines laterally to prevent penetration of the temporalis fascia into the temporalis muscle, which bleeds readily on incision. This suprapericranial plane may be dissected with ease. Incisions below the superior temporal line should be continuous with the subgaleal plane above the superior temporal line down to the level below the temporoparietal fascia just before the glistening superficial layer of temporal fascia, which blends with the pericranium. To maintain the correct plane below the superior temporal line, a curved scissors may be used to bluntly dissect a subgaleal plane toward the zygomatic arch.

After incision, the flap is elevated 1 to 2 cm anteriorly and posteriorly in the subgaleal plane. Hemostatic clips (Raney clips) are applied to the bleeding wound margins. Bleeding vessels may be cauterized; however, electrocautery should be discouraged owing to potential damage to hair follicles and subsequent alopecia. Bone wax or electrocautery may be used for bleeding emissary veins through the pericranium.

The flap may be elevated in the subgaleal plane with a scalpel (with dull end of blade resting on the pericranium, using the point of the blade to incise the subgaleal areolar tissue) or electrocautery, or with finger dissection. The scalpel method is useful in patients who have had previous coronal flaps with adhesions in the subgaleal layer. Anterior dissection is limited by the lateral extent of the incision and this should be released down to the temporalis fascia. Dissection should proceed anteriorly until it is possible to evert the flap so the galeal surface is superior.

The flap is dissected anteriorly until within 3 to 4 cm of the supraorbital rims. When a pericranial flap is not planned, after digital palpation of the supraorbital rims, an incision through pericranium is made between the superior temporal lines (**Fig. 9**). The incision is kept within the superior temporal lines to prevent unnecessary bleeding. After incision, a subperiosteal plane is developed toward the supraorbital rims. If the surgeon knows that a pericranial flap will not be used, then a subperiosteal plan may be developed posteriorly at the initial skin incision site. When planning to develop a vascularized pericranial flap, a suprapericranial (subgaleal) dissection is performed as described previously. Then an incision is made through pericranium from the most anterior aspect

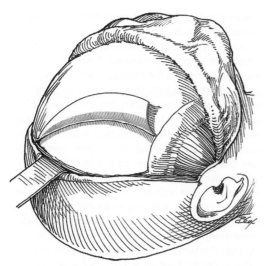

Fig. 9. If not using a pericranial flap, the incision through the pericranium may be made between the superior temporal lines just 3 to 4 cm above the supraorbital rims. (*From* Strong EB. Frontal sinus fractures. Operative Techniques in Otolaryngology 2008;19:151–60; with permission.)

to most posterior aspect of the incision just above the superior temporal lines (**Fig. 10**). A transverse incision through pericranium between the superior temporal lines is made, connecting the most posterior aspects of the sagittal incisions. Starting at the posterior aspect of the incision, pericranium is then elevated with a periosteal elevator (**Fig. 11**). Following elevation of the anteriorly based pericranial flap, a subperiosteal dissection is continued toward the supraorbital rims (**Fig. 12**).

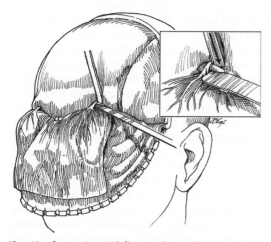

Fig. 10. If a pericranial flap is planned, an incision is made through pericranium from the most anterior aspect to most posterior aspect of the incision just above the superior temporal lines. (*From* Strong EB. Frontal sinus fractures. Operative Techniques in Otolaryngology 2008;19:151–60, with permission.)

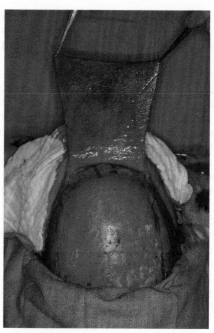

Fig. 11. A pericranial flap is reflected and kept moist on a wet surgical sponge.

Approaching the zygomatic arch

To expose the zygomatic arch, the coronal flap is developed laterally, staying superior to the glistening temporalis fascia to within 2 to 4 cm of the zygomatic arches and bodies.[10] The superficial layer of temporalis fascia is incised at the

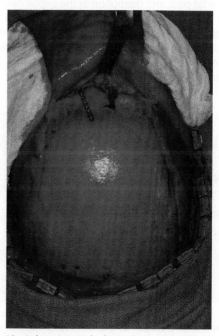

Fig. 12. Subpericranial dissection proceeds to the supraorbital rims.

root of the zygomatic arch just anterior to the ear and above the temporomandibular joint to the supraorbital rim in a vector paralleling the temporal branch of the facial nerve. The incision is continued superiorly at a 45-degree angle until combined with the transverse pericranial incision at the superior temporal line or where the pericranial flap has been elevated. On incision of the superficial layer of temporalis fascia, the superficial temporal fat pad (contained between superficial and deep temporalis fascia) may be exposed. Dissection proceeds immediately deep to the superficial layer of temporalis fascia, along the deep temporal fascia, or within the deep temporal fat pad to the level of the zygoma. The dense connective tissue at the lateral orbit is elevated to the periosteum of the zygomatic arch, which is then incised at the zygomatic arch and body (**Fig. 13**). A similar incision is made at the root of the zygoma and the 2 incisions are connected in a inferiosuperior plane of dissection. Of note, the temporal branch of the facial nerve should be contained within the temporoparietal layer, which is within the anteriorly everted coronal flap.

Many investigators have reported that exposure of the superficial temporal fat pad increases the incidence of hollowing of the temporal fossa and facial nerve damage.[28] The mechanism of temporal hollowing is thought to be multifocal and can be partially attributed to disruption of branching perforators from the middle and deep temporal arteries that transverse the substance of the fat pad, and disruption of the septal network that suspends the temporal fat pad from the anterior temporalis fascia.[28,29] Using magnetic resonance imaging to evaluate various incisions, Lacey and colleagues[30] demonstrated that it is diminution of the temporal fat pad, not the

temporalis muscles, that contributes to temporal hollowing following the coronal approach and recommended dissection immediately deep to the superficial layer of temporalis fascia to minimize dissection through the fat pad, rather than dissection over the superficial layer of the temporalis fascia or dissection within the substance of the superficial fat pad to prevent temporal hollowing. Matic and Kim[31] compared all 3 approaches and found that suprafascial dissection immediately over the superficial layer of the temporalis fascia with incision directly over the zygomatic arch was associated with less temporal hollowing and less damage to the zygomaticotemporal nerve and middle temporal artery (injured more in deep dissection) than deep dissection and dissection through the temporal fat pad. They also identified patient weight loss as a contributor to temporal hollowing. Baek and colleagues[32] recommended a similar approach superficial to the superficial layer of the temporalis fascia for exposure of the zygomatic arch in patients undergoing facial fracture and craniosynostosis repair, noting avoidance of the frontal branch of the facial nerve and temporal artery and subsequently decreased incidence of temporal hollowing with this approach. There was no incidence of facial nerve damage in either group. More recently, however, Steinbacher and colleagues[33] attempted to identify risk factors for temporal hollowing in infants undergoing unilateral fronto-orbital expansion for unicoronal synostosis. Using 3-dimensional (3D) computed tomography (CT) planning software (Materialise, Leuven, Belgium) to compare along the frontal bandeau and midline, temporal width, and temporalis muscle, superficial temporal fat pad, and cutaneous thickness between the operated and nonoperated sides and found that temporal hollowing was affected by bony constriction along the anterior frontal bandeau and decreased temporalis muscle thickness, and not change in superficial temporal fat pad thickness. However, these data are generalizable only to the unilateral craniosynostosis population, because the investigators used a dissection deep to the deep layer of temporalis fascia avoiding penetration of the superficial temporal pad and its septal attachments superiorly.

To access the superior orbits and nasal region, the supraorbital neurovascular bundle must be released. This is done by releasing a subperiosteal plane around the bundle and internal orbits and then either gently removing the bundle from the bony notch in the case when there is no inferior bone to the bundle, or using an osteotome to remove a bony ridge just inferior to the bundle in the case when there is a bony foramen (**Fig. 14**).

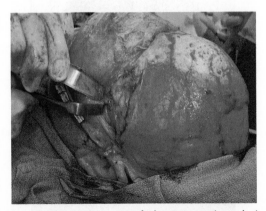

Fig. 13. The periosteum of the zygomatic arch is incised with a scalpel or electrocautery exposing the zygomatic arch and body and plated, usually with a miniplate.

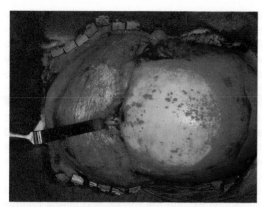

Fig. 14. After releasing a subperiosteal plane around the supraorbital nerve bundle, a bony notch is removed using an osteotome.

A subperiosteal dissection is then undertaken along the internal orbits. The tissues attached to the lateral orbital tubercle, as well the periosteum of the infraorbital rim, zygomatic arch, and body are released.

To access the nasal bones, a subperiosteal plane is dissected along the superior and medial orbital wall (**Fig. 15**). To dissect toward the dorsal nasal tip, the periosteum at the nasofrontal junction can be released. When dissecting the medial orbit, careful attention should be paid not to strip the medial canthal tendon from the anterior and

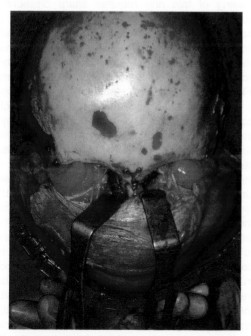

Fig. 15. Subperiosteal dissection proceeds throughout the medial orbits.

posterior lacrimal crests, which appear as dense fibrous attachments in the nasolacrimal fossa. As medial orbital wall dissection proceeds, the anterior and posterior ethmoidal arteries will be found approximately 25 mm and 35 mm anterior to the anterior lacrimal crest respectively. These vessels may be cauterized with bipolar electrocautery and transected with further posterior subperiosteal elevation. If necessary, the orbits may be dissected to their apex.

If access to the temporal fossa is needed, then by starting at its most anterior edge, the temporalis muscle is stripped subperiosteally from the temporal surfaces of the frontal, temporal, and zygomatic bones and temporal fossa. To access the temporomandibular joint (TMJ), mandibular condyle, and ramus, the inferior surface of the zygoma must be dissected subperiosteally. The lateral surface of the mandibular subcondylar region and ramus are exposed just lateral to the TMJ capsule. To expose the condylar neck, the periosteum is incised just inferior to the insertion of the TMJ capsule on the neck of the condyle. To achieve wider access below the zygomatic arch, the masseter muscle may be cut and released from its origin at the zygomatic arch and stripped away from the lateral mandibular ramus.[10] Alternatively, the zygomatic arch may be osteotomized with the masseter muscle attached. A plane between the masseter and temporalis may be developed, eventually exposing the lateral ramus of the mandible. Stripping of the masseter medially may severely affect function even after reapproximation, as the neurovascular supply from the masseteric artery and nerve that travels through the sigmoid notch into the masseter muscle is disturbed with this maneuver. Split-thickness and full-thickness calvarial bone grafts may be harvested with ease by either making a periosteal incision at the parietal budge,[10] or in the case when a pericranial flap is elevated, bone grafts may be harvested after posterior subperiosteal dissection from the initial incision. In the case of a separate periosteal incision, periosteal closure should precede scalp closure.

A closed suction drain may be left in place in the subgaleal plane exiting the scalp at a hair-bearing area. The soft tissues in the orbital and malar regions should be resuspended by 3-0 slow-resorbing or permanent sutures through the deep surface of the periosteum and pexing it to the temporalis, fascia, or other stable structure. Lateral canthopexy is also required if the lateral canthal tendon (buried in the deep surface of the coronal flap) was stripped from the lateral orbital tubercle. The lateral canthal tendon may be pexed to a hole drilled in the bone, a bone screw, or the temporalis fascia. To aid in preventing temporal hollowing, the temporalis muscle should be resuspended to the lateral orbit by running a 3-0 slow-resorbing suture from the anterior edge of the temporalis muscle to the posterior edge of the lateral orbital rim. A slow 4-0 resorbable suture is then used to close the periosteum around the lateral orbital rim and zygomatic arch. Suturing of the periosteum over the zygomatic arch may be difficult owing to limited availability of tissue and may risk damage to the frontal branch of the facial nerve, which is just superficial to the periosteum; therefore, oversuspension of the superficial layer of temporalis fascia is recommended.[10] This is done by running a horizontal 3-0 slow-resorbing suture starting the first stitch at the most inferior edge of temporalis facial and approximating it 1 cm superior to the superior edge of incised fascia. The horizontal pericranium incision superior to the supraorbital rims does not require closure because it is thin and does not hold sutures. The scalp incision is then closed in 2 layers using a slow-resorbing 2-0 suture to reapproximate galea and subcutaneous tissues and 2-0 skin sutures or staples to close skin.

Orbital exenteration Unlike other approaches for malignancy of the periorbita, for which there are many, orbital exenteration is a direct transcutaneous approach to the orbit that is indicated for removing malignant tumors arising from the globe with periorbital invasion, and for malignant tumors arising from the orbital adnexal structures, such as the periorbita, conjunctiva, bony orbital walls, and lacrimal apparatus.[34,35]

Technique The goal in orbital exenteration is to preserve as much periorbital skin as possible while maintaining tumor-free margins.[36] A circumferential incision from lateral to medial canthi should be marked just outside the tarsal margins but not through orbital septum (**Fig. 16**). Alternatively, if

the eyelids are involved, an incision may by marked around the margin of the bony orbital rim (**Fig. 17**). A modification of this technique is to extend the inferior tarsal margin incision inferiorly along the nasolabial fold to encompass skin overlying the lacrimal fossa and nasolacrimal duct. Injecting local anesthesia with vasoconstrictor will aid in hydro-dissecting a natural plane between skin and orbicularis oris. A scissors is then used to dissect a plane just superior to orbicularis oris in a vector toward the orbital rim (**Fig. 18**). A subperiosteal dissection of the orbital rim is performed. Points of resistance during subperiosteal dissection include the medial and lateral canthal tendons and trochlea of the anterosuperior aspect of the orbit. The canthal tendons are sharply dissected, and the trochlea and superior oblique muscle are dissected from the trochlear fossa. This will significantly free up the periorbita. Another point of resistance along the orbital floor will be at the infraorbital fissure. Sharp dissection may be needed to free up its contents. A subperiosteal dissection is then performed with electrocautery to the orbital apex. A right-angle clamp is then placed around the soft tissues of the orbital apex and is excised with a right-angle scissors (**Fig. 19**). A 3-0 silk suture is then used to ligate the remaining contents. This initial ligation usually encompasses tissue of the annulus of Zinn, or the annular tendon, which is the common tendinous fibrous ring surrounding the optic nerve and serves as the origin of the 6 extraocular muscles. Freeing of this ring requires sharp dissection from bone. After removal of the globe and its contents, the ophthalmic artery may be ligated. Remaining contents include the optic nerve stump, stump ends of the cranial nerves, and the ophthalmic vein in the superior orbital fissure (**Figs. 20** and **21**). If further posterior bone removal is needed to achieve adequate margins, the thick bone of the optic canal may be burred away, however this bone thins out as it transverses the superolateral wall of the sphenoid sinus. Dissection may be performed to the optic chiasm. If the tumor invades the lacrimal fossa, a power saw is then used to resect the lower medial orbital rim and the contents of the lacrimal fossa. The medial aspect of the bony orbital rim and the lateral aspect of the nasal bone are then divided to completely mobilize the bony lacrimal fossa in continuity with the orbital contents. The defect may then be reconstructed with a microvascular free flap, local or regional flaps, or a split-thickness skin graft with prosthesis at a later time.[37] The most common complication associated with orbital exenteration is fistula formation.[38] The coronal approach and Weber-Fergusson and

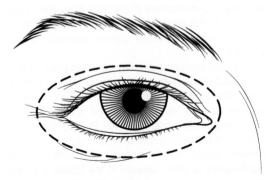

Fig. 16. A circumferential incision from lateral to medial canthi should be marked just outside the tarsal margins but not through orbital septum.

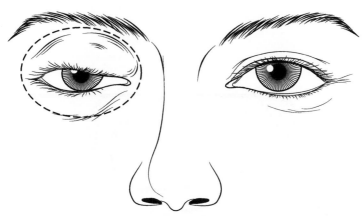

Fig. 17. If the eyelids are involved, an incision may by marked around the margin of the bony orbital rim.

lateral rhinotomy approaches, with periorbital extension, may be combined with orbital exenteration; however, these are beyond the scope of this article. Virtually any combination of the previously mentioned transcutaneous approaches may be used.[13]

Transconjunctival Approaches

Transconjunctival approach
The "conjunctival approach" was initially described by Bourguet in 1924, who used the technique to remove palpebral fat during lower eyelid blepharoplasty. Approximately 50 years later, the technique was described for access to small orbital floor fractures by Tenzel and Miller.[39]

Tessier popularized the technique for access to the orbit in patients with craniofacial dysostoses.[40] In addition, he also described its use with success in 3 patients with traumatic orbital injuries. Soon after, multiple reports described the conjunctival approach in traumatic orbital injuries.[3,41] Commonly referred to as the transconjunctival approach, this incision is useful to access the orbital floor and infraorbital rim. The primary advantage to this approach is that its scar is hidden in the conjunctiva and if performed correctly, is imperceptible and rarely results in complications.

Dissection may be performed in a preseptal or retroseptal fashion.[3] In a retroseptal approach, the conjunctiva is dissected from behind the

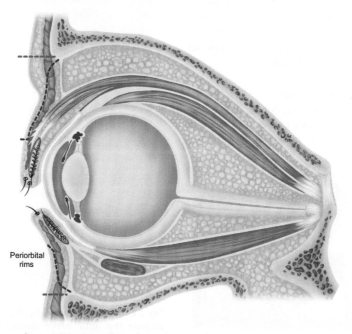

Periorbital rims

Fig. 18. Either a circumferential incision from lateral to medial canthi should marked just outside the tarsal margins (*purple*), or around the margin of the bony orbital rim may be made (*green*).

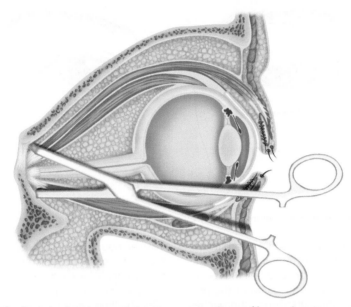

Fig. 19. A right angle clamp is placed around the common tendinous fibrous ring surrounding the optic nerve and serves as the origin of the 6 extraocular muscles.

orbital septum down to the bony orbit. In the preseptal approach (**Fig. 22**), the orbital septum is incised below the tarsus and is followed down to the orbital rim. The preseptal approach has been associated with an increased risk of entropion when compared with other approaches. Conversely, in the authors' experience, a retroseptal approach performed in the conjunctival fornix offers adequate access for most applications in the orbit and virtually eliminates the risk of entropion. The "fornix" postseptal transconjunctival incision is the senior author's (R.B.B.) preferred approach to the orbit (see **Fig. 22**).

Retroseptal (fornix) technique
Local anesthesia with vasoconstrictor is injected into the lower eyelid conjunctiva. A corneal protector is placed, as tarsorrhaphy sutures

cannot be used in this procedure. While everting the lower eyelid, several traction sutures may be placed from palpebral conjunctiva to skin at approximately 3 to 5 mm below the tarsal plate within. Then, using the traction sutures or a Demars retractor to evert the lower eyelid, a 15-blade or

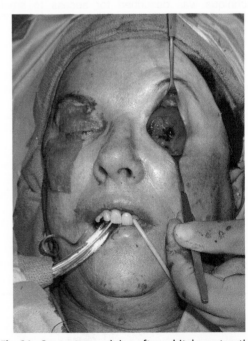

Fig. 21. Contents remaining after orbital exenteration include the optic nerve stump, stump ends of the cranial nerves, and the ophthalmic vein in the superior orbital fissure.

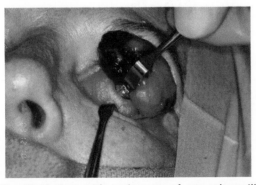

Fig. 20. Patient with melanoma of eye who will undergo orbital exenteration.

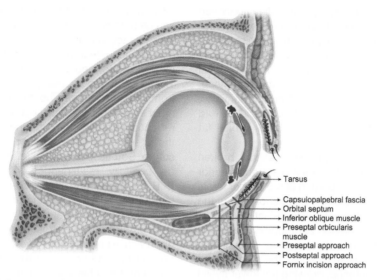

Fig. 22. Planes of dissection after transconjunctival incision may be preseptal or retroseptal.

Labels in figure:
- Tarsus
- Capsulopalpebral fascia
- Orbital septum
- Inferior oblique muscle
- Preseptal orbicularis muscle
- Preseptal approach
- Postseptal approach
- Fornix incision approach

fine-tipped electrocautery is used to make an incision through the conjunctiva at the arcuate line within the conjunctival fornix. Dissection will proceed posterior to the plane of the orbital septum, the lower eyelid retractors, or capsulopalpebral fascia, which contains the fascia extension of the inferior rectus, which are sympathetically mediated muscle fibers. The incision may extend as medial as the lacrimal sac. At this point, orbital fat and contents will extrude into the operative field and should be retracted superiorly. With a Demars retractor positioning the lower eyelid forward, an incision is then made through periosteum immediately posterior to the orbital rim. Periosteum is incised and a subperiosteal plane is then developed to access the orbital rim, anterior zygoma, and maxilla. Closure of the periosteum is optional. The authors, however, prefer to close the conjunctiva, which is facilitated with a running 6-0 plain gut suture with the ends of the suture buried to not irritate the globe.

Preseptal technique
Following local anesthesia with vasoconstrictor injection into the lower eyelid conjunctiva, a lateral canthotomy may or may not be performed depending on the need to access the lateral orbit.[42–44] After eversion of the lower eyelid, the conjunctiva is incised 2 to 3 mm below the tarsal plate in the mid-portion of the lower eyelid in a plane anterior to the orbital septum. Two retraction sutures are then used to retract the superior conjunctival flap superiorly. Using a scissors, the thin cranial part of the capsulopalpebral fascia is dissected above the lower lid retractor muscles

in a vector toward the orbital rim (see **Fig. 22**). The capsulopalpebral fascia has cranial attachments around the tarsal plate, inferior rectus muscle, and inferior oblique muscle. At the apex of the orbital fat, the capsulopalpebral fascia fuses with the orbital septum. The orbital septum is protected with a malleable retractor. Periosteum is incised and subperiosteal dissection is performed. As in the retroseptal approach, the periosteum does not need to be primarily closed. A running 6-0 fast gut suture may be used to close conjunctiva.

Transconjunctival approach with lateral canthotomy (disarticulation of the lower eyelid)
The addition of the lateral canthotomy incision to the transconjunctival approach allows wide access to the inferior and lateral orbit and complete disarticulation of the lower eyelid.[45–47] With one tip of a pointed scissors inserted into the palpebral fissure to the depth of the lateral orbital rim, the skin, orbicularis oculi, orbital septum, lateral canthal tendon, and conjunctiva are cut to a depth of approximately 7 to 10 mm.[10] The inferior limb of the lateral canthal tendon will most likely still be attached. Cantholysis of the inferior limb of the lateral canthal tendon should be performed vertically to completely free the eyelid from the lateral orbital rim. Tenotomy scissors are then used to create a pocket just posterior to the orbital septum, inferiorly to a point just posterior to the orbital rim. Then, while retracting the lower eyelid, the scissors are used to dissect and extend an incision made in the conjunctiva and

lower eyelid retractors to a point midway between the inferior part of the conjunctival fornix and inferior margin of the tarsal plate to a point as far medial as the lacrimal sac. A traction suture may then be placed in the most proximal conjunctival flap and used to hold the corneal shield in place. Following superior retraction of orbital contents, periosteum is then incised (**Fig. 23**). A broad malleable retractor is placed to block orbital fat extrusion.

To appropriately reapproximate the broken attachment between the tarsal plate and inferior canthal limb, the lateral portion of the inferior tarsal plate is then reattached to the superior limb of the lateral canthal tendon using a long-lasting resorbable suture. The inferior canthopexy suture is placed but not tied before closing conjunctiva. Following conjunctival closure, the canthopexy suture may be tightened, drawing the lower eyelid into a symmetric position with the contralateral eyelid, finally tying the suture into place. A running 6-0 fast gut subcutaneous stitch is then used to close the lateral canthotomy incision.

For access to the entire lateral orbital rim, the lateral canthotomy approach should be extended with undermining up to 1.0 to 1.5 cm in a natural skin crease. If no skin crease exists, then the incision may be extended laterally or superolaterally from the palpebral fissure. The superior limb of the lateral canthal tendon is then completely stripped from its attachment. Access up to 10 to

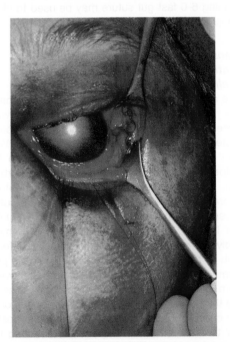

Fig. 23. Displays transconjunctival incision with lateral canthotomy (disarticulation of the lower eyelid).

12 mm superior to the zygomaticofrontal suture can be obtained via this approach. When attempting to access the zygomaticofrontal suture, a supraperiosteal dissection of the lateral rim may be performed to a point above the suture. The periosteum overlying the suture is incised from a point midway up the orbital rim to the most superior point of dissection. Orbital contents retraction is aided by a subperiosteal dissection of the lateral orbit to access the zygomaticofrontal suture. Soft tissues and the lateral canthus should be carefully resuspended. The senior author (R.B.B.) has found that, even in experienced hands, the lateral canthotomy results in an increase in entropion and rarely looks unoperated. By combining the retroseptal transconjunctival approach with an upper eyelid "blepharoplasty" approach, wide access to the inferior and lateral orbit can be achieved, obviating the need for the lateral canthotomy in most cases.

Transcaruncular (medial transconjunctival) approach

Lynch popularized traditional transcutaneous approaches to the medial orbit in 1921.[48] The Lynch incision courses midway between the medial canthus and the bridge of the nose and is associated with unsightly scar formation. Further refinements of the technique, such as z-plasty, still resulted in substantial scar formation.[49,50] The lid crease incision has a less noticeable scar than the Lynch incision; however, provides a limited view of the anterior and superior medial orbit.[51] Originally described by Garcia and colleagues,[52] and then soon after by Blach and colleagues,[53,54] the medial transconjunctival (transcaruncular) incision provides access to the medial orbital wall with no external scarring. Further investigations have since been reported on the approach with good success.[55-58]

Technique Pertinent anatomy in the region include the medial canthal ligament and associated fascia. It serves as the anterior insertion of Horner muscle, the medial orbital septum, the lower eyelid retractors (capsulopalpebral fascia), and anterior Tenon capsule (**Fig. 24**A, B).[53,59] Horner muscle is formed from posterior fibers of the pretarsal portion of the orbicularis oculi that line the posterior wall of the lacrimal sac to insert on the posterior lacrimal crest. The medial orbital septum also inserts onto the periosteum immediately posterior to the posterior lacrimal crest. The plica semilunaris, or semilunar fold, is a crescent-shaped fold of the medial conjunctiva, which is bordered laterally by the bular conjunctiva and inferomedially by the caruncle.[60] The lacrimal sac lies in a region

A

B

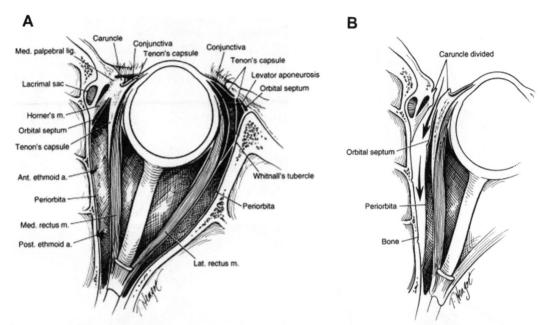

Fig. 24. Axial illustrations demonstrating Horner's muscle and the lacrimal sac lying outside the medial orbital septum, and insertion of Horner's muscle and the medial orbital septum into the periorbita immediately posterior to the posterior lacrimal crest (*A*). The plane of the dissection for the transcaruncular approach is lateral (posterior) to Horner's muscle and medial to the medial orbital septum (*B*). (*From* Shorr N, Baylis HI, Goldberg RA, et al. Transcaruncular approach to the medial orbit and orbital apex. Ophthalmology 2000;107(8):1459–63; with permission.)

between the anterior and posterior limbs of the medial canthal tendon known as the lacrimal fossa, which is bordered by the anterior and posterior lacrimal crests. Inferiorly, the fossa is contiguous with the nasolacrimal duct and superiorly the fossa extends just above the medial canthal tendon. The incision through the caruncle and dense fibrous condensation passes along a natural plane between Horner muscle and the medial orbital septum (posteriorly), medial rectus muscle (posterolaterally), and lacrimal drainage system (anteromedially) with buffering of Horner muscle of this safe and bloodless plane from the lacrimal sac. Detachment of Horner muscle may allow the medial eyelid to fall anteriorly away from the globe.

The medial orbital conjunctiva should be infiltrated with local anesthesia with vasoconstrictor. With gentle retraction of the globe, which flattens the caruncle and with a forceps grasping the semilunar fold posterior to the caruncle, an incision is made with either a Stevens or Westcott scissors or a fine-tipped electrocautery along the conjunctival groove just posterior to the lacrimal sac and medial to the levator aponeurosis with caution to avoid these structures (**Fig. 25**A, B). The posterior retraction of the globe will also force any extraconal fat posteriorly. It is important to note that the incision is made just posterior to the semilunar fold. The incision should extend approximately

12 mm just through the lateral one-third of the caruncle (see **Fig. 25**C). The dense fibrous layer deep to the caruncle is incised in a vector toward the posterior lacrimal crest. The lacrimal crest is palpated with a malleable retractor and held firmly against the medial orbit just posterior to the posterior lacrimal crest. The scissors are then spread to expose the cut periorbital edge posterior to the posterior lacrimal crest (see **Fig. 25**D). The dissection plane passes along the medial aspect of the medial orbital septum between the orbital septum and Horner muscle (see **Fig. 25**E). The periosteum along the posterior lacrimal crests in then incised with fine-tipped electrocautery or scalpel blade. Maintaining the periosteal incision posterior to the posterior lacrimal crest protects Horner muscle (inserts at lacrimal crest) and the lacrimal system from damage or detachment.[61] The dissection is continued posteriorly in the subperiorbital plane along the lateral and medial walls at the arcus marginalis (see **Fig. 25**F, H). The inferior oblique muscle may be divided if it hinders access (**Fig. 26**). After separate superior and inferior retraction of the periosteum, the anterior and posterior ethmoidal arteries are identified. They may be preserved or cauterized with bipolar electrocautery. The transcaruncular incision may be combined with a traditional transconjunctival incision for access to the orbital floor and medial wall.[62] No effort is made to reapproximate the inferior

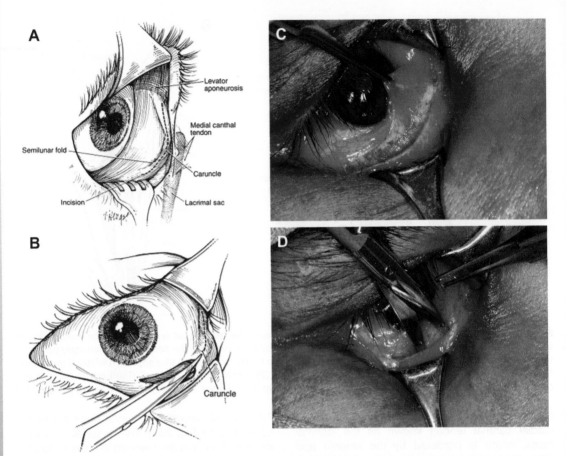

Fig. 25. An incision is made with either a Stevens or Westcott scissors or a fine tipped electrocautery along the conjunctival groove just posterior to the lacrimal sac and medial to the levator aponeurosis taken great caution to avoid these structures (*A, B*). During the approach, the semilunar fold is retracted, incising just between the caruncle and semilunar fold (*C*). A scissors is used to dissect the conjunctiva down to the medial orbit (*D*) The dissection plane passes along the medial aspect of the medial orbital septum between the orbital septum and Horner's muscle (*E*). The periosteum along the posterior lacrimal crest in then incised with fine tipped electrocautery or scalpel blade. Maintaining the periosteal incision posterior to the posterior lacrimal crest protects Horner's muscle (inserts at lacrimal crest) and the lacrimal system from damage or detachment (*F*). Dissection is continued posteriorly in the subperiorbital plane along the lateral and medial walls at the arcus marginalis (*G, H*). ([*C, D*] *Courtesy of* Edward E. Ellis, DDS, MS, San Antonio, TX. [*A, B, E, H*] *From* Shorr N, Baylis HI, Goldberg RA, et al. Transcaruncular approach to the medial orbit and orbital apex. Ophthalmology 2000;107(8):1459–63; with permission.)

oblique muscle if divided or stripped. The caruncular incision, however, must be closed with 6-0 gut sutures. Failure to adequately close the caruncular incision may result in symblepharon, pyogenic granuloma, or orbital fat prolapse.

Advantages of the transcaruncular approach are that it preserves the anterior and posterior ethmoidal arteries. This is in contrast to a Lynch incision in which these vessels are usually ligated.[48,63] In addition, the transcaruncular approach offers direct visualization of plate placement to the medial orbit and obviates the need for a coronal incision to access the superomedial orbit.

Combination of transconjunctival/ transcaruncular/lateral canthotomy approaches

The transcaruncular approach may be combined with a retroseptal transconjunctival approach for defects involving the media and inferior orbit. Additionally, if access to the lateral orbit is needed, a lateral canthotomy incision may be combined with medial and inferior transconjunctival approaches, which is often referred to as the C-shaped incision. This combination of approaches offers 270° of dissection along the medial, inferior, and lateral walls of the orbit along with the zygomaticofrontal suture.

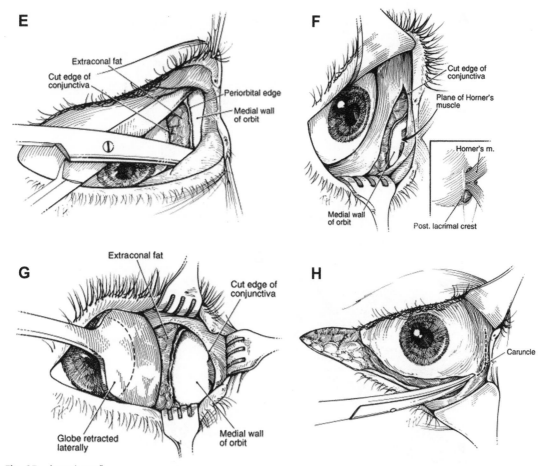

Fig. 25. (continued)

Technique If access to the lateral orbit is needed, lateral canthotomy should be performed before inferior or medial conjunctival incisions using previously discussed techniques.[55,62] The conjunctiva is then incised just lateral to the caruncle and dissection is continued superiorly to the levator aponeurosis. When encountering the inferior oblique muscle, it may be stripped from its origin or severed from its bony attachment leaving a small amount attached to bone for closure. The medial and inferior transconjunctival approach is then performed as previously described. Alternatively, the inferior orbital rim dissection may take place after the transcaruncular approach.[55] and/or lateral canthotomy approach for larger defects.

Transantral Approaches

Transantral endoscopic-assisted approach to the orbital floor

The transantral endoscopic-assisted approach to the orbit provides direct access to the orbital floor. The first report of orbital floor repair via a Caldwell-Luc approach was by Walter in 1972.[64] Although effective, this approach was abandoned for previously described transcutaneous and transconjunctival approaches for many years. Because of the discrete, but significant rate of complications associated with lower eyelid incision, however,

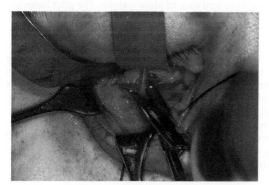

Fig. 26. If necessary, the inferior oblique muscle may be divided if it hinders access. (*Courtesy of* Edward E. Ellis, DDS, MS, San Antonio, TX.)

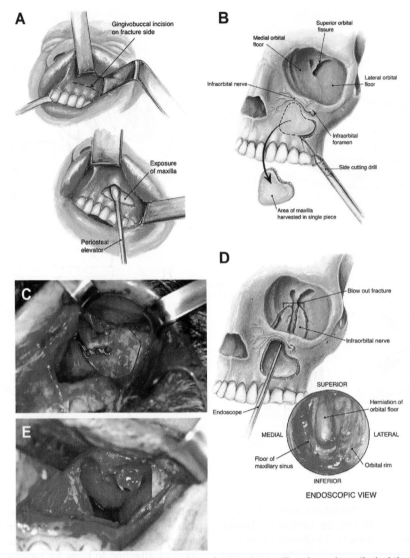

Fig. 27. A standard vestibular (Keen) incision is made in the upper maxillary buccal vestibule (*A*). A superior sub-periosteal dissection of the maxilla is carried out and a full-thickness mucoperiosteal flap is reflected. A large boney window is then outlined with pilot holes from a fine side cutting drill between the medial and lateral maxillary buttresses (*B*). A miniplate is then pre-bent and adapted to the proposed defect (*C*). The bony window is made as large as possible to allow large access to the orbital floor and ease of plate transfer. The pilot holes are connected and a window of bone is created with the rotary instrument into the maxillary antrum, which provides access to instrumentation and endoscopic visualization (*D*). The bony fragment is removed from the antral wall. Both 0- and 30-degree straight endoscopes are used to view the fracture through the bony window (**Fig. 26**d). Alternatively a flexible endoscope may be used.[67] The prolapsed orbital contents are visualized endoscopically (*E*) and a curved elevator is then used to elevate orbital contents superiorly into the orbit (*F, G, H*). The orbital periosteum is then elevated to approximately 5 mm around and beyond the entire fractured segment. If a trap door defect exists, the fracture's bony ledge should be elevate back to anatomic position with overlap of its edges on native orbital floor. MedPor (Porex surgical, Newnan, GA, USA) is used to reconstruct the orbital floor (*I–J*). by placing it through maxillary antral wall defect, rotating, and placed on the stable medial, lateral, and anterior orbital shelves (*K, L, M*). A postoperative forced duction test is then performed (*N*). (*Courtesy of* Mark E. Engelstad, DDS, MD, MHI, Portland, OR. [*A, B, D, F, K*] *From* Ducic Y, Verret DJ. Endoscopic transantral repair of orbital floor fractures. Otolaryngol Head Neck Surg 2009;140:849–54; with permission.)

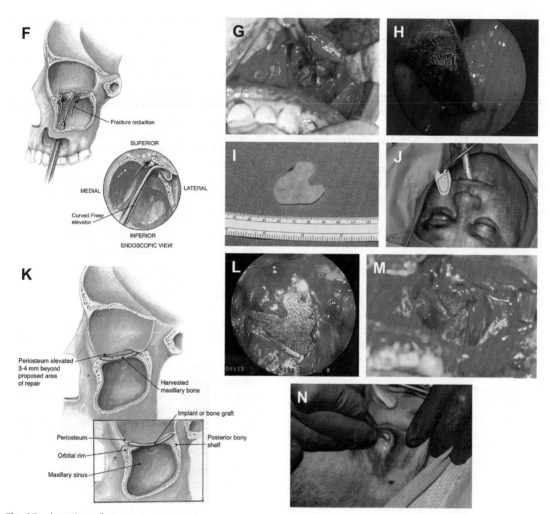

Fig. 27. (*continued*)

there has recently been a resurgence of enthusiasm for the transantral approach to the orbital floor.[65–73] Reported advantages of this approach include less scaring than subcutaneous approaches; a decreased incidence of postoperative lower lid malpositioning, entropion, and ectropion as compared with the transcutaneous approaches; and better visualization of the posterior orbit.[73] In addition, the transconjunctival approach is associated with increased scleral show, which does not occur in the transantral approach.

Technique Local anesthesia with vasoconstrictor is deposited into the maxillary buccal vestibule. Then a standard vestibular (Keen) incision is made in the upper maxillary buccal vestibule (**Fig. 27**A). A superior subperiosteal dissection of the maxilla is performed and a full-thickness mucoperiosteal flap is reflected. A large bony window is then outlined with pilot holes from

a fine side cutting drill between the medial and lateral maxillary buttresses (see **Fig. 27**B). One or 2 miniplates are then prebent and adapted to the proposed defect (see **Fig. 27**C). The bony window is made as large as possible to allow large access to the orbital floor and ease of plate transfer. The pilot holes are connected and a window of bone is created with the rotary instrument into the maxillary antrum, which provides access to instrumentation and endoscopic visualization. The bony fragment is removed from the antral wall. Both 0-degree and 30-degree straight endoscopes are used to view the fracture through the bony window (see **Fig. 27**D). Alternatively a flexible endoscope may be used.[67] The prolapsed orbital contents are visualized (see **Fig. 27**E) endoscopically and a curved elevator is then used to elevate orbital contents superiorly into the orbit (see **Fig. 27**F, H). The orbital periosteum is then elevated to approximately 5 mm around and beyond the entire fractured segment. If a trap door defect exists, the fracture's bony ledge should be elevated back to anatomic position with overlap of its edges on native orbital floor. If this is not possible, the segment should be removed for use as a bone graft at a later time. Alternatively, the orbital floor may be reconstructed with titanium mesh, MedPor (Porex Surgical, Newnan, GA), or the antral wall segment (see **Fig. 27**I, J).[68] The chosen material is introduced through maxillary antral wall defect, rotated, and placed on the stable medial, lateral, and anterior orbital shelves (see **Fig. 27**K, M). Fixation is not required if there is adequate stability of the bony shelves. If stability is inadequate, direct screw fixation can be performed from below.[69] Postoperative forced duction test is then performed (see **Fig. 27**N).

The senior author's (R.B.B.) preferred technique is to use a titanium plate that is inset into the posterior ledge (usually the orbital process of the palatine bone) and is stabilized with screws placed into the anterior maxillary wall. Anterior extensions of the plate are then brought through the antral window and the plate is stabilized with at least 2 screws placed on the facial surface of the maxilla. The bony window is then replaced with the removed antral wall segment and fixated with prebent plates. The vestibular incision may be closed with a running 3-0 gut or chromic gut suture. The transantral endoscopic approach has also been used to access tumors of the posterior orbit and orbital apex with successful removal.[74] In addition, the transantral approach may be combined with other approaches to the orbit.[75] Ultimately, in many instances, a combination of the previously described techniques will often be used for craniomaxillofacial reconstruction (**Figs. 28–33**).

CLINICAL OUTCOMES AND COMPLICATIONS

Relative indications for a cutaneous approach versus a transconjunctival approach include hypertrophy of the orbicularis oris, the presence of malar festoons, planned skin resection owing to lid laxity and adjunct cosmetic procedure, persistent chemosis, unstable or high-risk corneal or globe injury, such as traumatic hyphema, persistent globe edema, acute or chronic conjunctival disease, or the presence of a globe prosthesis.[12] However, when these conditions are not present, the literature suggests the use of a transconjunctival approach.

Wray and colleagues[5] found a higher incidence of ectropion in the subciliary group compared with the transconjunctival group; however, no difference was found in scar appearance, or incidence of entropion. Other reported advantages of transconjunctival with lateral canthotomy approach include less scarring and incidence of lagophthalmos, however. The combined transconjunctival with lateral canthotomy approach, however, is associated with higher incidence of canthal malposition.[76]

When using a subciliary approach, the advantages to the "stepped" skin-muscle flap technique include supreme esthetic outcomes compared with the "skin-only" and "non-stepped" skin-muscle techniques. The approach is technically easier than the other 2 modifications and has been associated with a lower incidence of skin necrosis, ecchymosis, and ectropion.[13,77,78] Disadvantages of the skin-muscle flap include lid retraction and pretarsal flattening.[79] Although the subciliary incision offers good visualization of the medial orbit, the transcaruncular approach is

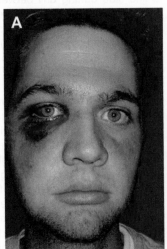
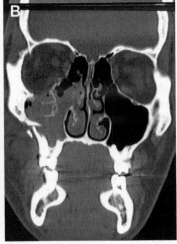

Fig. 28. Frontal photograph (*A*) and coronal view of preoperative CT (*B*) of a patient with a complex zygomaticomaxillary complex fracture.

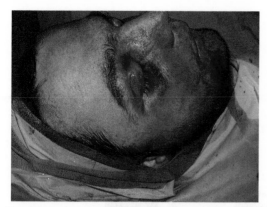

Fig. 29. Upper eyelid blepharoplasty incision made for approaching the frontozygomatic suture.

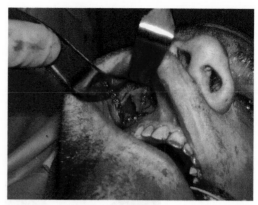

Fig. 31. Intraoral "Keen" incision for approaching the zygomaticomaxillary buttress.

associated with a lower incidence of postoperative ectropion. Although transconjunctival approaches of the lower fornix and transcaruncular approaches may be easily combined, Baumann and Ewers[61] have advised against this to reduce the incidence of symblepharon. Additionally the subciliary incision may lead to vertical shortening of the eyelid.

In a study assessing ideal placement for the subtarsal incision, to prevent the loss of lower eyelid height in the subtarsal approach, the investigators suggested that the incision must be below the tarsal plate but above the orbital-malar groove because cheek skin is thicker below this point and results in significantly more scarring than incisions in orbital skin. Their data also showed that incisions were less noticeable as they moved closer to the tarsal plate (6–7 mm inferior to the tarsal plate in younger patients and in a lower eyelid crease in elderly patients).[80]

Among 209 subjects undergoing a preseptal transconjunctival approach for orbital floor fractures, Schmal and colleagues[43,44] found that at

2-year follow-up, infraorbital dysesthesia was observed in only 3 subjects, and 4 subjects had persistently reduced motility and diplopia. In a cohort of 90 subjects undergoing preseptal transconjunctival approaches to the orbit, Baumann and Ewers[61] found an overall complication rate of 2%, with no evidence of permanent ectropion or entropion, 1 tarsal plate laceration, and 1 occurrence of temporary entropion after a primary subciliary incision.[43] Feldman and colleagues[80] argued that the major disadvantage of the transconjunctival approach when compared with the subtarsal approach is that when required, symmetric reapproximation after lateral canthotomy is difficult.

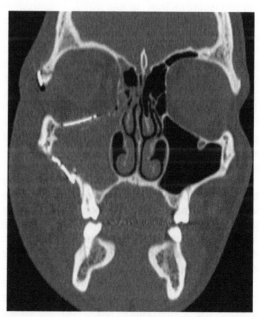

Fig. 32. Postoperative coronal view of CT displaying optimal restoration of the vertical dimension of the orbital floor.

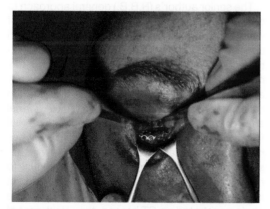

Fig. 30. Transconjunctival incision made for approaching the orbital floor component of the zygomatic fracture.

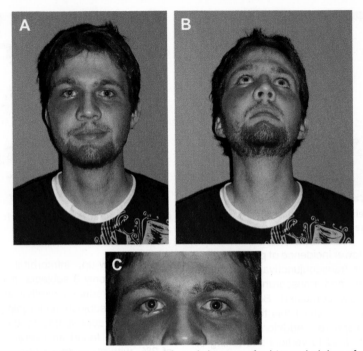

Fig. 33. Postoperative frontal (*A*), worm's-eye view (*B*), and close-up of orbits and globes of patient after reconstruction (*C*).

A review of the literature comparing subtarsal, subciliary, and transconjunctival incisions for orbital fracture repair found that the incidence of ectropion was highest in subciliary (12.5%), followed by subtarsal (2.7%), with none reported in the transconjunctival group (0%).[81] Entropion occurred only in the transconjunctival group (4.4%), whereas there were no occurrences in the subtarsal and subciliary groups. Hypertrophic scarring occurred the most in the subciliary group (3.6%), with only 1 occurrence in the subtarsal group and none in the transconjunctival group. These results are consistent with others, which have found as high as a 42% incidence of ectropion in those undergoing ectropion and ultimate esthetic outcome in those undergoing transconjunctival approaches.[2]

When faced with a pure orbital floor fracture, the transantral endoscopic-assisted approach may be less morbid than transcutaneous and transconjunctival approaches. The risk in the transantral approach is to the infraorbital nerve. A cadaveric study by Wallace and colleagues[70] compared the accuracy of endoscopic and transconjunctival approaches in restoring orbital volume in self-made orbital floor defects. Using a within-subjects design, the investigators found no significant difference in orbital volume restoration between endoscopic and transconjunctival approaches.

NAVIGATION-ASSISTED SURGICAL APPROACHES OF THE ORBIT
Treatment/Reconstructive Goals

The goal of orbital reconstruction is to return the patient to form and function by restoring external and internal orbital anatomy to its premorbid form and to prepare or reposition entrapped or injured soft tissues. Various approaches, techniques, and materials are used to achieve these purposes and there is no universal acceptance as to which approach, technique, or material is best in all instances.

The senior author's (R.B.B.) general approach to orbital injuries involves a multistep assessment of whether or not the patient's injury will result in either a functional or esthetic problem. If the external orbital injury is such that an esthetic deformity, such as cheek flattening, will be clinically apparent, then treatment is warranted. Once the external orbital frame is reduced into normal anatomic position and stabilized, rigid internal fixation is applied via the fewest approaches necessary. Internal orbital injuries are likewise assessed for ocular dysmotility or the potential to result in enophthalmos. If the orbital floor defect is greater than 3.4 cm^2 or 1.6 mL displaced volume as demonstrated on CT images, then treatment of the internal orbit is deemed necessary.[82] Furthermore, internal orbital disruptions posterior and/or medial to the equator of the globe are typically addressed unless the patient is completely devoid of symptoms.

In the authors' experience, most patients with low-velocity injuries involving the external orbital frame (eg, bare-fisted assault or ground-level falls) can be adequately restored to form and function without exploration or treatment of the internal orbit. Conversely, most high-velocity injuries, such as those occurring in motor vehicle collisions, result in a displacement of energy that causes significant internal orbital disruption and necessitates repair of the internal orbit regardless of the level of displacement seen on CT scan. This selective approach to repair of the internal orbit takes into consideration the patient's subjective symptoms (eg, blurred vision, diplopia), physical findings (eg, entrapment of the inferior rectus muscle), limitation and extraocular muscle movements, radiographic findings (linear defect greater than 3.5 cm^2 and volumetric displacement greater than 1.6) and mechanism of injury (ie, low velocity vs high velocity).

Complex, combined orbital fractures are some of the most challenging craniofacial injuries to manage. High-velocity trauma typically produces defects that affect 2, 3, or all 4 walls of the orbit. Such "shattered orbits" produce large volumetric increases intraorbitally, with massive herniation of periorbital contents into the surrounding anatomic spaces and occasional cranial neuropathies. Typically these defects extend into the orbital cone and may involve the optic canal. Their complex patterns and loss of posterior support in the posterior medial and posterior inferior bulges make restoration of normal orbital anatomy challenging. Although refinements of surgical approaches and the development of new biologic materials have improved our ability to more predictably restore these patients' form and function, a significant number of these individuals will still require revisional surgery despite the best efforts of an experienced surgeon.[15,17]

Four-walled fractures that involve the anterior skull base may require transcranial approaches, occasionally with the assistance of a neurosurgeon, and often involve management of the frontal sinus and occasionally the orbital apex. As the frontotemporal components are repositioned, the orbital roof must be restored with either titanium mesh or calvarial bone grafts, and the anterior skull base lined to prevent leak of cerebrospinal fluid.

When the entire orbit is disrupted and there are no posterior landmarks to guide the reconstruction, accurate positioning of bone grafts or titanium mesh becomes problematic (Fig. 34). There is difficulty in establishing proper orbital contour, volume, and medial bulge projection and there is risk to encroachment on the orbital apex and optic nerve. Presurgical computer planning to virtually reconstruct the affected orbit or orbits, stereolithographic models to establish proper plate contour, and the use of intraoperative navigation to ensure accurate and safe positioning of the plate in a poorly visualized anatomic region, has been described as a set of tools to improve the predictability of

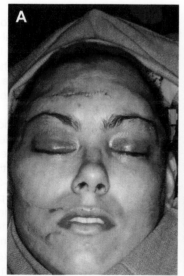 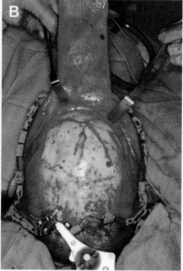

Fig. 34. Clinical photograph of a patient who suffered hard and soft tissue injuries of the maxillofacial skeleton including a bilateral orbital floor and medial wall fractures (A). (B) Skull fractures of coronal flap reflection.

accurate orbital reconstruction. The remaining section in this article addresses the specific work flow process relative to computer-aided orbital surgery.

Computer Aided Orbital Surgery: Work Flow Process

Despite the use of traditional approaches and reconstructive principles, functional and esthetic complications, such as enophthalmos, may persist following orbital reconstruction of posttraumatic and postablative defects.[83] This is especially true in the multiwalled injury in which accurate restoration of orbital volume may be difficult. The lack of reliable bony landmarks in these injuries makes the placement of bony plates and implants extremely difficult. Specific areas of difficulty are reestablishing proper orbital contour, volume, and the ethmoidal and antral bulges of the medial and inferior floors respectively, as well as plate adaptation around the orbital apex. Three-dimensional imaging has not only assisted preoperative planning of orbital defects, but intraoperative navigation has allowed increased precision of traditional reconstructive techniques, leading to a decrease in orbital volume and subsequent decrease in enophthalmos and more favorable position of the globe.[84–86]

Navigation-assisted computer-aided reconstruction can be divided into 4 phases: (1) the *data acquisition phase,* including visualization, orientation, and diagnosis of the orbital deformity, in which clinical and radiographic diagnosis is made, and a high-quality CT scan of the orbits with 1-mm slices is obtained; (2) the *manipulation (simulation) phase,* mirroring, segmentation, and virtual orbital implant insertion, in which CT data are imported into a proprietary software program for the purposes of virtual planning before surgery; (3) the *surgical phase,* which is performed using CAD/CAM-derived stereolithographic models, and/or custom orbital implant insertion using intraoperative navigation; and (4) *assessment phase,* in which the accuracy of the treatment plan transfer is evaluated using intraoperative (or postoperative CT imaging).[87,88]

Data acquisition

Data acquisition includes quantifying the orbital deformity clinically, acquiring a CT scan of the patient, and importing the Digital Imaging and Communications in Medicine (DICOM) data into the appropriate planning software.

Manipulation

Several software systems are not available for stimulation and manipulation of the virtual 3D facial skeleton using data derived from CT data-sets.[89–93] Once in the virtual 3D CT workspace, the orbit of the adjacent side (ideal dimensions) is measured and segmentalized. This "ideal" outline is then mirrored to the side of the orbital deformity. Virtual orbit implants may then be imported to the virtual environment and adapted to the orbital defect, restoring it to idea dimensions.[94,95]

Stereolithographic models (SLMs) of the craniomaxillofacial skeleton can be derived from high-resolution CT. SLMs allow the surgeon to visualize the entire anatomy of the orbits and defect. Stock or custom orbital implants may be adapted to the orbit in the preoperative period.[96] If placing autologous bone grafts, they may be adapted and pre-plated to the SLM intraoperatively.[85,97,98]

Several protocols have been developed to build custom plates specific to a patient's orbital defects.[96,99,100] Using an SLM derived from CT data, a plaster layer may be adapted to the orbital defect of the SLM and contoured to the anatomy of the orbit.[100] Using conventional techniques for denture fabrication, the plaster is then immersed in stone, and burnt out, leaving a template cast. Then, using traditional dental crown casting techniques, commercially annealed titanium is casted into the stone template making a custom titanium plate. Metzger and colleagues[99] developed a protocol that removes the SLM stage of the previously described technique. In their unique protocol, a custom plate is made virtually to the contours of the patient's orbit and transported directly to a template machine for fabrication of a custom titanium mesh.

Surgical

By importing DICOM CT data into navigation software, the surgeon may use "real-time" confirmation of an object's position in the maxillofacial skeleton and skull base.[101,102] There are 3 crucial components in the intraoperative navigation work flow: (1) a localizer, which is the camera or device that tracks the movements of the (2) surgical probe, which is the actual position of the patient currently on the operating table, and (3) a CT scan dataset, which is projected and confirms the position of the probe within the patient to the preoperative 3D image (**Figs. 35–38**). The localizer constantly records the patient's position in space by the placement of fiducial markers on stable and reliable anatomic points on the patient. Fiducial markers may be invasive and fixed, or non-invasive. Invasive fiducial markers are secured onto the patient's facial skeleton with screws via small incisions into the scalp or by a custom splint that is adapted to the patient's face. The patient's

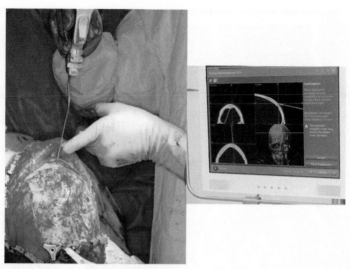

Fig. 35. Intraoperative navigation used to confirm placement of rigid fixation.

head must be immobilized by attaching it to a Mayfield headset when using invasive fiducial markers. Noninvasive (surface) fiducial markers are available in the form of individual adhesive markers, or a light-emitting diode (LED) mask. Noninvasive fiducial markers are much easier to use and are far less invasive than fixed techniques, offering a greater range of mobility of the patient during surgery. Disadvantages of noninvasive fiducial markers are that the mask is in the operating zone. An example of this in orbital surgery is when a coronal flap or transfacial approach, such as a Weber-Ferguson approach, is used. In this instance, the fixed technique should be used. A third, yet more time-consuming method, of fiducial markers placement is the "markerless" technique. This technique includes a set of points on the patient's face that are scanned and correlated with the CT dataset. The position of the surgical probe relative to the patient is determined by the computer using the "local rigid body" concept for which there must be at least 3 registration points (fiducial markers). A registration process is then undertaken in which the navigation software integrates the spatial information from the headset, surgical probe, and fiducial markers, and the end result is alignment of the Cartesian coordinates of the actual patient in the x, y, and z plane onto the computer monitor in comparison with the preoperative CT dataset.

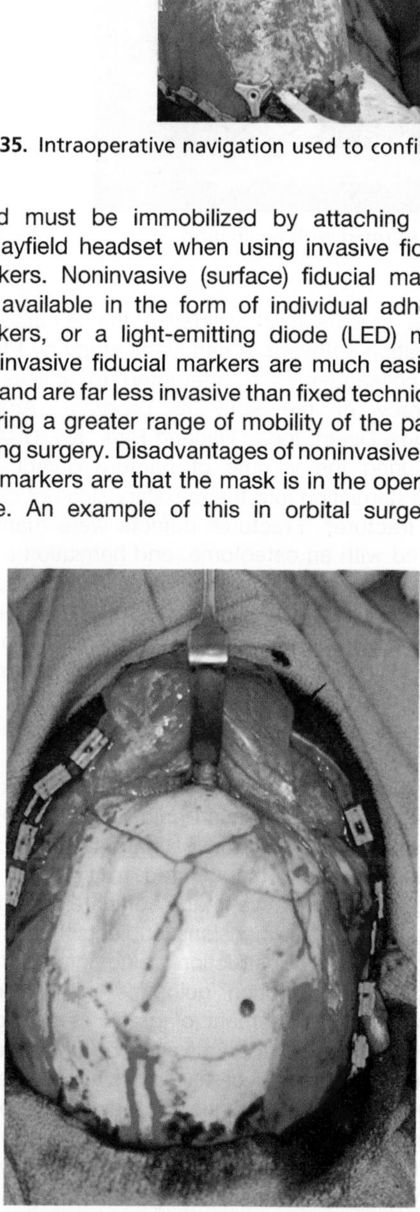

Fig. 36. Superior view of rigid fixation with intraorbital component placed under navigation guidance.

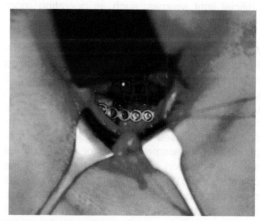

Fig. 37. Transconjunctival incision used to approach the orbital floor.

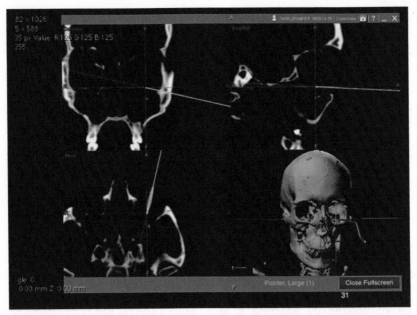

Fig. 38. Location within the clinically nonvisible orbital floor confirmed with navigation.

The most common type of tracking system is the optical tracking system designs, which are similar to the current motion activated gaming systems available today for the public. Optical tracking systems work by tracking LEDs and can be divided into 2 categories: active and passive trackers. Active trackers use battery-powered LEDs that are attached to the surgical probe. These probes can be placed anywhere in the body and tracked with a high degree of accuracy. Passive optical tacking systems have reflectors on the surgical probe that reflect light from the localizer, and carry the advantage of not needing electrical wires or batteries attached to the probe resulting in a lighter probe with more maneuverability. The major disadvantage of passive optical tacking systems is that artificial light sources, such as operating room lights, may interfere with tracking.

Assessment Once the virtual plan has been transferred to the patient by performing the planned reconstruction and insetting orbital implants and grafts, the accuracy of the surgery is then assessed using a portable CT scanner, which is available at many tertiary care facilities because this technology is often used by neurosurgeons.[103] Intraoperative CT assessment allows for any revision of the reconstruction before the patient leaves the operating room (**Fig. 39**). This is particularly useful in orbital reconstruction, where the surgical access and visualization is limited and the relationship of orbital implants and grafts relative to the orbital walls and apex is often misguided (**Fig. 40**).[97]

Few studies exist validating the accuracy of navigation software. A cadaveric study by Ploder and colleagues[104,105] attempted to assess the accuracy of the software program, Analyze (Analyze Direct, Inc., Overland Park, KS, USA), in measuring the volume of fracture defect, and tissue herniation into the maxillary sinus of orbital floor fractures. Fractures defects were manually created with an osteotome, and herniation of the orbital contents was simulated with silicone impression material. Both fracture size and volume of silicone were assessed by direct measurement, 3D CT volumetric measurement, and measurement using Analyze software. Both 3D CT and Analyze were very reliable when compared with direct measurements.

Gellrich and colleagues[85] initially developed a protocol for navigation-guided orbital reconstruction in which the investigators mirrored the unaffected orbit to the affected, traumatized orbit using 3D preoperative image software. Using this as "ideal" orbital dimensions, subjects then underwent orbital reconstruction using intraoperative navigation. Navigation guidance was used to confirm plate placement of grafts at the "goal" dimensions set preoperatively. The investigators found a significant decrease in orbital volume and increase in globe projection in their study cohort. Markiewicz and colleagues[97,106,107] performed a similar study, using the imaging software, Analyze, to assess the change in orbital volume and globe projection in a cohort of subjects with not only defects secondary to trauma, but tumor

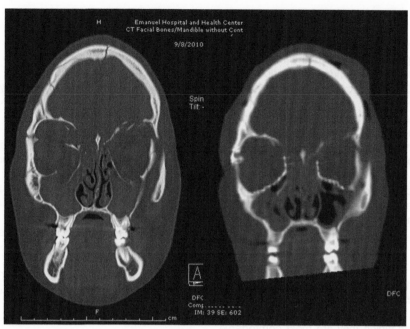

Fig. 39. Preoperative (*left*) and postoperative (*right*) coronal views of CT displaying defect and reconstruction respectively.

ablation as well. Similar results were seen in a study by Pham and colleagues,[94] in which using similar methods for reconstruction of zygomaticomaxillary complex fractures produced results to within 1 mm of the predicted position. Additionally, they used SLMs for preoperative graft contouring before surgery as well as confirming graft placement using intraoperative navigation. They found similar results to the study by Gellrich and colleagues[85]

with a significant decrease in orbital volume and increase in globe projection. In addition, they found a significant, linear correlation between goal and actual orbital volume and globe projection measurements following orbital reconstruction. In addition, Zizelmann and colleagues[95] found cone-beam CT to be just as accurate as traditional CT in computer-assisted navigation of the orbital floor. Studies comparing computer-assisted with

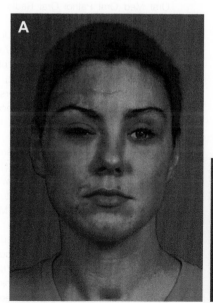

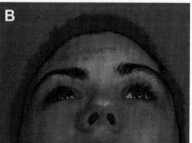

Fig. 40. Frontal (*A*) and worm's-eye view (*B*) of the patient postoperatively.

traditional orbital reconstruction, however, are lacking.

Nkenke and colleagues[108] compared postoperative globe position and enophthalmos between subjects undergoing secondary orbital floor reconstruction using either custom glass–bioceramic CAD/CAM-derived or titanium mesh implants. The investigators found that there was no difference in postoperative globe position and enophthalmos between either group at 365 days of follow-up. Other studies have shown promising results with custom implants; however, they did not have a control group, so therefore no inference can be made as to their superiority over traditional stock implants.[96,99,109–113]

SUMMARY

Numerous approaches to the orbit have been described and, although some have advantages over others, surgeons should generally use the approach with which they are most comfortable, that provides for optimal cosmesis, and that results in minimal complications. The authors' preferred approach for most isolated orbital fractures is a transconjunctival approach performed at the conjunctival fornix. A lateral canthotomy is not advised. Although once popular, our experience is that the lateral canthotomy combined with transconjunctival incision for disarticulation of the lower lid often results in an unnatural appearance even when closed by an experienced surgeon. An isolated transconjunctival fornix approach combined with upper lid blepharoplasty typically provides adequate access to the orbit for most applications. An alternative to a lower lid/transconjunctival approach is endoscopic-assisted transantral repair.

REFERENCES

1. Wright JE, Stewart WB, Krohel GB. Clinical presentation and management of lacrimal gland tumours. Br J Ophthalmol 1979;63(9):600–6.
2. Holtmann B, Wray RC, Little AG. A randomized comparison of four incisions for orbital fractures. Plast Reconstr Surg 1981;67(6):731–7.
3. Converse JM, Firmin F, Wood-Smith D, et al. The conjunctival approach in orbital fractures. Plast Reconstr Surg 1973;52(6):656–7.
4. Rohrich RJ, Janis JE, Adams WP Jr. Subciliary versus subtarsal approaches to orbitozygomatic fractures. Plast Reconstr Surg 2003;111(5):1708–14.
5. Wray RC, Holtmann B, Ribaudo JM, et al. A comparison of conjunctival and subciliary incisions for orbital fractures. Br J Plast Surg 1977;30(2):142–5.
6. McInnes AW, Burroughs JR, Anderson RL, et al. Temporary suture tarsorrhaphy. Am J Ophthalmol 2006;142(2):344–6.
7. Castillo GD, Remigio D. Temporary tarsorrhaphy during facial resurfacing surgery. Arch Facial Plast Surg 2001;3(4):280–1.
8. Gosain AK, Sewall SR, Yousif NJ. The temporal branch of the facial nerve: how reliably can we predict its path? Plast Reconstr Surg 1997;99(5):1224–33 [discussion: 1234–6].
9. Rice CD, Brodsky MC, Hembree K. Delayed tarsal eversion following periorbital trauma. Ophthalmic Surg 1995;26(4):372–3.
10. Ellis E, Zide MF. Surgical approaches to the facial skeleton. 2nd edition. Philadelphia: Lippincott Williams & Wilkins; 2006.
11. Bahr W, Bagambisa FB, Schlegel G, et al. Comparison of transcutaneous incisions used for exposure of the infraorbital rim and orbital floor: a retrospective study. Plast Reconstr Surg 1992;90(4):585–91.
12. Werther JR. Cutaneous approaches to the lower lid and orbit. J Oral Maxillofac Surg 1998;56(1):60–5.
13. Manson PN, Ruas E, Iliff N, et al. Single eyelid incision for exposure of the zygomatic bone and orbital reconstruction. Plast Reconstr Surg 1987;79(1):120–6.
14. Eppley BL, Custer PL, Sadove AM. Cutaneous approaches to the orbital skeleton and periorbital structures. J Oral Maxillofac Surg 1990;48(8):842–54.
15. Kung DS, Kaban LB. Supratarsal fold incision for approach to the superior lateral orbit. Oral Surg Oral Med Oral Pathol Oral Radiol Endod 1996;81(5):522–5.
16. Baker TJ, Gordon HL, Mosienko P. Upper lid blepharoplasty. Plast Reconstr Surg 1977;60(5):692–8.
17. Perman KI. Upper eyelid blepharoplasty. J Dermatol Surg Oncol 1992;18(12):1096–9.
18. Abubaker AO, Sotereanos G, Patterson GT. Use of the coronal surgical incision for reconstruction of severe craniomaxillofacial injuries. J Oral Maxillofac Surg 1990;48(6):579–86.
19. Matras H, Kuderna H. Combined cranio-facial fractures. J Maxillofac Surg 1980;8(1):52–9.
20. Luo W, Wang L, Jing W, et al. A new coronal scalp technique to treat craniofacial fracture: the supratemporalis approach. Oral Surg Oral Med Oral Pathol Oral Radiol 2012;113(2):177–82.
21. Al-Kayat A, Bramley P. A modified pre-auricular approach to the temporomandibular joint and malar arch. Br J Oral Surg 1979;17(2):91–103.
22. Furnas DW. Landmarks for the trunk and the temporofacial division of the facial nerve. Br J Surg 1965;52:694–6.

23. Stuzin JM, Wagstrom L, Kawamoto HK, et al. Anatomy of the frontal branch of the facial nerve: the significance of the temporal fat pad. Plast Reconstr Surg 1989;83(2):265–71.

24. Munro IR, Fearon JA. The coronal incision revisited. Plast Reconstr Surg 1994;93(1):185–7.

25. Fox AJ, Tatum SA. The coronal incision: sinusoidal, sawtooth, and postauricular techniques. Arch Facial Plast Surg 2003;5(3):259–62.

26. Akita S, Hirano A. Modified coronal incision: distribution of stress in the scalp and cranium. Cleft Palate Craniofac J 1993;30(4):382–6.

27. Posnick JC, Goldstein JA, Clokie C. Advantages of the postauricular coronal incision. Ann Plast Surg 1992;29(2):114–6.

28. Hanasono MM, Utley DS, Goode RL. The temporalis muscle flap for reconstruction after head and neck oncologic surgery. Laryngoscope 2001;111(10): 1719–25.

29. Kim S, Matic DB. The anatomy of temporal hollowing: the superficial temporal fat pad. J Craniofac Surg 2005;16(4):651–4.

30. Lacey M, Antonyshyn O, MacGregor JH. Temporal contour deformity after coronal flap elevation: an anatomical study. J Craniofac Surg 1994;5(4):223–7.

31. Matic DB, Kim S. Temporal hollowing following coronal incision: a prospective, randomized, controlled trial. Plast Reconstr Surg 2008;121(6): 379e–85e.

32. Baek RM, Heo CY, Lee SW. Temporal dissection technique that prevents temporal hollowing in coronal approach. J Craniofac Surg 2009;20(3): 748–51.

33. Steinbacher DM, Wink J, Bartlett SP. Temporal hollowing following surgical correction of unicoronal synostosis. Plast Reconstr Surg 2011;128(1):231–40.

34. Frezzotti R, Bonanni R, Nuti A, et al. Radical orbital resections. Adv Ophthalmic Plast Reconstr Surg 1992;9:175–92.

35. Rahman I, Cook AE, Leatherbarrow B. Orbital exenteration: a 13 year Manchester experience. Br J Ophthalmol 2005;89(10):1335–40.

36. Shields JA, Shields CL, Suvarnamani C, et al. Orbital exenteration with eyelid sparing: indications, technique, and results. Ophthalmic Surg 1991;22(5):292–7.

37. Nassab RS, Thomas SS, Murray D. Orbital exenteration for advanced periorbital skin cancers: 20 years experience. J Plast Reconstr Aesthet Surg 2007;60(10):1103–9.

38. Taylor A, Roberts F, Kemp EG. Orbital exenteration—a retrospective study over an 11 year period analyzing all cases from a single unit. Orbit 2006; 25(3):185–93.

39. Tenzel RR, Miller GR. Orbital blow-out fracture repair, conjunctival approach. Am J Ophthalmol 1971;71(5):1141–2.

40. Tessier P. The conjunctival approach to the orbital floor and maxilla in congenital malformation and trauma. J Maxillofac Surg 1973;1(1):3–8.

41. Lynch DJ, Lamp JC, Royster HP. The conjunctival approach for exploration of the orbital floor. Plast Reconstr Surg 1974;54(2):153–6.

42. de Chalain TM, Cohen SR, Burstein FD. Modification of the transconjunctival lower lid approach to the orbital floor: lateral paracanthal incision. Plast Reconstr Surg 1994;94(6):877–80.

43. Baumann A, Ewers R. Use of the preseptal transconjunctival approach in orbit reconstruction surgery. J Oral Maxillofac Surg 2001;59(3):287–91 [discussion: 291–2].

44. Schmal F, Basel T, Grenzebach UH, et al. Preseptal transconjunctival approach for orbital floor fracture repair: ophthalmologic results in 209 patients. Acta Otolaryngol 2006;126(4):381–9.

45. Stoll W, Busse H, Kroll P. Transconjunctival incision and lateral canthotomy. A suitable approach for orbital floor and zygomatic bone correction. Laryngol Rhinol Otol (Stuttg) 1984;63(2):45–7 [in German].

46. Ciarallo RL, Ziccardi VB, Ochs MW. Combined transconjunctival lateral canthotomy approach for infraorbital nerve exploration: report of a case. J Oral Maxillofac Surg 1994;52(1):79–81.

47. Hadeed H, Ziccardi VB, Sotereanos GC, et al. Lateral canthotomy transconjunctival approach to the orbit. Oral Surg Oral Med Oral Pathol 1992; 73(5):526–30.

48. Lynch RC. The technique of a radical frontal sinus operation which has given me the best results. Laryngoscope 1921;31:1–5.

49. Esclamado RM, Cummings CW. Z-plasty modification of the Lynch incision. Laryngoscope 1989; 99(9):986–7.

50. Neel HB 3rd, McDonald TJ, Facer GW. Modified Lynch procedure for chronic frontal sinus diseases: rationale, technique, and long-term results. Laryngoscope 1987;97(11):1274–9.

51. Katowitz JA, Welsh MG, Bersani TA. Lid crease approach for medial wall fracture repair. Ophthalmic Surg 1987;18(4):288–90.

52. Garcia GH, Goldberg RA, Shorr N. The transcaruncular approach in repair of orbital fractures: a retrospective study. J Craniomaxillofac Trauma 1998; 4(1):7–12.

53. Shorr N, Baylis HI, Goldberg RA, et al. Transcaruncular approach to the medial orbit and orbital apex. Ophthalmology 2000;107(8):1459–63.

54. Balch KC, Goldberg RA, Green JP, et al. The transcaruncular approach to the medial orbit and ethmoid sinus. A cosmetically superior option to the cutaneous (Lynch) incision. Facial Plast Surg Clin North Am 1998;6:71–7.

55. Scolozzi P. Reconstruction of severe medial orbital wall fractures using titanium mesh plates placed

using transcaruncular-transconjunctival approach: a successful combination of 2 techniques. J Oral Maxillofac Surg 2011;69(5):1415–20.

56. Edgin WA, Morgan-Marshall A, Fitzsimmons TD. Transcaruncular approach to medial orbital wall fractures. J Oral Maxillofac Surg 2007;65(11): 2345–9.

57. Graham SM, Thomas RD, Carter KD, et al. The transcaruncular approach to the medial orbital wall. Laryngoscope 2002;112(6):986–9.

58. Rodriguez J, Galan R, Forteza G, et al. Extended transcaruncular approach using detachment and repositioning of the inferior oblique muscle for the traumatic repair of the medial orbital wall. Craniomaxillofac Trauma Reconstr 2009;2(1): 35–40.

59. Kakizaki H, Valenzuela AA. Lacrimal caruncle: continuation to the lower eyelid retractors. Ophthal Plast Reconstr Surg 2011;27(3):198–200.

60. Demirci H, Hassan AS, Elner SG, et al. Comprehensive, combined anterior and transcaruncular orbital approach to medial canthal ligament plication. Ophthal Plast Reconstr Surg 2007;23(5): 384–8.

61. Baumann A, Ewers R. Transcaruncular approach for reconstruction of medial orbital wall fracture. Int J Oral Maxillofac Surg 2000;29(4):264–7.

62. Lee CS, Yoon JS, Lee SY. Combined transconjunctival and transcaruncular approach for repair of large medial orbital wall fractures. Arch Ophthalmol 2009;127(3):291–6.

63. Leone CR Jr, Lloyd WC 3rd, Rylander G. Surgical repair of medial wall fractures. Am J Ophthalmol 1984;97(3):349–56.

64. Walter WL. Early surgical repair of blowout fracture of the orbital floor by using the transantral approach. South Med J 1972;65(10):1229–43.

65. Cheong EC, Chen CT, Chen YR. Endoscopic management of orbital floor fractures. Facial Plast Surg 2009;25(1):8–16.

66. Ducic Y, Verret DJ. Endoscopic transantral repair of orbital floor fractures. Otolaryngol Head Neck Surg 2009;140(6):849–54.

67. Maturo SC, Wiseman J, Mair E. Transantral endoscopic repair of orbital floor fractures with the use of a flexible endoscope holder: a cadaver study. Ear Nose Throat J 2008;87(12):693–5.

68. Nishiike S, Nagai M, Nakagawa A, et al. Endoscopic transantral orbital floor repair with antral bone grafts. Arch Otolaryngol Head Neck Surg 2005;131(10):911–5.

69. Persons BL, Wong GB. Transantral endoscopic orbital floor repair using resorbable plate. J Craniofac Surg 2002;13(3):483–8 [discussion: 488–9].

70. Wallace TD, Moore CC, Bromwich MA, et al. Endoscopic repair of orbital floor fractures: computed tomographic analysis using a cadaveric model. J Otolaryngol 2006;35(1):1–7.

71. Strong EB. Endoscopic repair of orbital blow-out fractures. Facial Plast Surg 2004;20(3):223–30.

72. Strong EB, Kim KK, Diaz RC. Endoscopic approach to orbital blowout fracture repair. Otolaryngol Head Neck Surg 2004;131(5):683–95.

73. Farwell DG, Strong EB. Endoscopic repair of orbital floor fractures. Facial Plast Surg Clin North Am 2006;14(1):11–6.

74. Tsirbas A, Kazim M, Close L. Endoscopic approach to orbital apex lesions. Ophthal Plast Reconstr Surg 2005;21(4):271–5.

75. Livingston RJ, White NS, Catone GA, et al. Treatment of orbital fractures by an infraorbital-transantral approach. J Oral Surg 1975;33(8): 586–90.

76. De Riu G, Meloni SM, Gobbi R, et al. Subciliary versus swinging eyelid approach to the orbital floor. J Craniomaxillofac Surg 2008;36(8):439–42.

77. Pospisil OA, Fernando TD. Review of the lower blepharoplasty incision as a surgical approach to zygomatic-orbital fractures. Br J Oral Maxillofac Surg 1984;22(4):261–8.

78. Heckler FR, Songcharoen S, Sultani FA. Subciliary incision and skin-muscle eyelid flap for orbital fractures. Ann Plast Surg 1983;10(4): 309–13.

79. Kim YK, Kim JW. Evaluation of subciliary incision used in blowout fracture treatment: pretarsal flattening after lower eyelid surgery. Plast Reconstr Surg 2010;125(5):1479–84.

80. Feldman EM, Bruner TW, Sharabi SE, et al. The subtarsal incision: where should it be placed? J Oral Maxillofac Surg 2011;69(9):2419–23.

81. Ridgway EB, Chen C, Colakoglu S, et al. The incidence of lower eyelid malposition after facial fracture repair: a retrospective study and meta-analysis comparing subtarsal, subciliary, and transconjunctival incisions. Plast Reconstr Surg 2009;124(5):1578–86.

82. Ploder O, Klug C, Voracek M, et al. Evaluation of computer-based area and volume measurement from coronal computed tomography scans in isolated blowout fractures of the orbital floor. J Oral Maxillofac Surg 2002;60(11):1267–72 [discussion: 1273–4].

83. Hammer B, Kunz C, Schramm A, et al. Repair of complex orbital fractures: technical problems, state-of-the-art solutions and future perspectives. Ann Acad Med Singap 1999;28(5):687–91.

84. Yu H, Shen G, Wang X, et al. Navigation-guided reduction and orbital floor reconstruction in the treatment of zygomatic-orbital-maxillary complex fractures. J Oral Maxillofac Surg 2010;68(1):28–34.

85. Gellrich NC, Schramm A, Hammer B, et al. Computer-assisted secondary reconstruction of

unilateral posttraumatic orbital deformity. Plast Reconstr Surg 2002;110(6):1417–29.

86. He D, Li Z, Shi W, et al. Orbitozygomatic fractures with enophthalmos: analysis of 64 cases treated late. J Oral Maxillofac Surg 2012;70(3):562–76.

87. Markiewicz MR, Bell RB. The use of 3D imaging tools in facial plastic surgery. Facial Plast Surg Clin North Am 2011;19(4):655–82, ix.

88. Markiewicz MR, Bell RB. Modern concepts in computer-assisted craniomaxillofacial reconstruction. Curr Opin Otolaryngol Head Neck Surg 2011;19(4):295–301.

89. Altobelli DE, Kikinis R, Mulliken JB, et al. Computer-assisted three-dimensional planning in craniofacial surgery. Plast Reconstr Surg 1993;92(4):576–85 [discussion: 586–7].

90. Bohner P, Holler C, Hassfeld S. Operation planning in craniomaxillofacial surgery. Comput Aided Surg 1997;2(3–4):153–61.

91. Girod S, Keeve E, Girod B. Advances in interactive craniofacial surgery planning by 3D simulation and visualization. Int J Oral Maxillofac Surg 1995; 24(1 Pt 2):120–5.

92. Girod S, Teschner M, Schrell U, et al. Computer-aided 3-D simulation and prediction of craniofacial surgery: a new approach. J Maxillofac Surg 2001; 29(3):156–8.

93. Vannier MW, Marsh JL, Warren JO. Three dimensional CT reconstruction images for craniofacial surgical planning and evaluation. Radiology 1984; 150(1):179–84.

94. Pham AM, Rafii AA, Metzger MC, et al. Computer modeling and intraoperative navigation in maxillofacial surgery. Otolaryngol Head Neck Surg 2007; 137(4):624–31.

95. Zizelmann C, Gellrich NC, Metzger MC, et al. Computer-assisted reconstruction of orbital floor based on cone beam tomography. Br J Oral Maxillofac Surg 2007;45(1):79–80.

96. Metzger MC, Schon R, Schulze D, et al. Individual preformed titanium meshes for orbital fractures. Oral Surg Oral Med Oral Pathol Oral Radiol Endod 2006;102(4):442–7.

97. Bell RB, Markiewicz MR. Computer-assisted planning, stereolithographic modeling, and intraoperative navigation for complex orbital reconstruction: a descriptive study in a preliminary cohort. J Oral Maxillofac Surg 2009;67(12): 2559–70.

98. Schmelzeisen R, Gellrich NC, Schoen R, et al. Navigation-aided reconstruction of medial orbital wall and floor contour in cranio-maxillofacial reconstruction. Injury 2004;35(10):955–62.

99. Metzger MC, Schon R, Zizelmann C, et al. Semiautomatic procedure for individuals. Preforming of titanium meshes for orbital fractures. Plast Reconstr Surg 2007;119(3):969–76.

100. Lieger O, Richards R, Liu M, et al. Computer-assisted design and manufacture of implants in the late reconstruction of extensive orbital fractures. Arch Facial Plast Surg 2010;12(3):186–91.

101. Metzger MC, Schon R, Weyer N, et al. Computer-assisted extracorporeal orbital reconstruction after optic nerve decompression by removal of sphenoid bone. Ann Plast Surg 2006;57(2):223–7.

102. Schramm A, Suarez-Cunqueiro MM, Rucker M, et al. Computer-assisted therapy in orbital and mid-facial reconstructions. Int J Med Robot 2009; 5(2):111–24.

103. Metzger MC, Hohlweg-Majert B, Schon R, et al. Verification of clinical precision after computer-aided reconstruction in craniomaxillofacial surgery. Oral Surg Oral Med Oral Pathol Oral Radiol Endod 2007;104(4):e1–10.

104. Ploder O, Klug C, Backfrieder W, et al. 2D- and 3D-based measurements of orbital floor fractures from CT scans. J Craniomaxillofac Surg 2002; 30(3):153–9.

105. Ploder O, Klug C, Voracek M, et al. A computer-based method for calculation of orbital floor fractures from coronal computed tomography scans. J Oral Maxillofac Surg 2001;59(12):1437–42.

106. Markiewicz MR, Dierks EJ, Bell RB. Does intraoperative navigation restore orbital dimensions in traumatic and post-ablative defects? J Craniomaxillofac Surg 2012;40(2):142–8.

107. Markiewicz MR, Dierks EJ, Potter BE, et al. Reliability of intraoperative navigation in restoring normal orbital dimensions. J Oral Maxillofac Surg 2011;69(11):2833–40.

108. Nkenke E, Vairaktaris E, Spitzer M, et al. Secondary reconstruction of posttraumatic enophthalmos: prefabricated implants vs titanium mesh. Arch Facial Plast Surg 2011;13(4):271–7.

109. Chai G, Zhang Y, Ma X, et al. Reconstruction of fronto-orbital and nasal defects with compound epoxied maleic acrylate/hydroxyapatite implant prefabricated with a computer design program. Ann Plast Surg 2011;67(5):493–7.

110. Metzger MC, Gissler M, Asal M, et al. Simultaneous cutting of coupled tetrahedral and triangulated meshes and its application in orbital reconstruction. Int J Comput Assist Radiol Surg 2009;4(5):409–16.

111. Metzger MC, Schon R, Schmelzeisen R. Preformed titanium meshes: a new standard? Skull Base 2007; 17(4):269–72.

112. Schon R, Metzger MC, Zizelmann C, et al. Individually preformed titanium mesh implants for a true-to-original repair of orbital fractures. Int J Oral Maxillofac Surg 2006;35(11):990–5.

113. Metzger MC, Schon R, Weyer N, et al. Anatomical 3-dimensional pre-bent titanium implant for orbital floor fractures. Ophthalmology 2006; 113(10):1863–8.

Biomaterials for Reconstruction of the Internal Orbit

Jason K. Potter, MD, DDS[a],*, Michael Malmquist, DDS[b],
Edward Ellis III, DDS, MS[c]

KEYWORDS

- Orbital floor injury • Orbital reconstruction • Biomaterials • Bone grafts

KEY POINTS

- Orbital floor injuries, alone or combination with other facial fractures, are one of the most commonly encountered midface fractures.
- Techniques for orbital reconstruction have migrated away from autogenous bone grafts to well-tolerated alloplasts, such as titanium and Medpor.
- Material for reconstructing the orbit can then be selected based on requirements of the defect matched to the mechanical properties of the material.
- Material selection is largely and ultimately dependent upon surgeon preference.

INTRODUCTION

Orbital floor injuries, alone or combination with other facial fractures, are one of the most commonly encountered midface fractures. Significant complications can occur as a result of these injuries, including enophthalmos, persistent diplopia, vertical dystopia, and restriction of gaze. Appropriate repair is therefore critical. There is currently a greater understanding of the complex anatomy of the orbit and changes that occur within the orbit from disruption of its contents caused by trauma. The principal mechanism of posttraumatic enophthalmos has been shown to be displacement of the orbital soft tissues within an enlarged bony orbit.[1,2] Practitioners generally agree that the optimal treatment is to restore the normal bony architecture and reduce the herniated orbital tissues. Despite advances made in understanding of the injury, wide variation still exists in the method of reconstruction.[1–125]

Of all the considerations in orbital reconstruction, probably no topic has more differing opinions than the selection of biomaterial with which to reconstruct the orbital walls. This paper reviews the biomaterials currently available for internal orbital reconstruction and provides insight into their selection and application.

CHARACTERISTICS OF MATERIALS

Biomaterials include both naturally occurring and synthetic substances. They can be classified as alloplasts, allografts, autografts, and xenografts. The ideal material has physical properties that most closely replicate those of the tissue it replaces.

Portions of this article were previously published in: Potter JK, Ellis E. Biomaterials for reconstruction of the internal orbit. J Oral Maxillofac Surg 2004;62:1280–97; with permission.

[a] Department of Plastic Surgery, University of Texas Southwestern Medical Center, 8220 Walnut Hill Lane, Suite 206, Dallas, TX 75231, USA; [b] Department of Oral and Maxillofacial Surgery, Baylor College of Dentistry, Texas A&M Health Science Center, Dallas, TX, USA; [c] Department of Oral and Maxillofacial Surgery, University of Texas Health Science Center at San Antonio, San Antonio, TX, USA

* Corresponding author.

E-mail address: potterjason@verizon.net

Specific criteria for the ideal properties of a generic biomaterial have been established (**Box 1**). The material should be chemically inert, biocompatible, nonallergenic, and noncarcinogenic. If alloplastic, it should be cost-effective and capable of sterilization without deterioration of its chemical composition. The material should be easily cut and sized in the operating room, and be able to be shaped to fit orbital contours and retain its new form without memory. It should allow fixation to host bone using screws, wire, suture, or adhesive. It should not potentiate growth of microorganisms nor promote resorption of underlying bone or distortion of adjacent tissues. It should be radiopaque to allow radiographic evaluation. The material should be capable of removal without damage to surrounding tissues. The material should be permanently accepted and, if resorbable, completely resorb with replacement by host bone. Lastly, it should be readily available.[4–11] To date, no single material has been universally successful in meeting every one of these criteria. However, as materials science continues to advance, materials come to possess increasingly more of these qualities (**Fig. 1**). The clinician is responsible for recognizing the diversity of the available materials and selectively applying them to the appropriate clinical setting.

All of the characteristics listed in **Box 1** are important qualities of an implanted biomaterial; however, the interplay of the properties is what contributes to the most important aspect of an implanted material: its permanence. The long-term biocompatibility of a material is dependent on the dynamic relationship between host and implant and is influenced by many factors. Calnan[12] reported that alloplastic implants may initiate

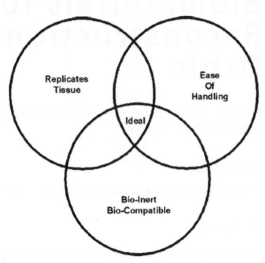

Fig. 1. Figure showing ideal properties of a generic biomaterial. (*From* Potter JK, Ellis E. Biomaterials for reconstruction of the internal orbit. J Oral Maxillofac Surg 2004;62:1280–97; with permission.)

6 different biologic reactions (**Box 2**). The cellular reaction to an implanted material, as described by Coleman and colleagues,[13] begins with an acute inflammatory reaction, with polymorphonuclear leukocytes being the predominant initial cell type. Lymphocytes and macrophages migrate into the area in an attempt to phagocytize the foreign material. Being unable to phagocytize the implant, a chronic inflammatory reaction ensues. This granulation tissue subsequently matures, and an encapsulating connective tissue sheath is formed, isolating the implant.

Once a fibrous capsule is established around the implant, it is generally well tolerated by the body; however, the relationship between host and implant can be altered by several factors.[7,12,14–17] These include various chemical, mechanical,

| Box 1 |
| **Ideal properties for generic biomaterial** |

Chemically inert

Biocompatible

Nonallergenic

Noncarcinogenic

Cost-effective

Sterilizable

Easy handling

Ability to stabilize

Radiopaque

Data from Potter JK, Ellis E. Biomaterials for reconstruction of the internal orbit. J Oral Maxillofac Surg 2004;62:1280–97.

| Box 2 |
| **Biologic reactions to foreign body** |

Immediate inflammation with early rejection

Delayed rejection

Fibrous encapsulation

Incomplete encapsulation with ongoing cellular reaction

Slow resorption

Incorporation

Data from Potter JK, Ellis E. Biomaterials for reconstruction of the internal orbit. J Oral Maxillofac Surg 2004;62:1280–97.

geometric, and physical factors. Chemical factors are associated with alterations in the composition of the material from degradation. Before the current implantable alloys, this was most problematic with corrosion of implanted metals. Most implanted polymers are regarded as chemically inert.[14]

Chemical factors have become a concern again in regard to resorbable biomaterials. All resorbable biomaterials undergo a breakdown reaction and provide the potential for a host's reaction to the breakdown products. Mechanical factors include chronic movement of the implant, discontinuity of the surrounding capsule, and chronic trauma to the implant site. In general, materials that are well tolerated (when implanted subcutaneously) show an increased host reaction if the implant is chronically mobile, subjected to repeated trauma, or insufficiently surrounded by host tissue (**Fig. 2**).[7] Each of these factors may lead to exposure of the implant, and once exposed, implants in humans practically never heal over.[7] Geometric and physical factors include size, shape, and form of the material. Studies have clearly shown that the physical form of a material can increase the host response to that material.[7,14–17] Porous materials allow for variable degrees of soft tissue ingrowth, decreased capsular contracture, and long-term immobility.[18] The acceptance of porous material is hypothesized to be through microscopic adherence of collagen fibrils and capillaries to the pores of the material.[14] Fibrovascular permeation of the implant by host tissue allows locally active immune defense and implant fixation.[19] The importance of

maintaining local immune defense to prevent late rejection of an implant is probably underestimated. Isolation of an implant by a thick fibrous capsule creates an avascular interface between host and implant. Bacterial seeding of the periimplant space is not accessible by the host immune defenses and can lead to abscess formation,[12] which ultimately will lead to failure of the implant. Optimal soft tissue compatibility is characterized by either a limited inflammatory reaction with thin fibrous encapsulation or mesenchymal ingrowth with minimal macrophage activity.[19] Small increases in the amount of host reaction to a given material directly affect the permanence of an implant. Davila and colleagues[16] observed that the encapsulating sheath can thicken and outstrip its blood supply, leading to inflammation, rupture of capillaries, and degeneration of the capsule. Realization of the important role of physical form and material biocompatibility have led to the development of the next generation of implantable materials that have the ultimate goal of incorporation into host tissue and not isolation from them.

CONSIDERATIONS FOR THE INTERNAL ORBIT

Several considerations unique to reconstruction of the internal orbit make the procedure particularly challenging for the development of an ideal biomaterial. Because of the diversity of problems that may present in orbital reconstruction, currently no single material is easily and successfully used in all situations. Clinicians must therefore be cognizant of the properties of the various biomaterials available and to which clinical situation each is best suited. Specific considerations in reconstruction of the internal orbit are presented in **Box 3**.

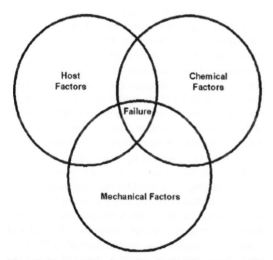

Fig. 2. Figure showing the interaction of major factors that can lead to failure of a biomaterial. (*From* Potter JK, Ellis E. Biomaterials for reconstruction of the internal orbit. J Oral Maxillofac Surg 2004;62:1280–97; with permission.)

Box 3
Factors influencing choice of biomaterial for use in the orbit

Size of defect

Involvement of multiple walls

Adaptation to internal contours

Restoration of proper volume

Presence of adjacent sinus cavity

Prevention of displacement

Risk of further trauma

Adhesions/restriction of ocular mobility

Early versus late repair

Data from Potter JK, Ellis E. Biomaterials for reconstruction of the internal orbit. J Oral Maxillofac Surg 2004;62:1280–97.

Size of the bony defect is important in considering a biomaterial for several reasons. As the size of the defect increases, the variability in shape of the defect increases as the involvement of multiple walls increases (**Fig. 3**). Failure to restore continuity to the walls of the orbital cavity inevitably leads to atrophy and cicatricial contraction of herniated or incarcerated intraorbital contents.[20] Therefore, materials to reconstruct larger defects ideally must be easy to size, shape, and contour to most accurately reconstruct the natural contours of the bony orbit. Dependence on the implant to support orbital soft tissues increases with increasing size of the defect. Consequently, more rigid materials are best suited for reconstruction of large defects to prevent sagging of the material or displacement into the maxillary antrum and/or ethmoid sinuses.[21]

The size of the defect can also be a reflection of the degree of trauma sustained and evidence of the disruption of the orbital ligament system. Disruption of this system has been implicated in the development of enophthalmos from the reshaping of orbital soft tissues that occurs from loss of ligament support.[22,23] Restoration of proper orbital volume and repositioning orbital soft tissues are of fundamental importance in orbital reconstruction.[2,18,22] Care must be taken to select a material that can reliably reconstruct orbital volume and reposition the soft tissues without significant resorption.

Displacement of the material is an unfortunate and preventable occurrence (**Fig. 4**). Converse and colleagues[6] theorized that implants become displaced on active rotation of the globe. The severity of this event depends on the direction and degree of displacement of the material. Extrusion, recurrent enophthalmos, restriction of gaze,

loss of vision, and lacrimal duct obstruction have all been reported in the literature as a result of displaced biomaterials in the orbit.[27–30] Displacement of the implant occurring before fibrous tissue becomes established across the defect provides a mechanism for recurrent prolapse of orbital contents into the paranasal sinus. These adverse effects underscore the importance of stabilizing biomaterials within the orbit. Browning[21] noted that large unfixed implants were more likely to become extruded than similar implants fixed in place with wire or suture. Many authors have advocated the routine use of fixation when placing biomaterials within the orbit. Fixation has been shown to reduce implant-associated complications[31]; therefore, migration should be considered a preventable complication. In a review of long-term stability of Teflon implants, Aronowitz and colleagues[31] reported no cases of migration or extrusion in 77 patients over a 16-year period when implants were stabilized. Several authors have reported that migration and displacement of an implant are directly related to the fixation modality.[3,21,31] Methods of fixation reported in the literature include nonresorbable suture, wire, adhesives, and screws.[3,32–34]

Preventing adhesions between orbital soft tissues and materials used for reconstruction is essential for restoring normal ocular function. Adhesions can lead to restriction of gaze and persistent diplopia. The primary function of the implant is to provide an inert nonadherent surface.[21] Browning and Walker[5] reported that interposition of a smooth inert floor plate between traumatized orbital soft tissues and the fragmented bony floor would prevent the development of motility-restricting adhesions. Concern about preventing adhesions has been most marked with metal implants, and several authors have recommended the placement of autogenous or alloplastic materials between the device and orbital tissues.[35] Adhesion to metal or other materials has been shown to not be a problem characteristic of the material[36,37] and is probably best prevented through meticulous handling of orbital soft tissues to prevent impingement by the implant.

Timing of the repair is a major consideration when selecting a material for reconstruction. Early repair of orbital fractures helps prevent long-term incarceration of orbital contents and more reliably restores proper orbital volume. Biomaterial selected for early repair should consist of the thinnest, least space-occupying material, because exophthalmos can result from overcorrection.[6] Soft tissue volume loss needs to be compensated for less in the acute setting. Browning[21] reported that small defects treated early may be adequately

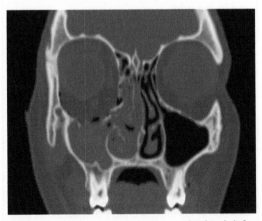

Fig. 3. CT scan showing a large internal orbital defect involving multiple walls.

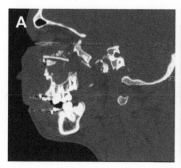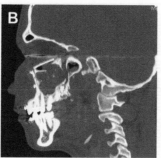

Fig. 4. (A) Sagittal CT scan showing displacement of bone graft requiring correction to prevent persistent deformity (B) Sagittal CT scan showing repositioned graft in correct position for reconstruction of large orbital floor defect.

reconstructed with thin (0.3–1 mm) materials because they need only provide a nonadherent surface. In contrast, late repair is much less predictable because atrophy and scar contracture often necessitate compensation for larger degrees of soft tissue loss and enlargement of orbital volumes (**Fig. 5**).[6] Except for titanium mesh, thin materials will not adequately correct globe dystopia and reduce orbital volume to correct cases of established enophthalmos.[21] Materials capable of occupying greater space and maintaining stability over time to maintain the appropriate orbital volume are usually necessary for late repair.

SELECTION OF A MATERIAL: AUTOGRAFT VERSUS ALLOPLASTIC MATERIALS

Selection of the source of material has been and remains an ongoing debate. Autogenous bone remains the standard against which other materials are compared, although its use has become less common over the past 2 decades. However, generally the material selected for orbital reconstruction is largely determined by the experience of the surgeon. Many authors have outlined the relative advantages and disadvantages of each class of material. These characteristics are based on concerns for donor site morbidity, complication rates, availability of the material, operating room

time, and stability of the material over time (**Table 1**).

AUTOGENOUS MATERIALS

Autogenous tissues were the first material used to reconstruct the internal orbit[6] and are still frequently used. They require a second operative site, which increases patient morbidity; require increased operative time to harvest; are limited in quantity; and are plagued by variable amounts of resorption over time. The variable resorption and potential for late-occurring enophthalmos are the most critical arguments against autogenous materials.

Autogenous Bone

The advantages of autogenous bone are its inherent strength, rigidity, and vascularization potential.[114] It also demonstrates a relative resistance to infection, incorporation by the host into new bone, lack of host response against the graft, and lack of concern for late extrusion. Foreign body reactions, such as infection, extrusion, collagenous capsule formation, and ocular tethering, are minimized. However, the use of autogenous bone is associated with several less favorable aspects, including donor site morbidity,

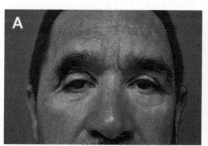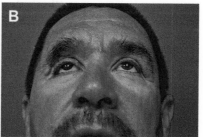

Fig. 5. (A, B) Patient with severe left enophthalmos 12 months after an internal orbital fracture that was not adequately treated.

Table 1
Attributes of materials for internal orbital reconstructions

Material	Biocompatible	Shape & Contour	Stiffness	Sterilizable	Ease of Stabilization	Maintains Volume	Resists Infection	Donor Morbidity	Visible on Imaging
Autologous bone	+++	-	+++	NA	++	-	+++	-	+++
Allogeneic bone	++	-	+++	++	++	-	++	NA	+++
Silicone	+	+++	-	+++	+	+++	-	NA	-
Teflon	+	+++	-	+++	+	+++	-	NA	-
Porous polyethylene	++	+++	+++	+++	+++	+++	+	NA	-
Metallic mesh	++	+++	+++	+++	+++	+++	+	NA	+++
Gelfilm	+	++	-	+++	-	-	-	NA	-
PGA/PLA/PDS	+	++	+	+++	+++	Unknown	-	NA	-

Symbols indication: -, poor; +, Fair; ++, good; +++, excellent. Abbreviations: NA, not applicable; PLA, polylactide; PGA, polyglactin; PDA, polydioxanone.
Data from Potter JK, Ellis E. Biomaterials for reconstruction of the internal orbit. J Oral Maxillofac Surg 2004;62:1280–97.

variable graft resorption, and limited ability to contour some types of bone (**Fig. 6**).

Endochondral and membranous bone sources are used in orbital reconstruction, with the major donor sites for each being iliac crest and calvarium, respectively. The technique of bone grafting in the internal orbit is most consistent with onlay grafting. All bone grafts undergo some degree of resorption and remodeling, although the degree to which each type of graft is affected remains unclear. Early studies showed that membranous bone maintained a greater volume of the original graft compared with endochondral bone when used as an onlay graft.[38–45] Resorption rates of up to 75% have been reported for endochondral,[39] and of 20% to 30%[19] for membranous bone grafts. In contrast, Ozaki and Buchman[46] showed that resorption is not a function of the embryonic origin of the graft, but instead depends on its microarchitecture. Separating the cortical and cancellous components of the grafts, these investigators found cortical grafts maintained their volume significantly better than cancellous grafts regardless of embryonic origin. Fixation of bone grafts has also been shown to reduce graft resorption when grafts are placed under mobile tissues (see **Fig. 6**).[38]

Resorption of graft volume is obviously a concern for the long-term success of reconstructions using autogenous bone. For this reason, calvarial bone is the primary choice for autogenous bone. It has the advantage of being located in the same operative field and provides a high volume of cortical bone. It is available in quantities sufficient for multiple grafts in bilateral orbital reconstructions and can be easily used in conjunction with rigid fixation.[10,48] It is also sufficiently available in children. Iliac crest and rib provide large quantities of bone, but show greater resorption because of the difference in microarchitecture, have potential for significant patient morbidity, and require a second operative field. Their primary advantage over cranial bone is the relative ease of shaping the graft.

Many alternative sources of autogenous bone have been anecdotally reported in the literature, including anterior maxillary wall, mandibular symphysis, ramus, lingual cortex, and coronoid process.[48–54] The main advantages reported for these sources are the ease of access and reduced donor site morbidity. These sources are extremely limited in quantity,[55] however, restricting their application to a narrow subset of internal orbital fractures.

Autogenous Cartilage

Autogenous cartilage grafts are the most frequently used material for nasal augmentation.[19] Their use for reconstructing orbital fractures, however, is not as prevalent. Proponents of autogenous cartilage tout its ease of harvest, flexibility, and limited donor site morbidity as its main advantages. Infection and resorption of autogenous cartilage grafts are rare.[19] Histologic studies have shown the survival of chondrocytes within normal matrix, and a general absence of fibrous ingrowth and resorption of the graft.[38,56–59] Investigators have postulated that cartilage grafts will calcify with time.[60]

The main sources of autogenous cartilage for orbital reconstruction are the cartilaginous nasal septum and conchal cartilage (**Fig. 7**). In general, both of these require contouring for accurate reconstruction of the internal orbit, which is problematic because cartilage possesses inherent

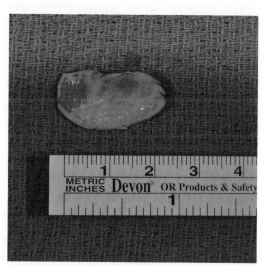

Fig. 7. Photograph of harvested conchal cartilage graft that can be used to reconstruct small internal orbital defects.

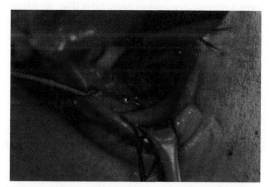

Fig. 6. Calvarial bone graft positioned over orbital floor defect and stabilized with a miniplate. Note that plate does not cross the orbital rim to reduce risk for scar adherence of lower lid to plate.

memory and a tendency to return to its previous shape.[56,61–64] Motoki and Mulliken[65] reported that cartilage will tend to return to its original shape unless maintained in the new shape for several months, which is difficult to accomplish within the confines of the internal orbit. Furthermore, carving necessary for contouring produces changes in the balance of intrinsic tensile and expansile forces, causing distortion of the cartilage shape.[65] Progressive changes in the shape of the graft can alter support and volume within the orbit, causing increased likelihood of late complications.

Patient selection is important because patients must be free of nasal symptoms, have no previous history of nasal surgery, and have a septum that is not complicated with significant deviation or spurs.[64] However, autogenous cartilage provides an easily harvested autogenous material for smaller defects in appropriately selected patients.

ALLOPLASTIC MATERIALS

Alloplasts have been gaining popularity for reconstruction of the internal orbit because of their ease of use and reduced surgical morbidity. Other benefits of alloplasts include decreased operative time, multitude of sizes and shapes available, and seemingly endless supply. The disadvantages of alloplasts have previously been outlined and stem from the fact that they are foreign bodies and elicit some degree of host reaction to the material (see **Box 2**). Many more products are available on the market today than ever before, some without long-term clinical outcome data. This lack of evidence is an obvious concern, because the literature contains many reports of implant complications occurring up to 20 years[27,30,55] after placement. The development of resorbable materials has renewed the interest in alloplastic materials. Resorbable materials are immune to many of the late-occurring complications; however, the literature reports several cases of inflammatory reactions to some of these products. The surgeon must bear in mind that alloplasts are not the panacea that some claim them to be, and that the risk for complications can be lifelong.

ALLOGENEIC MATERIALS

Allogeneic materials (allografts, homografts) and xenografts contain no living cells but, depending on the material, may possess osteoinductive and/or osteoconductive properties. These materials become incorporated into host tissues through providing a structural framework for ingrowth of host tissues. They do not require a second operative site, therefore require less operative time,

and are generally abundant in supply. Waite and Clantons[8] reported that allografts seem to give equally successful results as autografts for reconstruction of the orbital floor. Use of allogeneic materials, however, is marked by concern for antigenicity of the material and transmission of infectious disease.[68] Both xenograft and allogeneic materials are processed through various methods to reduce antigenicity. Xenografts possess more antigenic potential than homografts, and are therefore used less frequently and not recommended by the authors for internal orbital reconstruction. Before placement of xenografts, the surgeon should inquire about previous use of xenografts in the patient, because delayed hypersensitivity reactions have been reported.[8] The 2 most common allografts used for orbital reconstruction, namely homologous bone and cartilage, are discussed in the following sections.

Homologous Bone

Homologous bone provides a scaffold for new bone formation and has the same working properties of autogenous bone. In general, homologous bone is slower to become incorporated and revascularized than autogenous bone.[73] Studies have shown it to be associated with few complications when used for reconstructing the maxillofacial skeleton.[74] Homologous bone is uncommonly used in reconstructing the internal orbit because of reports that bone allografts have a greater tendency to resorb than autografts and are associated with more infections.[55] In a review of their use of homologous bone in the maxillofacial skeleton, Ellis and Sinn[74] reported few complications with its use and relative stability of volume with time. They also noted that, in several cases in which homologous bone was used to reconstruct the internal orbit, reexploration of those orbits showed that the material had undergone remodeling to form a normal-appearing bony orbit (**Fig. 8**). Abundant supply, rigidity, and incorporation into host tissue are characteristics of homologous bone that make it an acceptable material for reconstruction of the internal orbit.

Homologous Cartilage

Homologous cartilage has not been widely reported in the literature for reconstruction of the internal orbit. Chen and colleagues[70] reported their results with lyophilized fascia and cartilage over a 5-year period in 77 patients with isolated orbital floor fractures. Homologous fascia was used for minimally displaced fractures and defects smaller than 5 mm, and cartilage was used for moderately displaced fractures and defects larger

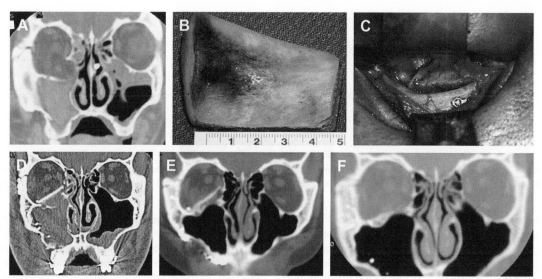

Fig. 8. Case of an internal orbital defect reconstructed with allogeneic bone. (*A*) CT showing orbital floor fracture. (*B*) Bicortical specimen of allogeneic ilium as obtained from bone bank. (*C*) Implant stabilized inside orbit using single bone screw. (*D*) Immediate postoperative CT scan showing position of bone graft. CT scans 1 (*E*) and 2 (*F*) years later showing maintenance of internal orbital volume. (*From* Potter JK, Ellis E. Biomaterials for reconstruction of the internal orbit. J Oral Maxillofac Surg 2004;62:1280–97; with permission.)

than 5 mm. Patients with severe displacement or other associated facial fractures were excluded. Only 11 patients were treated with homologous cartilage. Although the authors report a comparatively low complication rate for the overall study, how many complications were associated with the use of homologous cartilage is unclear.

Homologous cartilage has been shown to undergo ossification and calcification with time.[56,70] However, homologous cartilage has a greater tendency to undergo resorption and replacement with fibrous tissue than autogenous cartilage.[19,56–58] Preserved cartilage is reported to have significantly greater amounts of resorption and increased rates of infection.[19]

ALLOPLASTS

Alloplasts have been gaining popularity for reconstruction of the internal orbit because of their ease of use and reduction in surgical morbidity. Other benefits of alloplasts include decreased operative time, multitude of sizes and shapes available, and seemingly endless supply. The disadvantages of alloplasts have been outlined previously and stem from the fact that they are foreign bodies and elicit some degree of host reaction to the material (see **Box 2**). Alloplasts may be classified as nonresorbable or resorbable. Nonresorbable materials confer a lifelong risk for complications. Resorbable materials are immune to many of the late-occurring complications; however, the literature reports

several cases of inflammatory reactions to some of these products.

NONRESORBABLE MATERIALS
Metallic Mesh

Implantable metals and alloys have revolutionized the treatment of facial fractures through providing rigid internal fixation across fracture lines. As these systems have continued to evolve, the development of low-profile microplating systems has led to their acceptance in the treatment of orbital fractures. The earliest application of these materials in the orbit included rigid internal fixation of the fractured orbital skeleton and fixation of bone grafts within the orbit. Most recently, they have been adapted for reconstruction of the bony internal orbital walls and spanning large bony defects. Several different forms of these alloys are available for this purpose, including preformed orbital plating systems and mesh sheeting (**Fig. 9**). These materials are thin, easy to contour, easily stabilized, maintain their shape, and have the unique ability to compensate for volume when properly contoured, without the potential for resorption. They can easily span large defects to provide rigid support, are visible on radiographs, and are sterilizable. Titanium has the further advantage of producing fewer artifacts on CT than other metals.

Metallic mesh is used routinely to treat orbital fractures and has shown good success when used appropriately.[36,76,77] Rubin and colleagues[76]

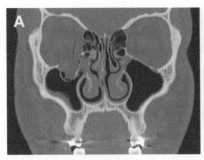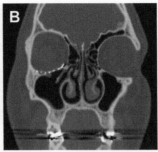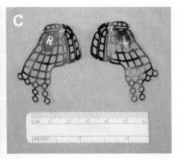

Fig. 9. Example of orbital floor fracture repaired with titanium mesh. (*A*) preoperative CT showing orbital floor blowout fracture. (*B*) Postoperative CT showing repair of defect with titanium mesh. (*C*) Examples of preformed titanium orbital implants.

compared the use of custom orbital floor titanium plates or vitallium mesh versus autologous bone grafts retained with either screw fixation or microplating techniques. They reported no significant complications related to the orbital implants and relative ease of use when compared with placing autologous bone grafts. In a review of 54 patients who underwent internal orbital reconstruction with vitallium mesh without bone grafts, Sargent and Fulks[36] reported excellent results, with no postoperative infections nor need for removal of the material in any case. Ellis and Tan[125] showed better overall reconstruction of orbital blowout fractures with titanium mesh compared with autogenous bone. Rubin and Yaremchuck,[4] in a comprehensive review of the implantable biomaterials literature, reported good results for both mesh and plate systems. Two studies with 69 total patients reported no complications, including infection or extrusion with titanium mesh. Range of follow-up was only 1 to 3 months. Four studies with 92 total patients reported an infection rate of 4.4% overall for metal plates, with 3.3% of implants requiring removal because of an implant-related complication. The range of follow-up was 6 months to 3 years.

Disadvantages of metal alloys include the risk of extrusion and infection, and the theoretical risk to the tissues of the orbital apex from another trauma. Removal of these materials when indicated may be extremely difficult because of fibrous ingrowth through holes machined into them, and also the possibility of osseous overgrowth/osseous integration of the material. Some investigators have also expressed concern that the presence of metal plates may lead to inflammation and adhesions, which contribute to ocular muscle restrictions (Paul Manson, MD, personal communication, 1998). Lee and Nunery[115] reviewed 10 patients with orbital fractures repaired using titanium mesh covering an orbital wall or a plate along the orbital rim who presented with orbital adherence syndrome. Of the 10 patients,

6 presented with cicatricial eyelid retraction, and 9 of 10 presented with extraocular motility restriction resulting in diplopia. During surgical repair, an intense fibrotic adherence was noted between the titanium implant within the orbit or periorbital tissues. All surgical patients with diplopia had improvement in extraocular motility after the titanium was removed and replaced with 0.4-mm nylon implants. They concluded that titanium implants may lead to the adherence of orbital and periorbital structures, resulting in restrictive diplopia and eyelid retraction.

High-density porous polyethylene

Polyethylene has been used as an implanted material for more than 40 years. High-density porous polyethylene (HDPE) has been commercially available as Medpore (Porex Surgical, College Park, GA) since 1985. HDPE is a pure polyethylene implant that is highly biocompatible and processed specifically to include and control pore size. It is insoluble in tissue fluids, does not resorb or degenerate, incites minimal surrounding soft tissue reactions, and possesses high tensile strength. Pore size is engineered to range in size from 100 to 200 μm, with greater than 50% being larger than 150 μm.[18] Pore size has been shown to directly influence the rate and amount of bony and fibrovascular ingrowth into the implant.[3] Animal studies[78] have shown that tissue ingrowth and formation of a mucosal lining occur even when the implant is placed over an open maxillary sinus. Fibrovascular ingrowth minimizes capsule formation; plays a vital role in maintaining the local host immune response within the implant, providing resistance to infection; and provides stability to the implant to prevent migration and exposure. Fibrovascular ingrowth has not been shown to cause extraocular muscle restriction through soft tissue adherence to the implant.[37]

HDPE is available in many different forms. Thin sheeting (0.85–3.0 mm) is most commonly used for internal orbit applications and is easily cut to form with scissors. The material should be soaked in an antibiotic solution before placement within the orbit. It is easily and reliably stabilized with screws.[3]

HDPE is widely accepted for its role in correcting acute injuries and late enophthalmos. Romano and colleagues[18] reviewed the use of HDPE in 140 patients with facial fractures, 128 of whom had implants placed within the orbit. They observed 1 instance of implant infection requiring removal and no cases of implant migration or extrusion. In a review of 21 patients who underwent late correction of enophthalmos using HDPE, Karesh and Horswell[79] observed no cases of infection or extrusion. In a report of 37 orbital reconstructions using HDPE, Rubin and colleagues[37] reported that 1 patient developed infection necessitating implant removal and a second patient had a palpable implant requiring revision 12 months later. Overall, their experience was favorable toward the use of HDPE within the orbit.

Lupi and colleagues[116] used porous HDPE to reconstruct the orbit floor in patients with posttraumatic (27 cases) and postoncologic (5 cases) injuries. No cases of implant migration, extrusion, or enophthalmos were seen; diplopia persisted in 2 patients after 6-month follow-up. The implant was considered safe and represented a stable platform for orbital soft tissues growth.

In 2008, Wang and colleagues[117] restored orbital floor fractures under the periosteum in 21 patients using shaped autogenous bone, titanium mesh, and porous polyethylene (Medpor). All patients had good results, including significant improvements in appearance and function after surgery, without exhibiting severe permanent complications. They suggested that porous polyethylene and titanium mesh may be preferable to autogenous bone because of decreased operative time and donor site morbidity.

Proponents of HDPE tout its technical ease of use for establishing precise 3-dimensional reconstructions and its biocompatibility, durability, and porous structure (allowing fibrovascular ingrowth).[18,35] Aside from being an alloplast, its main disadvantage for use in reconstructing the internal orbit is that it is not radiodense and therefore its position cannot be easily visualized on immediate postoperative CT scans (**Fig. 10**).

Medpor Titan

The Medpor Titan implant is a sheet of titanium mesh embedded in porous polyethylene and has gained much attention in the literature recently (**Fig. 11**). It has the strength, memory, and radiopacity of titanium and the potential for fibrous

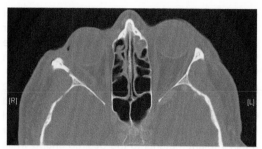

Fig. 10. Postoperative coronal CT after secondary reconstruction of the right orbit with HDPE. Implant is positioned on the lateral orbital wall; its position is difficult to discern because of its radiolucency (right lateral rectus muscle can be seen displaced slightly by the implant compared with the left side).

ingrowth of polyethylene. The new design provides a smooth surface on both sides of the implant; sharp edges of cut titanium are covered by the polyethylene layer, eliminating the need to burr down or smooth the edges to avoid abrasion. Tabrizi and colleagues[123] evaluated orbital floor reconstruction in 101 patients using different materials, including the Medpor Titan implant, concluding that Medpor Titan provided excellent structural support and stability within the orbit and in reconstruction of orbital volume. Both stability and orbital volume are important in resolving enophthalmos and diplopia. Garibaldi and colleagues[124] studied 100 patients who received Medpor Titan implants, 70% of which were fixated with a single screw. One case of orbital hemorrhage and overcorrection was

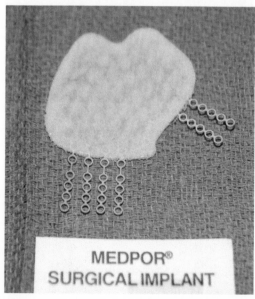

Fig. 11. Medpor/titanium-reinforced orbital implant.

reported, which was attributed to the thickness of the implant. They reported no cases of extrusion or infection. The Medpor Titan implant allows the surgeon to avoid the considerable tissue ingrowth through the holes that is seen with titanium mesh, preventing the tissue from adhering to the surface of the implant. Medpor Titan possesses improved handling characteristics compared with traditional Medpor, allowing the surgeon to bend and contour a thin implant material to the desired shape while providing the strength usually associated with a much thicker traditional Medpor implant.

Nylon SupraFoil

Smooth nylon foil is a nonabsorbable clear sheeting material manufactured from standard nylon suture (**Fig. 12**). Formerly known as Supramid, nylon foil has been used to repair orbital fractures since 1965. In 2007, Majmundar and Hamilton[118] examined 10 orbital floor fractures in 9 patients who were treated with smooth nylon foil from 2004 to 2006. They reported no incidences of implant extrusion, rejection, or infection, and concluded that SupraFoil was safe, easy to use, and reliable. In 2008, Numery and colleagues[119] reported excellent clinical outcomes obtained after implanting a single 0.4-mm thick nylon foil in 102 patients. They showed that 101 patients displayed normal globe position and full ocular motility without diplopia. One patient had persistent enophthalmos requiring a second procedure. Park and colleagues[120] reported a retrospective

Fig. 12. Smooth nylon foil for orbital reconstruction.

study of 181 patients having undergone repair of orbital fractures with nylon foil from 1995 to 2003. Repair of fractures consisted of nylon sheets of varying thickness using a transconjunctival approach with a single-screw fixation of the implant. They reported 1 case of orbital hemorrhage and 1 late infection. Results showed that smooth nylon foil implants are safe and effective in the repair of orbital fractures, and suggested that implant fixation may be instrumental in reducing the incidence of hemorrhage within the implant capsule in nonporous implants. Custer and colleagues[121] investigated complications of 41 orbital floor fractures repaired with Supramid implants. They concluded that insertion of larger implants (>600 mm^2) in late repair of orbital defects may predispose patients to hemorrhage or infection. Su and Harris[122] showed no complications in 19 repairs of combined floor and medial wall fractures using an implant 0.3-mm thick with prepunched holes to encourage fibrovascular ingrowth to aid in stabilization.

Hydroxyapatite

Hydroxyapatite [$Ca_{10}(PO4)_6(OH)_2$] is a calcium phosphate salt that is a major constituent of bone. Calcium phosphate ceramics can be produced through the fusion of calcium phosphate crystals. Several forms are available for reconstruction of the facial skeleton. Dense hydroxyapatite is produced synthetically through high-pressure compaction of calcium phosphate crystals, which are then sintered (fused) into a solid form. Porous hydroxyapatite can be produced synthetically or naturally. Various pore sizes may be engineered into the synthetically produced material. Porosity allows for bony and fibrovascular ingrowth.

Hydroxyapatite is highly biocompatible and causes minimal inflammatory response in the surrounding tissues. It produces a strong mechanical bond with host bone and allows ingrowth of host tissue, providing a scaffold for bone repair. It demonstrates limited resorption[80] and obviates a second surgical site. Hydroxyapatite (all types) has a favorable infection rate of 2.7% for craniofacial reconstruction.[4]

Block forms of hydroxyapatite are most commonly used within the internal orbital skeleton. Large blocks may be ground to the proper size for placement, or multiple small blocks may be placed.[81,82] Ease of use and limited mechanical qualities are the main disadvantages of hydroxyapatite.[83] Its low tensile strength and inflexibility make HA a poor bone substitute. It is brittle, and therefore challenging to contour for placement within the orbit. Hydroxyapatite is extremely difficult to stabilize because overtightening a screw will lead to fracture of the implant. Because of its limited adaptability and relative incompatibility with rigid fixation, hydroxyapatite is rarely used for primary treatment of orbital fractures.

Silicones and Polytetrafluoroethylene (Teflon)

These materials are included for discussion sake, but the current use of these materials is limited because of numerous reports of late complications arising as many as 20 years postoperatively.[5,14,21,25,27–31,50,85–92] Silicone rubber is a chemically inert material available in block and sheet (Silastic; Dow Corning, Midland, MI) forms (**Fig. 13**). Teflon is a long-chain halogenated carbon polymer produced by the polymerization of tetrafluoroethylene gas at high temperature and pressure. It is chemically inert with no known solvent, noncarcinogenic, and able to be sterilized. It is available in a felt-like sheet that is easily cut to size. Silicone and Teflon were the 2 earliest and most commonly used alloplasts for reconstruction of orbital defects. Both show excellent biocompatibility and ease of use. However, these materials histologically demonstrate fibrous encapsulation by the host, a mechanism that has been postulated to lead to failure.[16]

An overall rate of extrusion of 3.1% is reported for smooth silicone implants.[4] The infection rate reported in the literature for silicone implants in the orbit is 1.2%, and other complications include displacement (2%) and seroma (0.5%).[4] Morrison and colleagues[91] reported data on 302 patients treated over 20 years who had received silicone implants for treatment of orbital trauma. Of these patients, 41 (13%) required removal of the implant secondary to implant-related complications. Most complications associated with silicone implants can probably be attributed to their lack of stabilization that was characteristic of early techniques. Many reports have cited the lack of

fixation as a cause for a potentially preventable complication.[3,21,31]

Teflon implants have similarly been under scrutiny for potential late complications. Two reports have documented the long-term outcome with Teflon orbital implants. Aronowitz and colleagues[31] reported data on 35 implants in 31 patients treated over 16 years. The short-term and long-term complication rates were 3.9% and 2.8%, respectively. Antral packing was a clinically significant factor associated with implant failure. No cases of implant migration were seen with proper fixation. Polley and Ringler[25] reported data from a 20-year review of 230 Teflon implants, with a mean follow-up of 30 months. Only 10% of patients had fixation of the implant. No postoperative or long-term complications of extrusion, hemorrhage, or displacement of the implant were observed. One case of infection (0.4%) was reported. Despite these favorable reports, the literature is scattered, with case reports of Teflon implant complications resulting many years postoperatively.[30] These reports, combined with the development of more recent materials, have lead to the disfavor of Teflon for orbital reconstruction.

RESORBABLE ALLOPLASTS
Polylactide

Biodegradable fixation systems have been available for more than 10 years, and are gaining acceptance in many areas of facial reconstructive surgery. Advocates believe these systems perform comparably to metal fixation systems and that the resorbable systems possess a distinct advantage over the lifelong risk of complications characteristic of nonresorbable alloplasts. The development of a resorbable fixation system with mechanical properties similar to metal fixation systems is particularly enticing for use within the orbital skeleton.

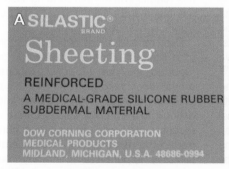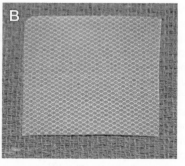

Fig. 13. (*A, B*) Silastic sheeting (reinforced).

Early systems consisted of high-molecular-weight polymerized poly(L-lactide) (PLLA). Initial animal studies reported the use of PLLA plating and screw systems for repair of mandibular fractures.[93] Another study showed the successful use of PLLA systems for the repair of zygomatic fractures in 10 patients.[94] A follow-up report to this study published 6 years later[95] reported that all of the patients developed swelling at the site of implantation approximately 3 years after placement. The cause of the late inflammatory reaction was attributed to the physical nature of the highly crystalline PLLA particles still present in large quantities in the tissues and the slow rate of PLLA degradation.

Animal studies investigating the use of PLLA within the orbit have been performed using a 0.4-mm thick PLLA implant in a goat model.[96] Clinical and microscopic evaluation showed good healing of the orbital defects, with formation of a mature connective tissue capsule and new bone on both antral and orbital sides of the implant. On the antral side, normal sinus mucosa was present across the implant surface. No inflammatory reactions were noted at longest follow-up (78 weeks); however, the implants had not fully resorbed at this time. In a 5-year follow-up to this study,[97] no complications related to the implants were seen in the remaining goats, and the implants were still present. The authors reported that the tissue reaction around the implants had not increased substantially, but the mass-loss seemed to be limited.

Lactosorb (Walter Lorenz Surgical, Jacksonville, FL) is a biodegradable copolymer of polylactic and polyglycolic acids that has been in use clinically for more than 10 years. Studies have shown that this copolymer formulation has a more rapid rate of degradation (9–15 months) compared with PLLA and therefore might be better suited for use as an orbital implant.[99] Clinical studies have shown good results with Lactosorb throughout the craniofacial skeleton.[99–101]

Polyglactin

Polyglactin 910, most commonly known as the suture material Vicryl, is a resorbable synthetic material composed of lactide and glycolide acids. Both film and mesh forms of polyglactin 910 have been reported for repair of orbital fractures.[101,102] In laboratory studies in a cat model, Morain and colleagues[102] showed that polyglactin 910 elicits the same tissue reaction adjacent to a paranasal sinus as the same control defect without an implant.[24] Mesh forms of the material elicit the same reaction, but the process of resorption may take longer compared with the film.[102]

Vicryl mesh is currently the most commonly used form of polyglactin 910 for repair of orbital fractures. Mauriello and colleagues[102] reported the use of Vicryl mesh for repair of orbital floor fractures in 28 patients over a 5-year period (median follow-up of 13 months). The mesh was folded in on itself to achieve the desired thickness (6–56 layers) and then cut to size. The most common complication reported was transient low-grade inflammation of the eyelid lasting up to 11 months. Mauriello and colleagues[102] believe Vicryl mesh has many advantages over other implants for use in the orbit, such as the fact that it is resorbable, it is layered and may be cut to the appropriate thickness at the time of surgery, it is soft and pliable, and therefore easily fits within the orbit and presents no risk to the tissues of the orbital apex; and it does not require fixation.

Vicryl mesh is too flimsy to function effectively as a material for orbital repair; this is best shown in the report by Mauriello and colleagues,[102] in which up to 56 layers of material were required to obtain the desired result. The bulk of material necessary for successful outcome may be the underlying cause of the low-grade inflammatory reactions seen; however, no mention is made of an association between the patients who developed inflammatory reactions and the amount of material used.

Polydioxanone Plates

Polydioxanone is a resorbable aliphatic polyester polymer. Degradation reportedly occurs through hydrolysis in 10 to 12 weeks, although animal models have demonstrated its persistence over 12 months. The use of polydioxanone plates for orbital fractures has been recommended for orbital defects of 1 to 2 cm.[103] Polydioxanone is available in preformed bowl-shaped plates that are easily cut to fit. It can be easily stabilized to adjacent host bone with screws, wires, or suture. Histologic studies have shown a wide range of host responses to the material, from minimal inflammatory reactions in the surrounding tissues[104] to fragmentation and dislocation of the material, causing significant tissue reaction.[105]

Early reports of use of polydioxanone within the orbit seemed favorable. Iizuka and colleagues[103] reported the use of polydioxanone plates for orbital floor reconstruction in 20 patients. All patients had a defect of 1 to 2 cm with communication into the maxillary sinus. Larger defects were reconstructed with homologous bone. They reported the material to be well tolerated, with no clinically apparent inflammatory reactions. The most common complication was inferior migration of globe position over time, for which the authors recommend routine overcorrection of globe position at surgery. Of the 20 patients in the study, 10 (50%) showed overcorrection postoperatively, 9 of which had transitory diplopia related to the degree of overcorrection. It resolved in all but 2 cases over an average of 29 days.

Other studies have shown a less favorable outcome. Kontio and colleagues[106] prospectively followed 16 patients treated with polydioxanone implants for internal orbital wall reconstruction. Postoperative evaluation consisted of clinical, CT, and MRI examination. Reconstructed orbital shape was unsatisfactory and proper orbital volume was not restored. MRI showed thick scar formation (37.5%). The investigators concluded that use of polydioxanone implants for internal orbital reconstruction is not advisable. de Roche and colleagues[105] compared the use of polydioxanone with polylactide in a sheep model. Histologic and radiologic findings at 4 and 12 months were reported for each material. The polydioxanone membranes showed fragmentation leading to severe fibrous tissue reaction, and demonstrated a greater tissue reaction than did polylactide membranes. Tissue reactions associated with polydioxanone led to significant postoperative sequelae, including sensory disturbances (59%), restriction of globe motility (38%), and enophthalmos (24%).[99] Currently, polydioxanone implants are not approved for internal orbital reconstruction in the United States.

DISCUSSION

Treatment of traumatic orbital injuries will continue to be a topic of considerable and evolving debate. The authors have witnessed significant change as techniques for orbital reconstruction have migrated away from autogenous bone grafts to well-tolerated alloplasts, such as titanium and Medpor. The ideal technique is influenced by many factors, including specific characteristics of the injury and the experience of the surgeon. The purpose of this paper was not to determine the ideal material for reconstruction of the internal orbit, but rather to outline the important factors of the most commonly used materials and a few of historical interest. Material for reconstructing the orbit can then be selected based on requirements of the defect matched to the mechanical properties of the material.

Autologous bone has persisted as a reliable, safe, and lifelong material for reconstruction of the orbit. Its use seems to depend on the experience of the surgeon. A wide variety of specialties, and therefore training backgrounds, are involved in the primary treatment of traumatic orbital injuries, which has significant impact on the selection of biomaterials for orbital reconstruction. Dr Anthony Wolfe stated at a symposium on biomaterials that alloplastic materials have been overused, because surgeons have not had adequate training to reach a level of comfort with the effective use of bone grafts.[109] The authors can echo this experience with residents in both oral and maxillofacial surgery and plastic surgery at their institution; few are comfortable with or have had any experience in harvesting cranial bone grafts during their training. In appropriate hands, harvesting autologous tissue results in minimal added morbidity to the patient, especially when it may be obtained within the same operative field, and is reasonably easy to mold and adapt for use within the orbit. No alloplastic material to date has been shown to be superior to fresh autogenous bone grafts. Autologous bone will remain the gold standard for reconstructing the bony defects characteristic of orbital injuries.

Resorbable materials may evolve into reliable materials for reconstruction of the orbit. However, biodegradable materials used in the orbital floor currently manifest an 8.3% incidence of inflammatory reactions.[4] This complication is the second most common when comparing all classes of orbital implants,[4] and therefore these materials should be used with appropriate caution.

After reviewing the literature, selection of biomaterial for reconstruction of the orbit becomes a topic mostly for academic discussion, because the literature shows that several easily available and user-friendly materials provide reliable outcomes for repair of most injuries. Knowledge of biomaterials prevents inappropriate application of materials and, it is hoped, will lower rates of complication. The literature also teaches one to be cautious when selecting from the ever-increasing number of alloplastic materials available. It may be many years before the newer en vogue materials begin to show possible complications. All materials should undergo thorough laboratory and clinical research, which should include clinical outcome data, before becoming a major constituent of one's surgical armamentarium.

REFERENCES

1. Manson PN, Grivas A, Rosenbaum A, et al. Studies on enophthalmos: II. The measurement of orbital injuries by quantitative computed tomography. Plast Reconstr Surg 1986;77(2):203.
2. Bite U, Jackson IT, Forbes GS, et al. Orbital volume measurements in enophthalmos using

three-dimensional CT imaging. Plast Reconstr Surg 1985;75:502–7.

3. Haug RH, Kimberly D, Bradick JP. A comparison of microscrew and suture fixation of porous high density polyethylene orbital floor implants. J Oral Maxillofac Surg 1993;51:1217–20.

4. Rubin PJ, Yaremchuck MJ. Complications and toxicities of implantable biomaterials used in facial reconstructive and aesthetic surgery: a comprehensive review of the literature. Plast Reconstr Surg 1997;100(5):1336–53.

5. Browning C, Walker RV. The use of alloplastics in 45 cases of orbital floor reconstruction. Am J Ophthalmol 1965;60:684–99.

6. Converse JM, Smith B, Obear MF, et al. Orbital blowout fractures: a ten year survey. Plast Reconstr Surg 1967;39(1):20–35.

7. Brown JB, Fryer MP, Ohliwiler DA. Study and use of synthetic materials such as silicone and Teflon as subcutaneous prostheses. Plast Reconstr Surg 1960;26:264.

8. Waite PD, Clantons JT. Orbital floor reconstruction with lyophilized dura. J Oral Maxillofac Surg 1988;46:727–30.

9. Hanson LJ, Donovan MG, Hellstein JW, et al. Experimental evaluation of expanded polytetrafluoroethylene for reconstruction of orbital floor defects. J Oral Maxillofac Surg 1994;52:1050–5.

10. Sugar AW, Kuriakose M, Walshaw ND. Titanium mesh in orbital wall reconstruction. Int J Oral Maxillofac Surg 1992;21:140–4.

11. Kazim M, Katowitz JA, Fallon M, et al. Evaluation of a collagen/hydroxylapatite implant for orbital reconstructive surgery. Ophthal Plast Reconstr Surg 1992;8(2):94–108.

12. Calnan J. The use of inert plastic material in reconstructive surgery. Br J Plast Surg 1963;16:1.

13. Coleman DL, King RN, Andrade JD. The foreign body reaction: a chronic inflammatory response. J Biomed Mater Res 1974;8:199.

14. Sewall SR, Pernoud FG, Pernoud MJ. Late reaction to silicone following reconstruction of an orbital floor fracture. J Oral Maxillofac Surg 1986;44:821–5.

15. Oppenheimer BS, Oppenheimer ET, Stout AP, et al. The latent period in carcinogenesis by plastics in rats and its relation to the presarcomatous stage. Cancer 1958;11:204.

16. Davila JC, Lautsch EV, Palmer TE. Some physical factors affecting the acceptance of synthetic materials as tissue implants. Ann N Y Acad Sci 1968;146:138.

17. Davila JC. Prostheses and living tissues. Ann Thorac Surg 1966;2:126.

18. Romano JJ, Iliff NT, Manson PN. Use of Medpor porous polyethylene implants in 140 patients with facial fractures. J Craniofac Surg 1993;4:142–7.

19. Vuyk HD, Adamson PA. Biomaterials in rhinoplasty. Clin Otolaryngol 1998;23:209–17.

20. Antonyshyn O, Gruss JS, Galbraith DJ, et al. Complex orbital fractures: a critical analysis of immediate bone graft reconstruction. Plast Reconstr Surg 1989;22(3):220–35.

21. Browning C. Alloplastic materials in orbital repair. Am J Ophthalmol 1967;63:955–61.

22. Manson PN, Clifford CM, Su CT, et al. Mechanisms of global support and posttraumatic enophthalmos: I. The anatomy of the ligament sling and its relation to intramuscular cone orbital fat. Plast Reconstr Surg 1986;77:193.

23. Koornneef L. Current concepts on the management of orbital blowout fractures. Ann Plast Surg 1982;9(3):185–200.

24. Morain WD, Colby ED, Stauffer ME, et al. Reconstruction of orbital wall fenestrations with polyglactin 910 film. Plast Reconstr Surg 1987;80(6):769–74.

25. Polley JW, Ringler SL. The use of Teflon in orbital floor reconstruction following blunt facial trauma: a 20 year experience. Plast Reconstr Surg 1987;79(1):39–43.

26. Constantian MB. Use of auricular cartilage in orbital floor reconstruction. Plast Reconstr Surg 1982;69:951.

27. Brown AE, Banks P. Late extrusion of alloplastic orbital floor implant. Br J Oral Maxillofac Surg 1993;31:154–7.

28. Wolfe SA. Correction of lower eyelid deformity caused by multiple extrusions of alloplastic orbital floor implants. Plast Reconstr Surg 1981;68:429.

29. Mauriello JA, Fiore PM, Kotch M. Late complication of orbital floor fracture with implant. Ophthalmology 1987;94(3):2248–50.

30. Mauriello JA, Flanagan JC, Peyster RG. An unusual late complication of orbital floor fracture repair. Ophthalmology 1984;91:102.

31. Aronowitz JA, Freeman BS, Spira M. Long term stability of Teflon orbital implants. Plast Reconstr Surg 1986;78(2):166–73.

32. Tse DT. Cyanoacrylate tissue adhesive in securing orbital implants. Ophthalmic Surg 1986;17:577–80.

33. Seiff SR. Cyanoacrylate fixed silicone sheet in medial blowout fracture repair. Ophthalmic Surg 1989;20(9):674–6.

34. Assael LA, Feineramn DM. Lag screw technique for orbital floor reconstruction with autologous bone grafts. J Oral Maxillofac Surg 1994;52:646–7.

35. Nguyen PN, Sullivan P. Advances in the management of orbital fractures. Clin Plast Surg 1992;19(1):87–98.

36. Sargent LA, Fulks DK. Reconstruction of internal orbital fractures with vitallium mesh. Plast Reconstr Surg 1991;88(1):31–8.

37. Rubin PA, Bilyk JR, Shore JW. Orbital reconstruction using porous polyethylene sheets. Ophthalmology 1994;101:1697–708.

38. Lin KY, Bartlett SP, Yaremchuck MJ, et al. The effect of rigid fixation on the survival of onlay bone graft: an experimental study. Plast Reconstr Surg 1990; 86:449.

39. Smith JD, Abramson M. Membranous bone versus endochondral bone autografts. Arch Otolaryngol 1974;99:203.

40. Zins JE, Whitaker LA. Membranous versus endochondral bone: implications for craniofacial reconstruction. Plast Reconstr Surg 1983;72:778.

41. Zins JE, Whitaker LA, Enlow DH. The influence of recipient site on bone grafts to the face. Plast Reconstr Surg 1984;73:371.

42. Phillip JH, Rahn BA. Fixation effects on membranous and endochondral onlay bone graft resorption. Plast Reconstr Surg 1988;82:872.

43. Kusiak JF, Zins JE, Whitaker LA. the early revascularization of membranous bone. Plast Reconstr Surg 1985;76(4):510–4.

44. Thompson N, Casson JA. Experimental onlay bone grafts to the jaws. A preliminary study on dogs. Plast Reconstr Surg 1970;46:341.

45. Knize DM. The influence of periosteum and calcitonin on onlay bone graft survival. A roentgenographic study. Plast Reconstr Surg 1974;53:190.

46. Ozaki W, Buchman SR. Volume maintenance of onlay bone grafts in the craniofacial skeleton: micro-architecture versus embryologic origin. Plast Reconstr Surg 1998;102(2):291–9.

47. Tovi F, Pitchazade N, Sidi J, et al. Healing of experimentally induced orbital floor defects. J Oral Maxillofac Surg 1983;41:385–8.

48. Sullivan PK, Rosenstein DA, Holmes RE, et al. Bone graft reconstruction of the monkey orbital floor with iliac grafts and titanium mesh plates: a histometric study. Plast Reconstr Surg 1993; 91(5):760–75.

49. Lee HH, Alcaraz N, Reino A, et al. Reconstruction of orbital floor fractures with maxillary bone. Arch Otolaryngol Head Neck Surg 1998;124:56–9.

50. Roncevic R, Malinger B. Experience with various procedures in the treatment of orbital floor fractures. J Maxillofac Surg 1981;9:81–4.

51. Bagatin M. Reconstruction of orbital defects with autogenous bone from mandibular symphysis. J Craniomaxillofac Surg 1987;15:103–5.

52. Girdler NM, Hosseini M. Orbital floor reconstruction with autogenous bone harvested from the mandibular lingual cortex. Br J Oral Maxillofac Surg 1992; 30:36–8.

53. Mintz SM, Ettinger A, Schmakel T, et al. Contralateral coronoid process bone grafts for orbital floor reconstruction: an anatomic and clinical study. J Oral Maxillofac Surg 1998;56:1140–4.

54. Krishnan V, Johnson JV. Orbital floor reconstruction with autogenous mandibular symphyseal bone grafts. J Oral Maxillofac Surg 1997;55:327–30.

55. Goldberg RA, Garbutt M, Shorr N. Oculoplastic uses of cranial bone grafts. Ophthalmic Surg 1993;24(3):190–6.

56. Peer LA. The fate of living and dead cartilage transplanted in humans. Surg Gynecol Obstet 1939;68: 603–10.

57. Peer LA. Diced cartilage grafts. Arch Otolaryngol 1943;38:156–65.

58. Peer LA. Cartilage grafting. Br J Plast Surg 1954;7: 250–62.

59. Ballantyne DL, Rees TD, Seidman I. Silicone fluid: response to massive subcutaneous injections of dimethylpolysiloxane fluid in animals. Plast Reconstr Surg 1965;36(3):330–8.

60. Werther JR. Not seeing eye to eye about septal grafts for orbital fractures [letter]. J Oral Maxillofac Surg 1998;56:906.

61. Ilankovan V, Jackson IT. Experience in the use of calvarial bone grafts in orbital reconstruction. Br J Oral Maxillofac Surg 1992;30:92–6.

62. Converse JM, Smith B. Reconstruction of the floor of the orbit by bone grafts. Arch Ophthalmol 1950;44(1):1–21.

63. Antonyshyn O, Gruss JS, Galbraith DJ, et al. Complex orbital fractures: a critical analysis of immediate bone graft reconstruction. Ann Plast Surg 1989;22:220.

64. Lai A, Gliklick RE, Rubin PA. Repair of orbital blowout fractures with nasoseptal cartilage. Laryngoscope 1998;108:645–50.

65. Motoki DS, Mulliken JB. The healing of bone and cartilage. Clin Plast Surg 1990;17:527–9.

66. Li KK. Repair of traumatic orbital wall defects with nasal septal cartilage: report of 5 cases. J Oral Maxillofac Surg 1997;55:1098–102.

67. Hendler BH, Gateno J, Smith BM. Use of auricular cartilage in the repair of orbital floor defects. Oral Surg Oral Med Oral Pathol 1992;74:719–22.

68. Prichard J, Thadani V, Kalb R, et al. Rapidly progressive dementia in a patient who received a cadaveric dura mater graft. JAMA 1987;257: 1036.

69. Friesenmecker J, Dammer R, Moritz M, et al. Long term results after primary restoration of the orbital floor. J Craniomaxillofac Surg 1995;23:31–3.

70. Chen JM, Zingg M, Laedrach K, et al. Early surgical intervention for orbital floor fractures: a clinical evaluation of lyophilized dura and cartilage reconstruction. J Oral Maxillofac Surg 1992;50: 935–41.

71. Celikoz B, Duman H, Selmanpakoglu N. Reconstruction of the orbital floor with lyophilized tensor fascia lata. J Oral Maxillofac Surg 1998; 55:240–4.

72. Bedrossian EH. Banked fascia lata as an orbital floor implant. Ophthal Plast Reconstr Surg 1993; 9(1):66–70.

73. Ellis E. Biology of bone grafting: an overview. Selected readings Oral Maxillofacial Surg 1991;1.

74. Ellis E, Sinn DP. Use of homologous bone in maxillofacial surgery. J Oral Maxillofac Surg 1993;51:1181–93.

75. Webster K. Orbital floor repair with lyophilized porcine dermis. Oral Surg Oral Med Oral Pathol 1988;65(2):161–4.

76. Rubin PA, Shore JW, Yaremchuck MJ. Complex orbital fracture repair using rigid fixation of the internal orbital skeleton. Ophthalmology 1992;99:553–9.

77. Yaremchuck MJ, Del Vecchio DA, Fiala TG, et al. Microfixation of acute orbital fractures. Ann Plast Surg 1993;30:385–97.

78. Dougherty WR, Wellisz T. The natural history of alloplastic implants in orbital floor reconstruction: an animal model. J Craniofac Surg 1994;5:26–32.

79. Karesh JW, Horswell BB. Correction of late enophthalmos with polyethylene implants. J Craniomaxillofac Trauma 1996;2:18–23.

80. Holmes R, Hagler H. Porous hydroxyapatite as a bone graft substitute in cranial reconstruction: a histometric study. Plast Reconstr Surg 1988;81:662.

81. Hes J, de Man K. Use of blocks of hydroxylapatite for secondary reconstruction of the orbital floor. Int J Oral Maxillofac Surg 1990;19:275–8.

82. Block MS, Kent JN. Correction of vertical orbital dystopia with a hydroxylapatite orbital floor graft. J Oral Maxillofac Surg 1988;46:420–5.

83. Zide MF. Late posttraumatic enophthalmos corrected by dense hydroxylapatite blocks. J Oral Maxillofac Surg 1986;44:804–6.

84. Ono I, Gunji H, Suda K, et al. Orbital reconstruction with hydroxyapatite ceramic implants. Scand J Plast Reconstr Hand Surg 1994;28:193–8.

85. Gamble J. Orbital floor implants. Arch Otolaryngol 1969;89:596–8.

86. Lipshutz H, Ardizone RA. Further observations on the use of silicones in the management of orbital fractures. J Trauma 1965;5:617.

87. Wolfe SA. Correction o persistent lower eyelid deformity caused by displaced orbital floor implant. Ann Plast Surg 1979;2:448.

88. Defresne CR, Manson PN, Iliff NT. Early and late complication of orbital fractures. Clin Plast Surg 1988;15(2):239–53.

89. Jordan DR, St. Onge P, Anderson RL, et al. Complications associated with alloplastic implants used in orbital fracture repair. Ophthalmol 1992;99:1600–8.

90. Stewart MG, Patrinely JR, Appling WD, et al. Late proptosis following orbital floor fracture repair. Arch Otolaryngol Head Neck Surg 1995;121:649–52.

91. Morrison AD, Sanderson RC, Moos KF. The use of silastic as an orbital implant for reconstructions of orbital wall defects: a review of 311 cases treated over 20 years. J Oral Maxillofac Surg 1995;53:412–7.

92. Marks MW, Yeatts RP. Hemorrhagic cyst of the orbit as a long-term complication of prosthetic orbital floor implants. Plast Reconstr Surg 1994;93(4):856–9.

93. Bos RR, Rozema FR, Boering G, et al. Bioabsorbable plates and screws for internal fixation of mandibular fractures. A study in six dogs. Int J Oral Maxillofac Surg 1989;18:365.

94. Bos RR, Rozema FR, Boering G, et al. Resorbable poly(L-lactide) plates and screws for the fixation of unstable zygomatic fractures. J Oral Maxillofac Surg 1987;45:751.

95. Bergsma EJ, Rozema FR, Bos RR, et al. Foreign body reactions to resorbable poly(L-lactide) bone plates and screws used for the fixation of unstable zygomatic fractures. J Oral Maxillofac Surg 1993;51:666–70.

96. Rozema FR, Bos RR, Pennings AJ, et al. Poly(L-lactide) implants in repair of defects of the orbital floor: an animal study. J Oral Maxillofac Surg 1990;48:1305–9.

97. Bergsma EJ, de Bruijn WC, Rozema FR, et al. Late degradation tissue response to poly(l-lactide) bone plates and screws. Biomater 1995;16:25–31.

98. Cordewener FW, Bos RR, Rozema FR, et al. Poly(L-lactide) implants for repair of human orbital floor defects: clinical and MRI evaluation of long term results. J Oral Maxillofac Surg 1996;54:9–13.

99. Enislidis G, Pichornes S, Kainberger F, et al. Lactosorb panel and screws for repair of large orbital floor defects. J Craniomaxillofac Surg 1997;25:316–21.

100. Ahu DK, Sims CD, Randolph MA, et al. Craniofacial skeletal fixation using biodegradable plates and cyanoacrylate glue. Plast Reconstr Surg 1997;99(6):1508–15.

101. Eppley BL, Sadove AM, Havlic RJ. Resorbable plate fixation in pediatric craniofacial surgery. Plast Reconstr Surg 1997;100(1):1–7.

102. Mauriello JA Jr, Wasserman B, Kraut R. Use of Vicryl (polyglactin 910) mesh implant for repair of orbital floor fracture causing diplopia: a study of 28 patients over 5 years. Ophthal Plast Reconstr Surg 1993;9(3):191–5.

103. Iizuka T, Mikkonen P, Paukku P, et al. Reconstruction of orbital floor with polydioxanone plate. Int J Oral Maxillofac Surg 1991;20:83–7.

104. Papgelopoulos PJ, Giannarakaos DG, Lyritis GP. Suitability of biodegradable polydioxanone materials for the internal fixation of fractures. Orthop Rev 1993;22:585.

105. de Roche R, Kuhn A, Adolphs N, et al. Reconstruction of critical size orbital defects in sheep using biodegradable implants: 12 months follow-up and conclusions for future clinical use in humans. Mund Kiefer Gesichtschir 2001;5: 49–56.

106. Kontio R, Suuronen R, Salonen O, et al. Effectiveness of operative treatment of internal orbital wall fracture with polydioxanone implant. Int J Oral Maxillofac Surg 2001;30:278–85.

107. Mermer RW, Orban RE. Repair of orbital floor fractures with absorbable gelatin film. J Craniomaxillofac Trauma 1995;1(4):30–4.

108. Levinson SR, Canalis RF. Experimental repair of orbital floor fracture. Arch Otolaryngol 1977;103: 188–91.

109. Gosain AK, Persing JA. Symposium: biomaterial in the face: benefits and risks. J Craniofac Surg 1999; 10(5):404–14.

110. Lang W. Traumatic enophthalmos with retention of perfect acuity vision. Trans Ophthalmol Soc U K 1889;9:41–5.

111. Fujino T. Mechanism of orbital blowout fracture. J Plast Surg 1974;17:427.

112. Smith B, Regan WF. Blow-out fractures of the orbit. Am J Ophthalmol 1957;44:733–9.

113. Goiato M, Demathe A, Suzuki T, et al. Management of orbital reconstruction. J Craniofac Surg 2010;21: 1834–6.

114. Chowdhury K, Krause GE. Selection of materials for orbital floor reconstruction. Arch Otolaryngol Head Neck Surg 1998;124:1398–401.

115. Lee H, Nunery W. Orbital adherence syndrome secondary to titanium implant material. Opthal Plast Reconstr Surg 2009;25:33–6.

116. Lupi E, Messi M, Ascani G, et al. Orbital floor repair using Medpor porous polyethylene implants. Invest Ophthamol Vis Sci 2004;45:E4700.

117. Wang S, Xiao J, Liu L, et al. Orbital floor reconstruction: a retrospective study of 21 cases. Oral Surg Oral Med Oral Pathol Oral Radiol Endod 2008; 106:324–30.

118. Majmundar M, Hamilton J. Repair of orbital floor fractures with SupraFOIL Smooth Nylon Foil. Arch Facial Plast Surg 2007;9:64–5.

119. Numery WR, Tao JP, Johl S. Nylon foil "wraparound" repair of combined orbital floor and medial wall fractures. Opthal Plast Reconstr Surg 2008;24:271–5.

120. Park DJ, Garibaldi DC, Lliff NT, et al. Smooth nylon foil (SupraFOIL) orbital implants in orbital fractures: a case series of 181 patients. Ophthal Plast Reconstr Surg 2008;24(4):266–70.

121. Custer P, Lind A, Trinkaus K. Complications of Supramid orbital implants. Opthal Plast Reconstr Surg 2003;19:62–7.

122. Su GW, Harris GJ. Combined inferior and medial surgical approaches and overlapping thin implants for orbital floor and medial wall fractures. Opthal Plast Surg 2006;22(6):420–3.

123. Tabrizi R, Ozkan TB, Mohammadinejad C, et al. Orbital floor reconstruction. J Craniofac Surg 2010;21:1142–6.

124. Garibaldi DC, Lliff NT, Grant MP, et al. Use of porous polyethylene with embedded titanium in orbital reconstruction: a review of 106 patients. Opthal Plast Reconstr Surg 2007;23(6):439–44.

125. Ellis E, Tan Y. Assessment of internal orbital reconstruction for pure blowout fractures; cranial bone versus titanium mesh. J Oral Maxillofac Surg 2003;61:442–53.

Orbital Trauma

Edward Ellis III, DDS, MS

KEYWORDS

- Orbit • Trauma • Blow-out

KEY POINTS

- Orbital trauma is the second leading cause of blindness, so the first priority for these injuries is the health of the globe.
- Clinical examination cannot thoroughly assess the presence and severity of internal orbital fractures; therefore, imaging is necessary and mandatory.
- The need for surgery and the timing of intervention for orbital injuries must be individualized.
- Accurate anatomic reconstruction of the orbit is more important that the particular biomaterial chosen.

INTRODUCTION

Orbital fractures are common facial injuries, occurring more often in men than in women. Orbital trauma is the second leading cause of blindness, so the first priority for these injuries is the health of the globe. There is also a high association with cerebral and ocular injuries.[1] Thus, triage dictates that treatment of orbital fractures can be delayed until more vital functions/structures have been managed.[2–4]

Types of Injuries

Many types of orbital fractures are possible, and they can be broadly broken into 2 main types: pure and impure. Impure orbital fractures are those that involve, in addition to the internal orbit, the orbital rim(s). Examples are zygomatico–orbital, naso–orbito–ethmoid, Le Fort maxillary, and supraorbital rim fractures. Impure orbital fractures are more common than pure, with fractures of the zygomatic complex being the most common orbital fracture.[1,5] Pure orbital fractures are also called blowout fractures. Blowout fractures are fractures of the internal orbital walls or floor without a concomitant fracture of the orbital rim(s). Most orbital blowout fractures occur along the floor and/or medial walls of the orbit, where the walls are the thinnest.

The remainder of this article will focus on isolated fractures of the internal orbit (ie, blowout fractures), because the treatment of the internal orbital in cases of impure orbital fractures is essentially the same. The main difference is that when treating impure orbital fractures, the orbital rims (eg, zygoma, maxilla) must first be placed into proper position before internal orbital reconstruction.

Mechanism of Injuries

The physical mechanism of orbital blowout fractures has been debated for years by ophthalmologists, otolaryngologists, plastic surgeons, and maxillofacial surgeons. Because it occurs behind the rim of the orbit, a direct contact of the bony walls with an external object does not occur. Blowout fractures therefore occur indirectly. Most opinions about the mechanism of blowout fractures fall into 3 main theories: the hydraulic theory, the globe-to-wall contact theory, and the bone conduction theory.

The hydraulic theory was first proposed by King in 1944 when he wrote, "The most ready

Disclosures: None.
Department of Oral and Maxillofacial Surgery, University of Texas, Health Science Center, 7703 Floyd Curl Drive, MC 7908, San Antonio, TX 78229–3900, USA
E-mail address: Ellise3@uthscsa.edu

Oral Maxillofacial Surg Clin N Am 24 (2012) 629–648
http://dx.doi.org/10.1016/j.coms.2012.07.006
1042-3699/12/$ – see front matter © 2012 Elsevier Inc. All rights reserved.

oralmaxsurgery.theclinics.com

explanation [for orbital blowout fractures] is trauma transmitted through the eye to the orbital floor."[6] Smith and Regan in 1957 were advocates of this theory, stating that blowout fractures were caused by a generalized increase in orbital soft tissue pressure resulting from the globe being pushed posteriorly from contact with an object.[7] The posterior displacement of the globe increases pressure within the orbit, resulting in fracture of the thin-walled orbital floor and/or medial wall. The hydraulic mechanism for blowout fractures is supported by many other authors.[8–12]

The globe-to-wall contact theory proposed by Raymond Pfeiffer in 1943 states that a force is delivered to the globe, pushing it backward into the orbit, causing it to strike and fracture the bony walls.[8] It is based on common sense and practical deduction from radiologic analysis, but lack of experimental evidence. However, Erling and colleagues[13] found the size of the orbital wall defect exactly fits the size of the globe in many cases of blowout fractures analyzed with computed tomography (CT) scans. They stated that it is the displacement of the globe that directly causes many orbital wall fractures.

An alternate theory for the cause of blowout fractures was proposed by Le Fort in 1901[14] and Lagrange in 1917.[15] The bone conduction hypothesis states that a force is delivered to the orbital rim, which temporarily deforms, or buckles without grossly fracturing. The posterior movement of the orbital rim during that split second causes fracture along the orbital floor and/or medial wall. The orbital rim then springs back into position without any evidence of a complete fracture. This possibility was experimentally demonstrated by Fujino.[16–19] This mechanism is also supported by several others.[20–23] People who disagree with this theory point out that if it were true, the complication of extraocular muscle entrapment would be much less common.[24–26] This theory would not explain all floor fractures and would certainly not play a large role in the commonly observed medial wall fracture.[24,26]

Because of the large variety of blowout fractures that are seen, it is presumptuous to believe that 1 theory may explain all types of fractures completely. It is likely that more than 1 mechanism occurs simultaneously.[27]

Ocular Examination

The status of the eye is the first priority for any periorbital injury, and it is wise to have ophthalmologic consultation on all internal orbital fractures. Studies have shown that an ophthalmologist can discover injuries that are not recognized by nonophthalmologists.[28,29]

A thorough periocular and ocular examination should be performed, looking for foreign bodies, laceration/rupture of the globe, retinal detachment, lens dislocation, and other signs. The mobility of the globe is important, because there is always the possibility that the extraocular muscles and periocular tissues can be incarcerated into the fracture lines or by jagged pieces of bone. Visual acuity, pupillary response, and fundoscopic examinations are mandatory.

Given the mechanisms of blowout fractures discussed previously, one would expect that there should be a large association between the blowout fractures and traumatically induced ocular injuries, especially with the hydraulic and the globe-to-wall theories, because in both, the force is delivered directly to the ocular globe. Surprisingly, studies have shown that this is not the case. In 1 recent study, blowout fractures were associated with traumatic optic neuropathy in only 3% of cases.[27] The incidence of ocular injuries associated with blowout fractures is usually reported in the 20% to 30% range, but most of these are minor.[27,28,30–33] The most common ocular findings, such as commotio retinae, traumatic mydriasis and traumatic iritis, by themselves or in combination, are usually self-limiting and would not usually prohibit the repair of orbital fractures soon after the injury.

Diagnosis

Anyone with a history of blunt trauma to the middle or upper face should be suspected of having an orbital fracture. As with all facial injuries, the diagnosis and severity of orbital fractures are based on clinical and imaging findings. Of note is that diagnosis of orbital injury is not always obvious in the acute scenario. Orbital fractures are commonly missed in unconscious, traumatized patients.[34] Almost half of these undiagnosed fractures require surgical intervention.[35]

Clinical Findings

Most of the clinical findings for patients with blowout fractures are nonspecific and are similar to other fractures involving the orbit (impure). Periorbital swelling may be severe and can hinder a good clinical examination (**Fig. 1**). Even palpation of the orbital rims can be difficult in patients with marked swelling and tenderness.

Subconjunctival ecchymosis is a nonspecific finding that is of little value. Orbital emphysema is common with internal orbital fractures, especially those involving the medial wall (**Fig. 2**). Infraorbital nerve dysfunction is extremely common with zygomatico–orbital, Le Fort, and pure internal

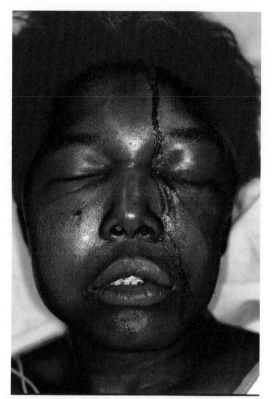

Fig. 1. Photograph of a patient who sustained a left internal orbital fracture. Note the intense edema that can accompany this injury. This makes the clinical examination extremely difficult.

orbital fractures. This can be 1 of the easiest things for an emergency room physician to check on a patient with a history of being struck in the eye. If their infraorbital nerve is dysfunctional, it is almost certain that there is a fracture of the floor of the orbit.[36]

The most important portion of the clinical examination is the ocular examination. Limitation in the ability to move the eye can make one suspect that there is an orbital fracture. Whether a muscle is incarcerated is not usually possible to determine

by simply asking the patient to move the eye. A forced duction test is the most useful method to make this determination, but it is often not easily performed or diagnostic in the awake patient (**Fig. 3**).

Unfortunately, the clinical examination cannot thoroughly assess the presence and severity of internal orbital fractures. For this reason, imaging is necessary and mandatory.

Imaging

CT is the gold standard for assessing the status of the bony orbit. It is much more sensitive than the clinical examination for assessing the bony walls of the internal orbit. Fine cuts (1–2 mm) are required for a thorough analysis of the orbit. Coronal CTs provide the best view of the internal orbit, but sagittal cuts are also very useful when assessing the status of the orbital floor (**Fig. 4**). Sagittal cuts are ideal for orbital floor fractures (see **Fig. 4**B). Axial cuts are ideal for evaluating the medial wall (see **Fig. 4**B). Bone windows can show fractures, but the soft tissue window is best for evaluating the position of the ocular muscles and their relationship to the fracture line(s) (see **Fig. 4**D).

The most common error made when treating orbital fractures is not appreciating the full extent of the injury! Therefore, one should obtain and thoroughly study the CT scans.

WHICH INTERNAL ORBITAL FRACTURES REQUIRE TREATMENT?

An often-debated topic is which internal orbital fractures require treatment. While opinions vary, there are 2 major reasons why these fractures are treated: globe malposition and diplopia. Globe malposition from a pure blowout fracture will manifest as enophthalmos and/or hypophthalmos and has been shown to be the result of changes in the volume of the orbit.[37–39] Studies have shown that most patients will notice once there is 2 to

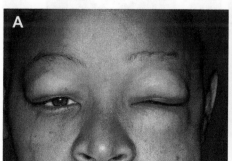
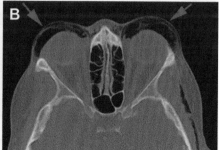

Fig. 2. (A) Photograph of a patient with a, internal orbital fractures who blew her nose and immediately developed air emphysema of the eyelids and orbit. (B) CT scan showing air emphysema of her eyelids.

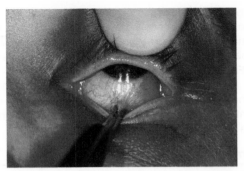

Fig. 3. Photograph showing forced duction test being used to check for incarceration of tissues below the globe. The forceps grasp the insertion of the inferior rectus muscle, and the eyeball is rolled upward. In this case, the test is negative, meaning that the eye moves fine. A positive forced duction test is a test in which the eye does not move properly. The movement of the eye can be checked in all directions by grasping the other rectus muscles and rolling the eye in other directions.

4 mm of globe malposition.[40–42] Just how much internal orbital disruption is necessary to cause clinically apparent enophthalmos and/or hypophthalmos has been the subject of several studies. The studies have also shown that the amount of internal orbital disruption is related to the amount

of globe malposition that may become manifest.[37–39,43–49] However, it is clear that it is not just the amount of orbit involved with the fracture or defect but also the location of the defect and the amount of periorbital soft tissue herniation that are important for the development of clinically obvious enophthalmos.

In particular, defects that are located at the junction of the floor and medial wall of the orbit are those most prone to cause enophthalmos.[1,50] This is the area of convergence of the floor and medial wall and is a convex surface just behind the globe (**Fig. 5**). Anatomically it is the upward bulge of the maxillary sinus and is critical in maintaining the forward position of the globe. When this area is comminuted, the patient will likely have some globe malposition after healing.[1,50]

Studies have shown that anywhere from 0.5 cc to 1 cc of increase in orbital volume will create approximately 1 mm of enophthalmos.[43,46,47,49,51] Unfortunately, it is not easy for most clinicians to calculate orbital volumes, because software to automate this process is not readily available. Therefore the clinician is left to make decisions based on the size, position and extent of the defect, and the amount of soft tissue herniation. Compounding the decision about which orbital fractures require reconstruction is that globe

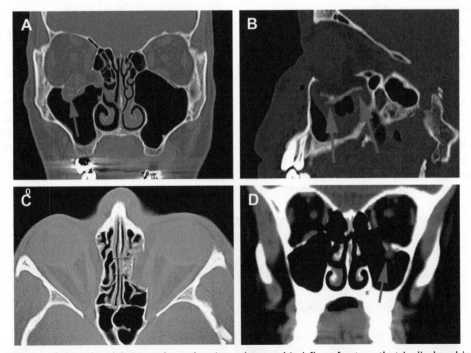

Fig. 4. CT scans of the orbit. (*A*) Coronal cut showing a large orbital floor fracture that is displaced inferiorly (*arrows*). (*B*) Sagittal cut showing a large orbital floor fracture that is displaced inferiorly (*arrows*). (*C*) Axial cut showing a medial blowout fracture (*arrows*). (*D*) Soft tissue window showing the inferior rectus muscle entrapped in an orbital floor fracture. Soft tissue windows show the muscles much better than bony windows.

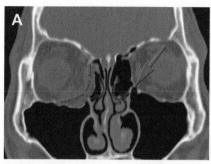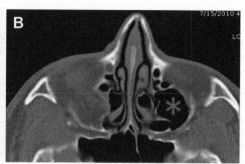

Fig. 5. CTs showing the location of the transition zone between the floor and the medial wall. (*A*) Coronal CT of a combined medial wall/orbital floor fracture of the right orbit demonstrating the great gain in orbital volume by blowout of the transition zone (*dashed lines* indicate normal anatomy). The arrow on the uninjured (*left*) orbit demonstrated the location of the transition zone. (*B*) Axial CT scan showing the location of the upward bulge of the maxillary sinus of the left orbit (*asterisk*) and its loss on the right orbit, where a fracture of the transition zone has blown out this area.

malposition is not common immediately after injury because of associated orbital hemorrhage and swelling that commonly occurs. For acute injuries, imaging findings are a more sensitive method of evaluating the extent of injury than the clinical examination of globe position. For assessment of ocular position before the onset or after the resolution of edema, an exophthalmometer is the best way to clinically measure the relative anteroposterior position of the globes (**Fig. 6**).

The second potential reason to reconstruct the internal orbit is to prevent or treat diplopia. However, binocular diplopia is not a sensitive indicator for the need for internal orbital reconstruction early after injury. Most patients will have diplopia immediately after an orbital fracture secondary to intraorbital edema. However, persistent diplopia may be 1 reason for performing reconstruction of the internal orbit, because it may be the result of soft tissue entrapment (muscle or periorbita), displacement of the globe, and displacement of

the origin of extraocular muscles. In such cases, surgical dissection and freeing the soft tissues from bone fragments and reconstruction of the bony orbit may improve diplopia. However, one would never operate based solely on the symptom of diplopia. Imaging evidence of a fracture or defect would also be necessary.

Determining which orbital fractures require treatment is very important, because the problem associated with not treating some is deformity such as globe malposition, and possibly diplopia. However, the potential benefits of internal orbital reconstruction have to be weighed against the possible iatrogenic injuries that attend surgical correction. Asymmetries of the palpebral fissure secondary to surgical intervention have been demonstrated in up to 20% of surgical approaches to the orbit.[52] Iatrogenic injuries to the infraorbital nerve and intraorbital contents can also occur.

There are factors that are useful in deciding on whether a pure blowout fracture requires internal orbital surgery, and these can be broken down into the following indications:

Absolute indications such as acute enophthalmos and/or hypoglobus or mechanical restriction of ocular motility

Relative indications such as conditions likely to cause enophthalmos and/or hypoglobus or persistence of diplopia

Relative contraindications such as ocular injuries (eg, hyphema, retinal tears, lens displacement) or the fracture has occurred in the only seeing eye

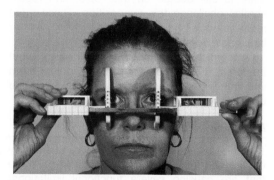

Fig. 6. Photograph showing use of the Naugle exophthalmometer (Richmond Products, Albuquerque, NM), which uses the forehead and infraorbital areas as stable landmarks onto which the device can rest. Measurements of the relative anteroposterior position of the ocular globes are then made.

Absolute Indications

If a patient with a fresh injury presents with acute enophthalmos and/or hypophthalmos, it is almost certain that he or she has a very large internal orbital defect. CT confirmation is necessary, but it will be very unlikely to show anything less than a huge defect with periorbital soft tissue herniation into adjacent sinuses.

If a patient has severe restriction of ocular motility, it is likely that he or she has incarceration of periorbital soft tissues into the fracture line. This can sometimes be verified with CT (see **Fig. 4**D), but a forced duction test is the best method for diagnosis (see **Fig. 3**). In such cases, surgery to free the soft tissue and reconstruct the orbital defect(s) will be necessary.

Relative Indications

Conditions likely to cause enophthalmos and/or hypoglobus are a relative indication for surgery. Conditions likely to cause orbital malposition are large internal orbital defect(s) and can be identified with CT scans. Thus, when a patient is seen with defects of the internal orbit, especially those with fractures in the critical area at the junction of the floor and medial wall (see **Fig. 5**), reconstruction of the internal orbit is often recommended to prevent the development of globe malposition. The other relative indication for surgery is a nonresolving diplopia, especially when the diplopia is in a cardinal field of gaze (forward, downward) and especially when correlated with CT evidence of orbital soft tissues disrupted and extending into the disrupted orbital wall.

Relative Contraindications

Vision is much more important to the patient than the position of the globe within the orbit. Therefore, any condition that puts the globe in jeopardy may be a contraindication to internal orbital reconstruction. For instance, a lacerated globe or hyphema may put the globe at further risk by the retraction necessary to perform internal orbital surgery. In such cases, the ophthalmologist will be the individual to make the recommendation about if and when surgery of the internal orbit might be performed. The other thing that must be considered is the status of the noninjured eye. If the patient has no sight in the other eye, one has to be very careful about recommending surgery of the only seeing eye to help prevent globe malposition. Diplopia (binocular) would not be possible in such a patient, so the only reason to perform surgery other than severe restriction of globe motion secondary to incarceration of soft tissues would be to prevent globe malposition. Certainly, in cases when the fracture involves the only seeing eye, the patient must be the one who decides about the worth of internal orbital reconstruction.

TIMING OF TREATMENT

While deciding on which orbits require reconstruction is an important task, deciding on the timing of repair is another. In the 1960s, orbital blowout fractures were considered medical emergencies and so were treated early. A landmark study in 1974 by Putterman and colleagues[53] completely changed the thinking about timing and even the worth of treatment. They followed 57 patients with orbital blowout fractures rather than operate on them. At 4 to 6 months, 80% of patients had resolution of their diplopia, and the other 20% had diplopia only in extreme upward gaze. Analysis of globe position showed 20% to have enophthalmos, but all were less than 3 mm and were cosmetically acceptable to the patients. The infraorbital nerve dysfunction had also resolved in all patients. The recommendation from Putterman was that orbital blowout fractures should not have any internal orbital reconstruction for 4 to 6 months. The results of this study changed the recommendations about treatment of orbital blowout fractures for the next 20 years.

One must recall that Putterman's study was in the days before CT scanning, so the amount of internal orbital disruption could not be accurately assessed. Once CT scanning became available and surgeons were able to clearly see the amount of internal orbital disruption, the thinking about which fractures should be treated and their timing changed. Some felt that if it was likely that internal orbital reconstruction would be necessary (see previously described indications), then early treatment would provide better outcomes than later treatment.

Several reports suggest that late repairs, beyond 2 to 3 months, result in worse outcomes than early surgery (within 14 days).[54–59] However, there is still debate on this topic, and recent studies challenge this supposition. These more recent studies showed that results from early or late repair were comparable.[60–62]

Concerning the timing of repair of blowout fractures, it may be useful to categorize them into immediate repair, repair within 2 weeks, and observation with the possibility of later repair.

Immediate Repair

There is 1 condition that would mandate early repair—entrapped tissues within the fracture line that are causing severe functional limitations/problems—especially and predominantly in children. In 1965, Soll and Poley published a paper on 4 young patients with a history of orbital trauma with minimal evidence of injury on imaging (tomography).[63] During surgery, they noted orbital tissues trapped within linear or wedge-shaped floor fractures. This report was the first to demonstrate that the internal orbital fractures in children are different than those in adults. Whereas adults have comminution, pediatric orbital fractures, with children's more flexible bones, tend to sustain linear and/or trapdoor fractures. The next paper on this topic was published in 1991 by DeMan and colleagues[64] that included 50 patients with blowout fractures. Fifteen of these were in children, and in 14 of them, orbital soft tissues were trapped and strangulated within the trapdoor fractures. They were the first to recommend immediate surgery in young patients with positive forced duction tests to free the trapped tissues. In 1998, Jordan and colleagues[65] published a similar paper and gave the condition a name: white-eyed blowout fracture. They are white-eyed, because there is no subconjunctival ecchymosis (**Fig. 7**). The eye looks uninjured; however, the patient will have severe restriction of gaze secondary to entrapped tissue in a fracture line that may be so small that there is no CT evidence of a fracture (see **Fig. 7**C, D). They also recommended early (within 1–2 days) surgery to free the entrapped tissue. Sometimes the CT will show no obvious fracture, but the involved rectus muscle is not within

the orbit, instead being found within the sinus (**Fig. 8**).[66] The so-called missing muscle syndrome is also usually found in pediatric patients, and urgent surgery is required to prevent necrosis of the muscle.[56,64,65]

The mechanism by which these injuries occurs is an increase in intraorbital pressure from the traumatizing force, which creates a linear or trapdoor fracture of the bony floor or wall. As the fracture opens, the periorbital soft tissues are pushed through the open space. Because the bones in children are elastic, the bone snaps back into position very quickly, much faster than the soft tissues can recoil, and the bony edges of the fracture incarcerate the trapped soft tissue, strangulating it. Over time, the muscle undergoes avascular necrosis and is permanently damaged. Just how long this takes is not known, but most feel that pediatric blowout fractures with entrapment of soft tissues should be considered medical emergencies and treated as soon as possible.

The other problems that entrapped periorbital soft tissues can cause are bradycardia, heart block, nausea, vomiting, and syncope, occurring almost exclusively in young patients. A nonresolving oculocardiac reflex with CT evidence of entrapped soft tissues within a linear or trapdoor

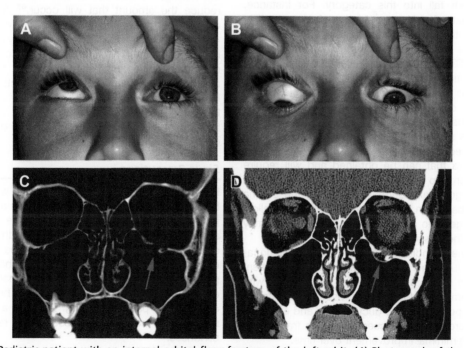

Fig. 7. Pediatric patient with an internal orbital floor fracture of the left orbit. (*A*) Photograph of the patient trying to look up. Note that there is no subconjunctival ecchymosis or other external indication that an orbital fracture has occurred. However, when attempting to look upwards, the left globe does not move. (*B*) Photograph of the patient trying to look down. Note that the left globe does not move. (*C*) Coronal CT bone window cut showing small orbital floor fracture. (*D*) Coronal CT soft tissue window cut showing the inferior rectus muscle entrapped in a small orbital floor fracture.

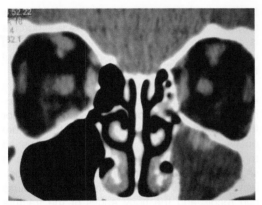

Fig. 8. Coronal CT scan showing lack of the inferior rectus muscle within the left orbit. It is not clearly visible in the sinus because of sinus engorgement with blood/mucus.

fracture is another reason for urgent surgery for the same reasons as discussed previously.[58,67] Certainly, medication with anticholinergics (eg, atropine or glycopyrrolate) to alleviate the intense vagal effects of the oculocardiac reflex are indicated until surgery is possible.

Repair within 2 Weeks

Most adult orbital blowout fractures that require treatment fall into this category. For instance, those patients with no restriction of ocular motility (or negative forced duction test) but acute enophthalmos and/or hypophthalmos, or those orbits whose CT shows that they will likely develop globe malposition if not treated, fall into this category. There is no urgency to repair the defect, and surgery can be deferred until periorbital edema has subsided and/or the patient's medical condition is stable. One should remember that intraorbital edema will limit the amount of surgical exposure that can be obtained and will require more force to be placed on the globe in an effort to get good exposure. Waiting until the edema has subsided in such cases not only may allow the surgeon to attain a better repair, but it may lessen the possibility of globe injury.

Another condition that can be treated nonacutely but within the first few weeks is a patient with an adult orbital fracture associated with symptomatic diplopia, some restriction of motion and/or positive forced duction test, and evidence of periorobital soft tissues within the fracture on CT with minimal improvement over time.

Observation with the Possibility of Later Repair

Patients with orbital fractures associated with minimal diplopia (none in primary or down

gaze), good ocular motility, no significant enophthalmos and/or hypophthalmos, and a CT scan that shows a defect not likely to result in enophthalmos and/or hypophthalmos can be observed. Should symptoms and/or globe position become problematic, intervention can proceed at that time. Many patients in clinical practice fall into this category. Their orbital defects are small; they have minimal functional problems acutely, and those they do have resolve over the first few weeks.

MEDICAL MANAGEMENT OF INTERNAL ORBITAL FRACTURES

Patients who present with internal orbital fractures should be managed medically whether or not they are going to undergo surgical repair. There are several considerations.

Periorbital Swelling

Any patient who has had a force applied to the periorbital region will develop edema that can often be severe. All measures to help reduce this should be attempted to make the patient more comfortable and to facilitate surgical exposure of the orbit. If the patient is seen before the onset of swelling, steroids can be administered to help reduce the amount that will occur.[68] An initial dose of 8 mg of dexamethasone followed by 4 mg every 8 hours for 1 day after surgery is useful in this situation. The intermittent application of cold compresses can also be useful. Steroids and cold compresses are probably of little value if the patient is already maximally swollen. However, a head-up position while in bed will help promote the resolution of edema over the course of days.

Sinus Precautions

Patients with an internal orbital fracture will likely have a fracture between the orbit and an adjacent perinasal sinus. The patient should be told to avoid blowing their nose; not only can this force sinus bacteria into the periorbital tissues, but an immediate air emphysema of the orbital and periorbital soft tissues can occur. The ballooning of the eyelids from air emphysema can be frightening to the patient (see **Fig. 2**). Such a severe increase in intraorbital pressure can result in blindness.[69–74]

Antibiotics

There is no convincing evidence that antibiotics are of any value for orbital fractures, and therefore they should be used with discretion.

Blood Pressure

The blood pressure should be managed if it is high, because this can lead to increased bleeding into the orbital and periorbital compartments.

Anticholinergics

Any patient who has severe bradycardia when attempting to move the eye should have an anticholinergic administered until the trapped periorbita can be freed with surgery. Assuming there are no contraindications to this medication, 0.01 to 0.015 mg/kg of atropine or 0.007 mg/kg of glycopyrrolate should be adequate.

Ocular Pressures

An increase in ocular pressure is usually medically managed by the ophthalmologist. If the intraocular pressure is less than 30, medical treatment may be helpful (ie, steroids, acetazolamide, mannitol, or topical timolol). When the intraocular pressure is higher, immediate surgical decompression is indicated (ie, lateral canthotomy with inferior cantholysis, incision, and drainage).

Coagulation/Clotting

Patients should not be placed on aspirin or other medications that interfere with clotting. Patients already on anticoagulant/antiplatelet medication must be watched carefully for signs of orbital or periorbital hematoma.

INTERNAL ORBITAL RECONSTRUCTION

If surgery is necessary, there are several intraoperative considerations that should be mentioned. They are discussed in the following sections.

Fluid Management

The anesthesiologist should understand that the patient undergoing orbital reconstruction should be medically managed like a neurosurgical patient. The surgeon should discuss with the anesthesiologist the ill effects of liberal fluid management on surgical access and the amount of force of retraction that will be required during surgery. For patients in good health, a minimum of intraoperative fluid instillation is ideal.

Ventilation

The anesthesiologist should avoid or minimize the ventilation provided by facemask during the intubation to prevent air emphysema of the orbital and periorbital compartments.

Anticholinergic Medication

The surgeon should mention to the anesthesiologist that during deep orbital dissection, it is possible that the patient may develop sudden bradycardia. This happens more often in the pediatric population than in adults. Should that happen, the anesthesiologist should notify the surgeon so the retraction of the orbital contents can be immediately withdrawn. Removal of the pressure from the orbital contents will usually quickly reverse the bradycardia. However, it may be beneficial for the patient to receive an anticholinergic (eg, atropine or glycopyrrolate) for the remainder of the surgery if not contraindicated to block the oculocardiac reflex.

Globe Protection

The surgeon must always be cognizant to protect the cornea. There are many methods to do so, and they will vary depending on the surgical approach used. A temporary tarsorraphy is useful when transcutaneous approaches to the orbit are used. A suture through the bulbar conjunctiva to retract the flap upward over the cornea is useful when using a transconjunctival approach. One can also use scleral shields in either approach.

Retraction

One of the most important considerations during surgery is to be cognizant of the amount of force one is applying to the periorbital soft tissues when retracting. The deeper the dissection into the orbit, the more retraction necessary. Recall that the force is being applied to a smaller portion of the periorbita as one reaches the depths of the orbit.

INTERNAL ORBITAL DISSECTION
Orbital Floor

No matter which surgical approach one uses to gain access to the orbital floor, the internal orbital dissection is the same. The pertinent anatomy for orbital floor reconstruction is the inferior orbital fissure and the infraorbital nerve and its canal/groove (**Fig. 9**). Dissection begins by subperiosteal exposure of the infra orbital rim and the ledge of orbital floor just behind it. When dissecting the floor, 2 structures will come into view. One is the fracture, and the other is the inferior orbital fissure. The fracture may or may not extend into the inferior orbital fissure. Often there is a bridge of bone medial to the inferior orbital fissure remaining. In either case, however, the key to an adequate internal orbital dissection for exposure of the floor of the orbit is the complete amputation of any and

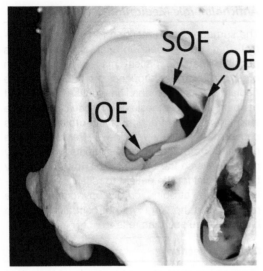

Fig. 9. Right orbit showing the location of the inferior orbital fissure (IOF), the superior orbital fissure (SOF) and the optic foramen (OF).

ascends at a 30° slope from the midaxial plane (**Fig. 11**). One should be especially cognizant of this fact when trying to locate the posterior ledge of bone behind the defect. The tendency is to dissect into the maxillary sinus unless one is always ascending as one dissects posteriorly. The best way to clearly identify the defect is to elevate the periosteum from sound bone completely around the defect. Because the periosteum in the region of the fracture will be fragmented, the only structure along the floor to help guide the path of dissection will be the infraorbital nerve. The periorbital fat will have engulfed the nerve, but this hearty structure provides the best path for dissection; everything above the nerve stays within the orbit (**Fig. 12**). The periorbital soft tissues can be dissected off the nerve (loop magnification is helpful), and the nerve can be followed posteriorly to the point where it meets the posterior aspect of the inferior orbital fissure. The most important structure to locate is the posterior ledge of bone on which a reconstruction material can rest. Anatomically, this is the orbital plate of the palatine bone, a very solid piece of bone, supported by the lesser wing of the sphenoid (**Fig. 13**). It is rarely injured but can be difficult to find when dissecting from anterior to posterior over the fracture defect. It is easy to find if one has completely incised the structures from the inferior orbital fissure. The lateral wall of the orbit can be followed medially and the inferior orbital fissure followed as it converges to the posterior orbit at the same position as the posterior ledge of bone (see **Fig. 13**).

The medial extent of the fracture must also be dissected, and this usually requires subperiosteal elevation along the medial orbital wall, beginning anterior and encircling the defect toward the posterior. Once the defect has been completely dissected and sound bony margins located, a piece of radiographic film or other similar sheet-like material that is a bit larger than the defect can be inserted so that edges of the film or foil are resting on sound bone (**Fig. 14**). This helps

all structures that traverse the inferior orbital fissure. As the fissure is encountered, the periosteum of the orbital floor turns into the fissure. The same thing occurs from the periosteum along the lateral wall of the orbit. The invagination of the periosteum into the fissure limits the amount of exposure one can obtain within the orbit. Structures traversing the inferior orbital fissure are unimportant and can be severed with no functional impairment. The fissure contents should undergo bipolar cauterization and incision (**Fig. 10**), allowing dissection from the floor up the lateral orbital wall as far as necessary. The ability to lift the periorbital tissues superiorly from the floor to the lateral wall provides the needed exposure to fully expose the posterior orbital floor and the junction of the floor with the medial wall, where most of the significant defects will be located.

As subperiosteal exposure continues posteriorly, one must keep in mind that the orbital floor

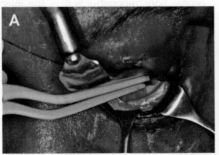
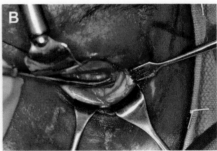

Fig. 10. Photographs showing dissection through the contents of the IOF. (*A*) Bipolar cautery used to coagulate any vessels traversing the IOF. (*B*) Contents of the IOF being severed with scissors after coagulation.

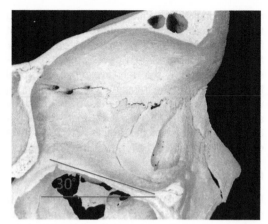

Fig. 11. Photograph of a sagittal section of right orbit demonstrating how the floor of the orbit ascends approximately 30° from the anterior to the posterior orbit.

confine the orbital fat so that a suitable retractor can be used to provide visualization of the defect. A suitable reconstructive material can then be used to span the defect.

Medial Wall

The medial wall is usually approached through a transconjunctival incision that extends through or behind the caruncle and superiorly, to a point at least the halfway up the medial orbital rim. The medial wall of the orbit is almost completely straight in the sagittal plane. Therefore, dissection is straight posteriorly (**Fig. 15**). As one dissects posterior to the lacrimal fossa, there are only 3 anatomic structures that are important. The first is the anterior ethmoidal vessel, which arises through the frontoethmoidal suture approximately 25 mm posterior to the orbital rim (**Fig. 16**). It is a small vessel but important, because if lacerated, it can retract into the periorbita and continue to

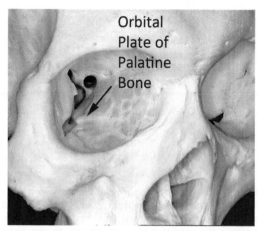

Fig. 13. Photograph of the right orbit showing the location of the orbital plate of the palatine bone, which is the posterior ledge onto which an orbital implant should rest. One must dissect the periorbita until this landmark is identified.

bleed. This vessel will almost always need to be cauterized and cut for blowout fractures of the medial wall. The best way to do so is to strip the periosteum of the orbit superior and inferior to the frontoethmoid suture. Retracting the periosteum will stretch the vessel and make it available for bipolar cautery. It can then be cut, and dissection can proceed posteriorly. As one dissects the medial wall, it is important to point out that the frontoethmoid suture is the same level as the cribriform plate (see **Fig. 16**). If one inadvertently pokes through the thin frontal bone just above the suture line, one can enter the anterior cranial fossa depending on the position in the orbit and the development of the ethmoid sinus. Care must therefore be taken.

Large fractures of the medial wall will almost always extend posteriorly to the level of the posterior ethmoidal vessels, which like the anterior

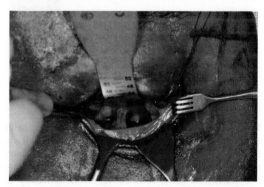

Fig. 12. Photograph showing an orbital floor fracture after dissection of the periorbita off the infraorbital nerve.

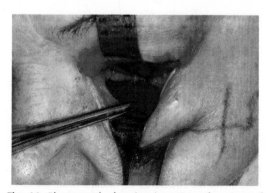

Fig. 14. Photograph showing insertion of a piece of radiographic film into the orbit to help confine the periorbital contents.

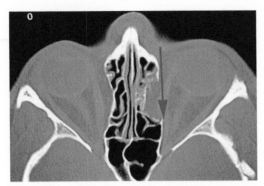

Fig. 15. Axial CT showing medial wall blowout fracture. Note that dissection of the medial wall is almost straight posteriorly (*arrow*). One has to be careful, because the medial wall leads directly to the optic foramen.

ethmoidal vessels, exit the anterior cranial fossa through the frontoethmoidal suture. The importance of the posterior ethmoidal vessel is that it is only 7 mm to 10 mm from the optic foramen. Therefore, one must be extremely careful when dissecting and retracting tissues in the posterior orbit. The posterior ethmoidal vessel does not often need to be cauterized, because the fractures usually end just short of it.

Most isolated medial wall fractures can be adequately visualized using ribbon retractors. When combined with fractures of the floor, 2 retractors may be required, 1 along the floor and another along the medial wall.

Access to fractures the orbital floor and medial wall have traditionally been via various lower eyelid incisions. A transantral approach to the orbital floor was attempted as early as the 1950s, when Converse and Smith[9,54,75] advocated palpating the orbital floor through the antrum before deciding on the need for formal open exploration of the orbital floor. Walter also described using the transmaxillary route, with the aid of a headlight for the visualization and repair of orbital floor fractures.[76] With the rapid development in endoscope technology, the definitive repair of orbital floor fractures via the transantral route and medial wall fractures via the nose has been used by some surgeons.[77–85] However, that subject is beyond the scope of this article and will not be dealt with further.

INTERNAL ORBITAL RECONSTRUCTION

Reconstruction of the internal orbit, with a few exceptions, is treated very differently than other facial fractures. Because of the thinness of the bony orbital walls, the bone usually shatters when injured, so one cannot simply reduce the bones of the orbit. The bones are missing or non-useable. Instead, one must reconstruct the orbital walls. Therefore, instead of using bone plates to hold the bone fragments into a particular position, sheets of bone or another biomaterial are required to replace the bony walls. The goal is to restore the pretrauma anatomy, and this is not as simple as it might sound. The internal orbit is complex in shape (**Fig. 17**), and an almost perfect reconstruction is required for restoration of globe position. The choice of the material one uses to reconstruct the internal orbit is much less important than the adequacy of restoring the anatomy.

The only exception is with linear or trapdoor fractures, usually in the pediatric patient. Because of the elasticity of bone, linear or trap-door

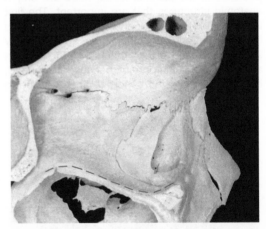

Fig. 17. Photograph of a sagittal section of right orbit demonstrating the lazy S shape of the orbital floor. Note that in the anterior, just behind the orbital rim, the floor is concave, whereas posteriorly, near the transition zone, it is convex. This convexity or upward bulge of the maxillary sinus is important to reconstruct, because it helps maintain the anterior position of the globe.

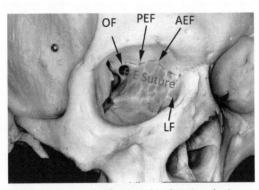

Fig. 16. Photograph of right orbit showing the important anatomic structures for medial wall fractures. Abbreviations: AEF, anterior ethmoid foramen; F-E, frontoethmoid suture (*dashed line*); LF, lacrimal fossa; OF, optic foramen; PEF, posterior ethmoid foramen.

fractures in the young are common. When exposing these fractures, one will notice that the periorbital soft tissue is pinched into a crack in the orbital floor (**Fig. 18**). It is important to not further damage these delicate tissues by trying to pull them out of the fracture defect. Instead, one should try to push the trapdoor downward to see if it flexes and releases the incarcerated periorbital soft tissues (see **Fig. 18**D). If that is not possible, one should make the fracture defect larger by removing bone around the defect (**Fig. 19**). The soft tissues can then be gently lifted out. Once the soft tissues have been carefully removed from the fracture, the defect may or may not require reconstruction. If the defect has been made larger, reconstructing it with whatever biomaterial the surgeon chooses may be necessary (see **Figs. 18**G and **19**E). If the defect was a trapdoor, and it does not stay in a properly reduced position, a small bone plate can be used to maintain it in its proper position (**Fig. 20**).

When placing bone or a biomaterial to reconstruct a missing orbital wall, there are several principles that one could list:

1. When the defect is large, use a thin, rigid material. Maintenance of the orbital shape that is established during the surgery is critical. If a material is not rigid, it may sag into the adjacent perinasal sinuses. For instance, consider the use of a thin sheet of silicone to span a large defect. It does not have the inherent rigidity to maintain the shape and will certainly bulge into the sinus. The only way to counteract that tendency is to use a much thicker piece of silicone. However, doing so may elevate the globe. Therefore, one should only use thin, rigid materials when performing primary reconstruction of internal orbital defects. One should also use a material that will maintain its shape forever. Therefore, the use of bioabsorbable materials for reconstruction of large internal

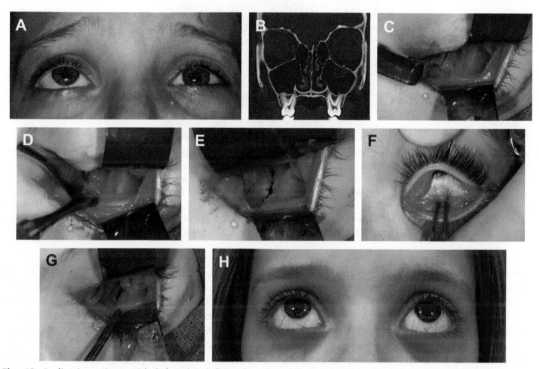

Fig. 18. Pediatric patient with left orbital floor fracture. (*A*) Photograph showing patient looking upwards. Notice that the patient has no subconjunctival ecchymosis or other external indication that a fracture exists. However, the patient's left globe does not rotate upwards. (*B*) Coronal CT scan showing no obvious fracture but soft tissue hanging from the orbital roof into the maxillary sinus. (*C*) Intraoperative photograph showing periorbital soft tissues incarcerated in a linear orbital floor trapdoor fracture. (*D*) Intraoperative photograph showing the use of a periosteal elevator to depress the trapdoor to release the periorbital soft tissues. (*E*) Intraoperative photograph after release of the periorbital soft tissues. Note the linear defect in the orbital floor. (*F*) Intraoperative forced duction test is now negative. (*G*) Intraoperative photograph showing a sheet of gelatin film being placed over the orbital floor defect to prevent periorbital soft tissues from falling into the defect. (*H*) Photograph of patient looking upward 6 weeks after surgery, demonstrating that her globe mobility has been restored.

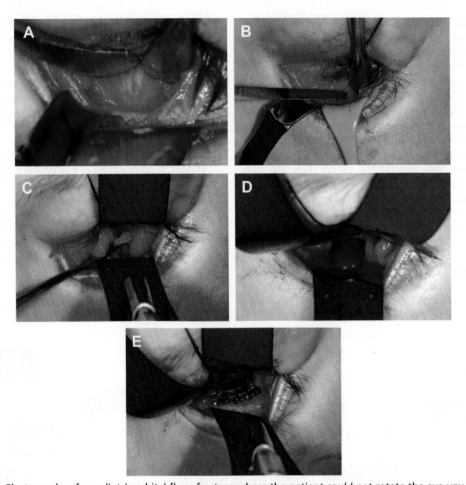

Fig. 19. Photographs of a pediatric orbital floor fracture where the patient could not rotate the eye upward. (*A*) Intraoperative photograph showing a large amount of periorbital soft tissue caught in a linear, nontrapdoor fracture. (*B*) Intraoperative photograph showing the creation of an osteotomy around the entrapped soft tissue using an osteotome. (*C*) Intraoperative photograph showing removal of the bone freed by the osteotomy. (*D*) Intraoperative photograph showing the orbit after the soft tissues have been removed. Note the defect, which was made larger in an attempt to atraumatically free the entrapped periorbital tissues. (*E*) Intraoperative photograph showing the reconstruction of the orbital floor defect with titanium mesh.

orbital defects is not recommended, as they have been shown to be dimensionally unstable over time.[86–88]

2. Use the minimum size necessary. The material used to replace the missing wall should span the entire defect, all edges resting on sound bone to assure the internal orbital is properly reconstructed. However, one also does not want to damage vital structures, especially those at the apex of the orbit. Therefore, the material should be just slightly larger than the size of the defect.

3. Properly shape the material prior to insertion. Small defects may not require much shaping of the material chosen for internal orbital reconstruction. However, large defects of the internal orbit, especially those that involve more than 1 wall, must be properly contoured to recreate the normal anatomy of the internal orbit (**Fig. 21**). This can be very difficult without using surgical aids. A simple technique that can be used is having a sterile artificial skull available in the operating room on which one can shape an implant before placing it into the patient's orbit (**Fig. 22**). The shape provided, while not patient-specific, is usually adequate to recreate the anatomy. Another technique that can be used to help re-create the normal internal orbital anatomy is to use preformed implants (MatrixMIDFACE Preformed Orbital Plate; Synthes Maxillofacial, Paoli, Pennsylvania) (**Fig. 23**). These are especially useful when reconstructing combined floor or medial wall fractures, because the complex shapes of the floor,

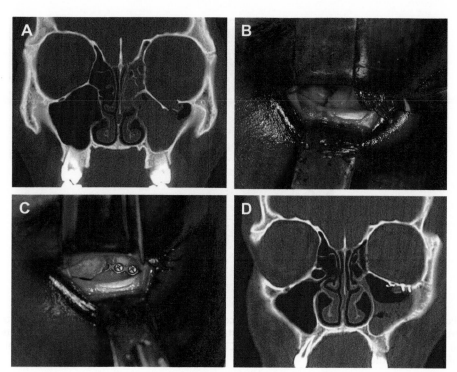

Fig. 20. Photographs of an adult trapdoor fracture. (*A*) Coronal CT scan showing large trapdoor fracture of left orbital floor. (*B*) Intraoperative photograph showing defect after dissection of the periorbital soft tissues. Note the trapdoor tilted downward into the maxillary sinus. (*C*) Intraoperative photograph showing the use of a small bone plate inserted underneath the trapdoor to hold the bone in place. (*D*) Postoperative coronal CT scan showing the reconstruction.

transition zone, and medial wall have been prefabricated into the implants. Two sizes are available for each orbit, and the appropriate size can be made preoperatively using CT scans or intraoperatively using measurements taken of the defect.

4. Tension-free placement should be employed. One can easily trap periorbital soft tissues between the edges of the reconstruction material and the bony walls, especially deep inside the orbit. This can restrict ocular motility and cause persistent diplopia. Therefore, it is imperative that the material be placed in a tension-free manner. The best way to do this is by performing serial forced duction tests throughout the surgery. The first should be performed as soon as the patient is anesthetized and prepared for surgery. The surgeon will get a sense of ocular motility, and it should be compared with the opposite (uninjured) side. As soon as the orbital dissection has been performed, another forced duction test should be performed. There will often be more mobility than before dissection from the freeing of the soft tissues from the bony edges of the defect. Immediately after any reconstruction material has been placed into the orbit, another forced

duction test must be performed to assure that the material has not impinged on or trapped periorbital tissues and restricted globe mobility. If restricted, the material should be removed and replaced until globe motility by forced duction testing is passive.

5. Stabilize the material. While there are differing opinions about this, one should at least consider stabilizing the material within the orbit by securing it to the adjacent orbital floor, orbital rim, or other location with a screw. Mobile materials cause inflammation and infection. If the material is not stable by virtue of its placement within the orbit, it should be stabilized before closure.

6. Adequacy of reconstruction should be verified. The only way to know that the reconstruction has been adequate is to have verification that the reconstructed orbit has the proper shape and volume. There are different methods of doing this. The first is with a postoperative CT scan (see **Fig. 21**). A postoperative CT scan allows the surgeon to critically evaluate his or her ability to reconstruct the orbit. Obviously, to evaluate the reconstruction means that a material that is radiopaque has to be used. The main negative of getting a postoperative CT scan is that if the reconstruction has not

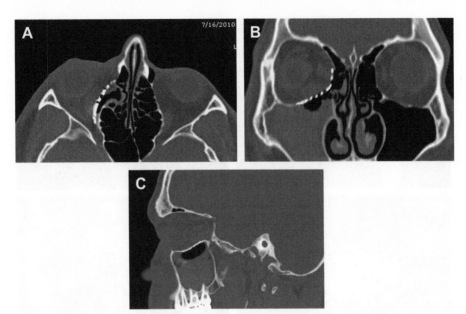

Fig. 21. Postoperative CT scans after internal orbital reconstruction. (*A*) Axial CT scan showing reconstruction of medial orbital wall. (*B*) Coronal CT scan showing reconstruction of both the medial wall and floor. Note that the transition zone has been re-established. (*C*) Sagittal CT scan showing reconstruction of the normal contours (lazy S) of the floor of the orbit.

been performed well, the patient either has to live with an inadequate reconstruction, or the surgeon has to take the patient back to surgery. This has several ramifications that are all negative for the patient. The ideal time to obtain verification of the adequacy of reconstruction is intraoperatively. If the reconstruction is not ideal, it can be repeated without having to bring the patient back to the operating room. There are 2 methods that are available to intraoperatively verify the adequacy of reconstruction. The first is with an intraoperative CT scan. Portable cone–beam C-arm and ring CT scanners are now available for use in operating rooms. The second method that can be used to help position the reconstructive material

and then verify its position is using intraoperative navigation. This is discussed elsewhere in this issue by Potter et al.

POSTOPERATIVE CONSIDERATIONS

As with any surgery, the postoperative management of the patient is important. There are several

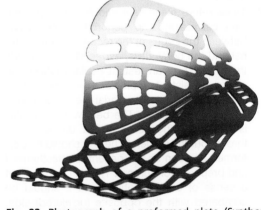

Fig. 23. Photograph of a preformed plate (Synthes Maxillofacial, Paoli, Pennsylvania). It is designed to span defects of the floor and medial walls. Note the complex contours that have been built into the implant. Also note that tabs of material along the medial wall and the posterior edge can be trimmed off for customizing the implant to the patient's defect.

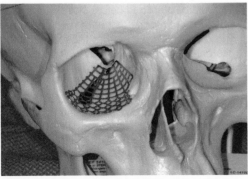

Fig. 22. Photograph of a sterile skull being used to shape an implant for use inside the orbit.

considerations, which will be discussed in the following sections.

Eye Examinations

After the surgery has been completed and the patient taken to the recovery area, one should perform a basic ocular examination as soon as the patient is sufficiently awake. It should include an assessment of visual acuity and eye motility, and this should be documented in the patient's chart. Orders should be written for a vision assessment every hour for the first 6 hours, then every shift. Whether a formal ophthalmologic examination is obtained should be individualized for the patient and will depend on many factors including the preoperative ophthalmologic examination findings, the type of surgery, and the patient's signs and symptoms. The patient should be told that any diplopia may take several months to resolve.[89]

Positioning

Patients should be told to keep the head elevated above the level of their heart until the surgical edema resolves. Doing so will help promote resolution of the edema.

Sinus Precautions

Patients should be told to avoid blowing their nose or performing a valsalva maneuver for at least 2 weeks after surgery for the same reasons as outlined previously.

Steroids

Administration of steroids after surgery may help minimize postoperative periorbital edema.[68] Dexamethasone at a dose of 4 mg every 8 hours for 3 to 4 doses is probably adequate.

Antibiotics

There is no convincing evidence that antibiotics are of any value for orbital fractures, even though bone grafting or alloplastic implantation has been used; they therefore should be used with discretion.

Nasal Decongestants

The value of nasal decongestants is not proven, but the surgeon may wish to consider their use to help promote drainage of the sinuses, which are usually filled with blood after orbital surgery.

Prevention of Barotrauma

A question that is often asked by the patient is when it is safe to fly in a commercial airplane or to go scuba diving. Boyle's law (pressure = 1/volume × constant) describes the relationship between a gas' volume at different pressures. It states that the volume of a gas is inversely proportional to its pressure. The greater the pressure, the less the volume; the lower the pressure, the greater the volume. Therefore, any patient who may have some air inside his or her orbit can have the potential of that air expanding if he or she is in a low-pressure environment, such as climbing in altitude. Doing so expands the volume of air inside the orbit. This can be a potential problem for the patient, and there are some reports of patients having orbital pain and even going blind from ascending in altitude when air was present in the orbit.[70,90–93] If a person with air in their orbit ascends in a commercial aircraft, it is only rarely problematic, because commercial aircraft are pressurized to the atmospheric pressure at 8000 ft. That may cause some discomfort in the eye for some patients, but most do not complain of this. For those who have discomfort, when the plane descends for landing, the pressure increases, the volume of air decreases, and the pain resolves. Patients should be cautioned, however, to not perform valsalva maneuvers in an attempt to equalize pressure in the middle ear because they can force more air into their orbits.

A bigger potential problem is for those who scuba dive. During descending into the water, frequent valsalva maneuvers are performed to equalize the pressure in the middle ear. This can force air from the sinuses into the orbit, which is 1 problem from the standpoint of Boyle's law. Another problem, however, is that valsalva maneuvers can cause temporary or permanent blindness in patients.[69–74] Any air present in the orbit will not have any effect on the diver when he or she is descending, because the atmospheric pressure increases greatly as they descend, increasing 1 atm (760 mm Hg) for every 33 ft they descend. This increase in pressure decreases the volume of air in his or her orbit. However, as the diver ascends to the surface, the pressure decreases, and the volume of air in their orbits increase, sometimes dramatically if a large amount of air has been forced into the orbit by valsalva maneuvers. The increase in volume of air can cause severe pain and has even caused proptosis and blindness from ischemic optic neuropathy or central retinal occlusion.[69–74,94,95] A diver encountering orbital pain and visual changes on ascent should consider the possibility of orbital emphysema. If the situation permits, the diver should re-descend to a depth where the symptoms are minimized, and then begin a slow ascent in an attempt to allow the compressed orbital air to equilibrate with sinus air pressure as the diver rises through the water. A decompression chamber may be required should this not be effective. So when is it safe to scuba dive after an orbital fracture or fracture reconstruction? The answer is not clear, because it has been shown that air can be forced into the orbit for up to 8 weeks in some patients.[70] The best evidence available comes from the military's recommendation that any of their pilots who have undergone functional endoscopic sinus surgery not fly military aircraft for 8 weeks.[96] By that time, the sinus defects will probably have remucosalized, sealing the sinuses from the adjacent orbits. The same 8-week recommendation for scuba diving seems prudent.

REFERENCES

1. Hammer B. Orbital fractures: diagnosis, operative treatment, secondary corrections. Seattle (WA): Hogrefe & Huber Publishers; 1995.
2. Robotti E, Forcht Dagi T, Ravegnani M, et al. A new prospect on the approach to open, complex, craniofacial trauma. J Neurosurg Sci 1992;36:89–99.
3. Piotrowski WP. The primary treatment of frontobasal and midfacial fractures in patients with head injuries. J Oral Maxillofac Surg 1992;50:1264–8.
4. Seider N, Gilboa M, Miller B, et al. Orbital fractures complicated by late enophthalmos: higher prevalence in patients with multiple trauma. Ophthal Plast Reconstr Surg 2007;23:115–8.
5. Ellis E, El-Attar A, Moos K. An analysis of 2067 cases of zygomatico–orbital fracture. J Oral Maxillofac Surg 1985;43:417–28.
6. King EF. Fractures of the orbit. Trans Ophthalmol Soc U K 1944;64:134–8.
7. Smith B, Regan W. Blowout fractures of the orbit. Am J Ophthalmol 1957;44:733–9.
8. Pfeiffer RL. Traumatic enophthalmos. Arch Ophthalmol 1943;30:718–24.
9. Converse JM, Smith B. Enophthalmos and diplopia in fracture of the orbital floor. Br J Plast Surg 1957;9:265–9.
10. Bessiere E, Depaulis J, Verein P, et al. Quelques considerations anatomo–pathologiques et physiopathologiques sur les "blow-out fractures". J Med Bord 1964;141:227–33 [in French].
11. Jones DE, Evans JN. Blow-out fractures of the orbit: an investigation into their anatomical basis. J Laryngol Otol 1967;81:1109–15.
12. Green RP, Peters DR, Shore JW, et al. Force necessary to fracture the orbital floor. Ophthal Plast Reconstr Surg 1990;6:211–7.
13. Erling BF, Iliff N, Robertson B, et al. Footprints of the globe: a practical look at the mechanism of orbital blowout fractures, with a revisit to the work of Raymond Pfeiffer Plast. Plast Reconstr Surg 1999;103:1313–9.
14. Le Fort R. Etude experimentale sur les fractures de la machoire superiure. Rev Chir 1901;23:208–27 [in French].
15. Lagrange F. Les fractures de l'orbite. Paris: Masson & Cie; 1917. p. 22 [in French].
16. Fujino T. Experimental "blowout" fracture of the orbit. Plast Reconstr Surg 1974;54:81–92.
17. Tajima S, Fujino T, Oshiro T. Mechanism of orbital blowout fracture I: stress coat test. Keio J Med 1974;23:71–8.
18. Fujino T, Sugimoto C, Tajima S, et al. Mechanism of orbital blowout fracture II: analysis by high speed camera in two dimensional eye model. Keio J Med 1974;23:115–21.
19. Fujino T, Sato TB. Mechanisms, tolerance limit curve and theoretical analysis in blow-out fractures of two and three-dimensional orbital wall models. In: Anderson RL, editor. Proceedings of the 3rd international symposium on orbital disorders. Amsterdam (Holland): Excerpta Medica; 1977. p. 240–7.
20. McCoy FJ, Chandler RA, Magnan CG, et al. An analysis of facial fractures and their complications. Plast Reconstr Surg 1962;29:381–90.
21. Kulwin DR, Leadbetter MG. Orbital rim trauma causing a blowout fracture. Plast Reconstr Surg 1984;74:969–74.
22. Phalen JJ, Baumel JJ, Kaplan PA. Orbital floor fractures: a reassessment of pathogenesis. Nebr Med J 1990;5:100–3.
23. Kersten RC. Blow-out fracture of the orbital floor with entrapment caused by isolated trauma to the orbital rim. Am J Ophthalmol 1987;103:215–8.
24. Converse JM. The blowout fracture of the orbit: some common sense. In: Brockhurst RJ, editor. Controversy in ophthalmology. Philadelphia: Saunders; 1977. p. 201.
25. Converse JM, Smith B. On the treatment of blowout fractures of the orbit. Plast Reconstr Surg 1978;62:100–3.
26. Fujino T, Makino K, Converse JM. Discussion of: entrapment mechanism and ocular injury in orbital blowout fracture. Plast Reconstr Surg 1980;65:575–6.
27. He D, Blomquist PH, Ellis E. Association between ocular injuries and internal orbital fractures. J Oral Maxillofac Surg 2007;65:713–20.
28. Jabaley ME, Lerman M, Sanders HJ. Ocular injuries in orbital fractures. Plast Reconstr Surg 1975;56:410–4.
29. Cook T. Ocular and periocular injuries from orbital fractures. J Am Coll Surg 2002;195:831–4.
30. Milauskas AT, Fueger GF. Serious ocular complications associated with blowout orbital fractures of the orbit. Am J Ophthalmol 1966;62:670–3.
31. Miller G, Tenzel R. Ocular complication of midface fractures. Plast Reconstr Surg 1967;39:37–41.
32. Brown MS, Ky W, Lisman RD. Concomitant ocular injuries with orbital fractures. J Craniomaxillofac Trauma 1999;5:41–4.

33. Kreidl KO, Kim DY, Mansour SE. Prevalence of significant intraocular sequelae in blunt orbital trauma. Am J Emerg Med 2003;21:525–30.

34. Holmgren EP, Dierks EJ, Homer LD, et al. Facial computed tomography use in trauma patients who require a head computed tomogram. J Oral Maxillofac Surg 2004;62:913–8.

35. Rehm CG, Ross SE. Diagnosis of unsuspected facial fractures on routine head computerized tomographic scans in the unconscious multiply injured patient. J Oral Maxillofac Surg 1995;53:522–4.

36. Ellis E, Scott K. Assessment of patients with facial fractures. Emerg Med Clin North Am 2000;18:411–48.

37. Bite U, Jackson IT, Forbes GS, et al. Orbital volume measurements in enophthalmos using three-dimensional CT imaging. Plast Reconstr Surg 1985;75:502–7.

38. Manson PN, Clifford CM, Su CT, et al. Mechanisms of global support and post-traumatic enophthalmos: I. The anatomy of the ligament sling and its relation intramuscular cone orbital fat. Plast Reconstr Surg 1986;77:193–202.

39. Manson PN, Grivas A, Rosenbaum A, et al. Studies on enophthalmos: II. The measurement of orbital injuries and their treatment by quantitative computed tomography. Plast Reconstr Surg 1986;77:203–14.

40. Dulley B, Fells P. Long-term follow up of orbital blowout fracture with or without surgery. Mod Probl Ophthalmol 1975;19:467–70.

41. Osguthorpe JD. Orbital wall fractures: evaluation and management. Otolaryngol Head Neck Surg 1991;105:702–7.

42. Koo L, Hatton MP, Rubin PA. When is enophthalmos "significant"? Ophthal Plast Reconstr Surg 2006;22:274–7.

43. Whitehouse RW, Batterbury M, Jackson A, et al. Prediction of enophthalmos by computed tomography after 'blow out' orbital fractures. Br J Ophthalmol 1994;78:618–20.

44. Schuknecht B, Carls F, Valavanis A, et al. CT assessment of orbital volume in late post-traumatic enophthalmos. Neuroradiology 1996;38:470–5.

45. Yab K, Tajima S, Ohba S. Displacements of eyeball in orbital blowout fractures. Plast Reconstr Surg 1997;100:1409–17.

46. Raskin EM, Millman AL, Lubkin V, et al. Prediction of late enophthalmos by volumetric analysis of orbital fractures. Ophthal Plast Reconstr Surg 1998;14:19–26.

47. Ploder O, Klug C, Voracek M, et al. Evaluation of computer-based area and volume measurement from coronary computed tomography scans in isolated blowout fractures of the orbital floor. J Oral Maxillofac Surg 2002;60:1267–72.

48. Kolk A, Pautke C, Schott V, et al. Secondary post-traumatic enophthalmos: high-resolution magnetic resonance imaging compared with multislice computed tomography in postoperative orbital volume measurement. J Oral Maxillofac Surg 2007;65:1926–34.

49. Ahn HB, Ryu WY, Yoo KW, et al. Prediction of enophthalmos by computer-based volume measurement of orbital fractures in a Korean population. Ophthal Plast Reconstr Surg 2008;24:36–9.

50. Burm JS, Chung CH, Oh SJ. Pure orbital blowout fracture: new concepts and importance of medial orbital blowout fracture. Plast Reconstr Surg 1999;103:1839–49.

51. Fan X, Li J, Zhu J, et al. Computer-assisted orbital volume measurement in the surgical correction of late enophthalmos caused by blowout fractures. Ophthal Plast Reconstr Surg 2003;19:207–11.

52. Ellis E, Kittidumkerng W. Analysis of treatment for isolated zygomaticomaxillary complex fractures. J Oral Maxillofac Surg 1996;54:386–400.

53. Putterman AM, Stevens T, Urist MJ. Nonsurgical management of blow-out fractures of the orbital floor. Am J Ophthalmol 1974;77:232–9.

54. Converse JM, Smith B, Obear MF, et al. Orbital blowout fractures: a ten-year survey. Plast Reconstr Surg 1967;39:20–36.

55. Hawes MJ, Dortzbach RK. Surgery on orbital floor fractures. Influence of time or repair and fracture size. Ophthalmology 1983;90:1066–70.

56. Egbert JE, May K, Kersten RC, et al. Pediatric orbital floor fracture: direct extraocular muscle involvement. Ophthalmology 2000;107:1875–9.

57. Brady SM, McMann MA, Mazzoli RA, et al. The diagnosis and management of orbital blowout fractures: update 2001. Am J Emerg Med 2001;19:147–54.

58. Burnstine MA. Clinical recommendations for repair of isolated orbital floor fractures. Ophthalmology 2002;109:1207–10.

59. Hosal BM, Beatty RL. Diplopia and enophthalmos after surgical repair of blowout fracture. Orbit 2002;21:27–33.

60. Dal Canto AJ, Linberg JV. Comparison of orbital fracture repair performed within 14 days versus 15 to 29 days after trauma. Ophthal Plast Reconstr Surg 2008;24:437–43.

61. Simon GJ, Syed HM, McCann JD, et al. Early versus late repair of orbital blowout fractures. Ophthalmic Surg Lasers Imaging 2009;40:141–8.

62. Amrith S, Almousa R, Wong WL, et al. Blowout fractures: surgical outcome in relation to age, time of intervention, and other preoperative risk factors. Craniomaxillofac Trauma Reconstr 2010;3:131–6.

63. Soll DB, Poley BJ. Trapdoor variety of blowout fracture of the orbital floor. Am J Ophthalmol 1965;60:269–72.

64. de Man K, Wijngaarde R, Hes J, et al. Influence of age on the management of blow-out fractures of the orbital floor. Int J Oral Maxillofac Surg 1991;20:330.

65. Jordan DR, Allen LH, White J, et al. Intervention within days for some orbital floor fractures: the white-eyed blowout. Ophthal Plast Reconstr Surg 1998;14:379–90.

66. Wachler BS, Holds JB. The missing muscle syndrome in blowout fractures: an indication for urgent surgery. Ophthal Plast Reconstr Surg 1998;14:17–22.

67. Cohen SM, Garrett CG. Pediatric orbital floor fractures: nausea/vomiting as signs of entrapment. Otolaryngol Head Neck Surg 2003;129:43–7.

68. Flood TR, McManners J, El Attar A, et al. Randomized prospective study on the influence of steroids on postoperative eye opening after exploration of the orbital floor. Br J Oral Maxillofac Surg 1999;37:312–5.

69. Linberg JV. Orbital emphysema complicated by acute central retinal artery occlusion: case report and treatment. Ann Ophthalmol 1982;14:747–9.

70. Seiff SR. Atmospheric pressure changes and the orbit. Recommendations for patients after orbital trauma or surgery. Ophthal Plast Reconstr Surg 2002;18:239–41.

71. Harmer SG, Ethunandan M, Zaki GA, et al. Sudden transient complete loss of vision caused by nose blowing after a fracture of the orbital floor. Br J Oral Maxillofac Surg 2007;45:154–5.

72. Singh M, Phua VM, Sundar G. Sight-threatening orbital emphysema treated with needle decompression. Clin Experiment Ophthalmol 2007;35:386–7.

73. Furlani BA, Diniz B, Bitelli LG, et al. Envisema orbitario compressivo apos asseio nasal: relato de caso. Arq Bras Oftalmol 2009;72:251–3.

74. Peters N, Holtmannspotter, Buttner U. Valsalva maneuver-induced recurrent transient bilateral visual loss. Clin Neurol Neurosurg 2011;113:150–2.

75. Converse JM, Smith B. Blowout fracture of the floor of the orbit. Trans Am Acad Ophthalmol Otolaryngol 1960;64:676–81.

76. Walter WL. Early surgical repair of blowout fracture of the orbital floor by using the transantral approach. South Med J 1972;65:1229–33.

77. Saunders CJ, Whetzel TP, Stokes RB, et al. Transantral endoscopic orbital floor exploration: a cadaver and clinical study. Plast Reconstr Surg 1997;100:575–80.

78. Mohammad JA, Warnke PH, Shenaq SM. Endoscopic exploration of the orbital floor: a technique for transantral grafting of floor blowout fractures. J Craniomaxillofac Trauma 1998;4:16–22.

79. Forrest CR. Application of endoscope-assisted minimal access techniques in orbitozygomatic complex, orbital floor, and frontal sinus fractures. J Craniomaxillofac Trauma 1999;5:7–13.

80. Chen CT, Chen YR, Tung TC, et al. Endoscopically assisted reconstruction of orbital medial wall fractures. Plast Reconstr Surg 1999;103:714–8.

81. Chen CT, Chen YR. Endoscopically assisted repair of orbital floor fractures. Plast Reconstr Surg 2001;108:2011–9.

82. Chen CT, Chen YR. Application of endoscope in orbital fractures. Semin Plast Surg 2002;16:241–7.

83. Han K, Choi JH, Choi TH, et al. Comparison of endoscopic endonasal reduction and transcaruncular reduction for the treatment of medial orbital wall fractures. Ann Plast Surg 2009;62:258–64.

84. Ducic Y, Verret DJ. Endoscopic transantral repair of orbital floor fractures. Otolaryngol Head Neck Surg 2009;140:849–54.

85. Cheong EC, Chen CT, Chen YR. Broad application of the endoscope for orbital floor reconstruction: long-term follow-up results. Plast Reconstr Surg 2010;125:969–78.

86. Kontio R, Suuronen R, Salonen O, et al. Effectiveness of operative treatment of internal orbital wall fracture with polydioxanone implant. Int J Oral Maxillofac Surg 2001;30:278–85.

87. Baumann A, Burggasser G, Gaus N, et al. Orbital floor reconstruction with an alloplastic resorbable polydioxanone sheet. Int J Oral Maxillofac Surg 2002;31:367–73.

88. Kontio R, Suuronen R, Konttinen YT, et al. Orbital floor reconstruction with poly-L/D-lactide implants: clinical, radiological and immunohistochemical study in sheep. Int J Oral Maxillofac Surg 2004;33:361–8.

89. Sleep TJ, Evans BT, Webb AA. Resolution of diplopia after repair of the deep orbit. Br J Oral Maxillofac Surg 2007;45:190–6.

90. Wood BJ, Mirvis SE, Shanmuganathan K. Tension pneumocephalus and tension orbital emphysema following blunt trauma. Ann Emerg Med 1996;28:446–9.

91. Dickinson J. Transient monocular amaurosis at high altitude. High Alt Med Biol 2001;2:75–9.

92. Shiramizu KM, Okada AA, Hirakata A. Transient amaurosis associated with intraocular gas during ascending high-speed train travel. Retina 2001;21:528–9.

93. Polk JD, Rugaber C, Kohn G, et al. Central retinal artery occlusion by proxy: a cause of sudden blindness in an airline passenger. Aviat Space Environ Med 2002;73:385–7.

94. Butler FK. Diving and hyperbaric ophthalmology. Surv Ophthalmol 1995;39:347–66.

95. Senn P, Helfenstein U, Senn ML, et al. Oculare druckbelastung und barotrauma. Studie an 15 Sporttauchern. Klin Monbl Augenheikd 2001;218:232–6 [in German].

96. Bolger WE, Parsons DS, Matson RE. Functional endoscopic sinus surgery in aviators with recurrent sinus barotrauma. Aviat Space Environ Med 1990;61:148–59.

Late Correction of Orbital Deformities

Celso F. Palmieri Jr, DDS*, G.E. Ghali, DDS, MD

KEYWORDS

- Blow-out • Orbital surgery • Orbital reconstruction • Fracture of orbit • Bone graft

KEY POINTS

- The treatment of orbital fractures includes repairing the bone anatomy, correcting functional disturbances, and restoring the cosmetics of the face.
- Any delay of the treatment of orbital fractures will have an impact on the final result; for that reason, the diagnosis, timing, and treatment plan are critical to obtain an optimal result.
- Late orbital reconstruction is sometimes necessary for inadequate primary reconstruction or for severe injuries with adequate primary reconstruction.
- There are different materials available for orbital reconstruction, and there is no consensus about which is best.
- Early surgical intervention may improve the ultimate outcome, but identifying patients at risk of late complications is often difficult.

Orbital fractures are some of the most challenging injuries the oral surgeon deals with on a daily basis. As part of the most prominent bone of the face, even small defects, asymmetries, or deviations may be noticed by the patients.

Delaying the treatment of the orbital fractures may have a huge impact on the final result, making the diagnosis, timing, and treatment plan critical to obtaining an optimal result.

Most orbital fractures are caused by assault or motor vehicle accidents.[1] Isolated orbital fractures account for 4% to 16% of all facial fractures. If zygomatic complex (ZMC) and naso-orbito-ethmoid fractures are included, then this accounts for 30% to 55% of all facial fractures.[2]

The most common ophthalmic complications in midfacial reconstruction are diplopia, enophthalmos, and, on rare occasions, blindness. Binocular diplopia is by far the most common complication in midfacial trauma involving the orbit. This finding may be temporary or permanent if not treated.

Rehabilitation of patients requires an understanding of the alteration in form and function of the orbit, including the intraorbital and intraocular tissues, and the materials and methods available for repair.[3]

Late orbital reconstruction is sometimes necessary for inadequate primary reconstruction, for severe injuries with adequate primary reconstruction, or for orbital injuries that were missed or for which no medical evaluation was sought. Healing and wound contraction make the identification and mobilization of orbital structures difficult in secondary reconstructions. As a result, secondary orbital reconstruction can be technically demanding, require more extensive soft tissue dissection, and often produce compromised results. The types of deformities that can present secondarily include cosmetic ones, such as enophthalmos, hypo-opthalmos, telecanthus, contour abnormalities, and eyelid deformities. Functional deformities, including restricted ocular motility and diplopia, may also occur.[4]

The authors have nothing to disclose.
Department of Oral and Maxillofacial Surgery, Louisiana State University Health Sciences Center at Shreveport, 1501 Kings Highway, Shreveport, LA 71103, USA
* Corresponding author.
E-mail address: cpalmi@lsuhsc.edu

Oral Maxillofacial Surg Clin N Am 24 (2012) 649–663
http://dx.doi.org/10.1016/j.coms.2012.08.002
1042-3699/12/$ – see front matter © 2012 Published by Elsevier Inc.

Incorrectly restored orbital fractures can result in unpleasant and handicapping functional and cosmetic results. The final goal of all orbital fracture repairs must be the primary restoration of the preoperative bony orbital volume and shape.[5]

ORBITAL ANATOMY

The orbit is the bony vault that houses and protects the eyeball (or globe). It is a quadrangular-based pyramid that has its peak at the orbital apex. The average adult orbit has a volume of 30 mL, and the globe averages 7 mL. By 5 years of age, orbital growth is 85% complete, and it is finalized between 7 years of age and puberty.[2]

Seven bones contribute to the formation of the orbit: maxillary, zygomatic, frontal, ethmoidal, lacrimal, palatine, and sphenoid.

The orbital rim is comprised of dense cortical bone that protects the orbital contents and globe from direct blunt trauma. The orbital walls vary considerably in their thickness. The superior lateral and inferior rim tend to be rather thick, whereas the bones just posterior to these and the medial rim are usually fairly thin (<1 mm). The orbital floor and medial wall are most frequently fractured owing to their thinness and lack of support.

The orbital roof consists mainly of the frontal bone, with the anterior cranial fossa superior to it. The lesser wing of the sphenoid has a minor contribution posteriorly. The superior orbital rim is generally rather thick and then rapidly becomes quite thin (<1 mm) posterior from the edge. In elderly patients, the orbital roof may be resorbed in selected areas, allowing the dura to become confluent with the periorbita. Anterolaterally, there is a smooth broad fossa that houses the lacrimal gland.

The orbital floor is bordered laterally by the inferior orbital fissure, and there is no distinct border medially. It is formed primarily by the orbital process of the maxilla, anterolaterally by a portion of the zygomatic bone, and posteriorly by a small portion of the palatine bone. The maxillary sinuses are present at birth and reach the orbital floor and the infraorbital canal by 2 years of age. The inferior orbital fissure gives rise to the infraorbital groove from its midportion, which is about 2.5 to 3.0 cm from the infraorbital rim. The infraorbital fissure converts to a canal halfway forward, carrying the infraorbital nerve and vessels and opening approximately 5 mm below the rim of the maxilla at the infraorbital foramen. The orbital floor can be as thin as 0.5 mm, with its weakest portion just medial to the infraorbital groove and canal. This dimension explains the phenomenon that most blunt traumas resulting in orbital floor blow-out fractures are manifested primarily with injury and sagging of the medial orbital floor contents into the underlying maxillary sinus.

The lateral wall of the orbit is formed mainly by the greater wing of the sphenoid and portions of the zygoma. Although this tends to be the strongest wall, it is fairly commonly fractured along the frontozygomatic junction, extending slightly posteriorly, and then running vertically along the thinnest portion of the suture line where the greater wing of the sphenoid and zygoma meet. The lateral orbital walls, if they were to be extended posteriorly, would form a 90° angle to each other. Each lateral orbital wall forms a 45° angle at the orbital apex with its medial wall counterpart.

The superior orbital fissure separates the greater and the lesser wings of the sphenoid and serves as the delineation between the orbital roof and the lateral wall.

The medial wall of the orbit is by far the most complex and potentially problematic to manage in severe trauma. The medial orbital wall is comprised anteroposteriorly by a portion of the maxillary, lacrimal, ethmoid, and sphenoid bones. Most of the medial wall is formed by the extremely thin (0.2–0.4 mm) lamina papyracea of the ethmoid bone. The anterior ethmoidal foramen is 20 to 25 mm behind the medial orbital rim, and the posterior ethmoidal foramen is 12 mm beyond this. The foramina can be found approximately two-thirds of the way up the medial orbital wall, within the frontoethmoidal suture line, and serves as an important surgical landmark identifying the level of the corresponding cribriform plate.

The anterior boundary of the orbit is defined by the orbital septum. The upper and lower eyelids are anatomically similar in their composition, with corresponding layers anteriorly to posteriorly. The orbicularis oculi has 2 distinct layers: the outer superficial fibers (orbital portion) and the deeper fibers (palpebral portion). The upper and lower lids should form a 30 to 40° angle at the lateral canthus, which is situated 1 cm below the frontozygomatic suture. Typically, the lateral canthus is situated 2 to 4 mm above the medial canthus.

The orbital septum is just posterior to the orbicularis oculi. The orbital septum is continuous with the orbital periosteum and the periosteum of the facial bones overlying the rim. The distal edges of the orbital septum insert into the superior edge of the tarsal plates. The orbital septum prevents the preaponeurotic orbital fat from herniating out into the eyelids. Superiorly, there is a central and medial fat pad; and there are 3 distinct fat pads inferiorly (medial, central, and lateral).

The tarsal plate is formed by dense fibrous connective tissue and is primarily responsible for the convex form of each of the lids. The tarsal border parallels the free margin of the eyelid. The horizontal length of each tarsus is approximately 30 mm. The height of the upper tarsus is 10 mm, and it is 4 mm in the lower lid.

The palpebral portion of the orbicularis oculi has dense intertwined insertions that envelop the lacrimal sac. The lacrimal sac is 1 cm in length and 5 mm in diameter. Inferiorly, the sac drains into the nasolacrimal duct, which has a 12-mm intrabony canal coursing inferiorly and posteriorly that opens into the inferior meatus of the nasal cavity below the inferior concha. This opening is 30 to 35 mm from the edge of the external nares.

THE DEEP ORBIT

Dissection deep within the orbit is a concern for surgeons because of the risks of injuring critical structures, including the contents of the superior orbital fissure and the optic nerve. Dissection in the posterior orbit may have to be compromised rather than placing these structures at risk, even though the traumatic defects will be inadequately treated.[6]

The anatomic landmarks of the deep orbit are both hard and soft tissue structures: the infraorbital nerve, the inferior orbital fissure, the greater wing of the sphenoid, and the orbital plate of the palatine bone.

THE INFRAORBITAL NERVE

The infraorbital nerve is a particularly useful landmark in high-energy injuries and in old injuries in which the orbital periosteum and, therefore, the subperiosteal plane of dissection may not be identifiable with certainty. It provides the surgeon with an excellent guide both to the depth of dissection and the direction along the floor of the orbit.[6]

THE INFERIOR ORBITAL FISSURE

The contents of the inferior orbital fissure can be safely divided because there are no critical neurovascular structures that pass from the infratemporal fossa or pterygopalatine fossa into the orbit through the fissure. If the infraorbital nerve has not already been identified in the floor of the orbit, care must be taken as the dissection is developed further medially along the fissure because the infraorbital nerve becomes more superficial in the posterior orbit. Sectioning the contents of the inferior orbital fissure allows the surgeon to develop the dissection safely in both the lateral orbit to the orbital plate of the greater wing of the sphenoid and along the orbital floor. If the dissection is continued medially above the infraorbital nerve,

the landmark of the orbital plate of the palatine bone is immediately apparent.[6]

GREATER WING OF THE SPHENOID

The orbital plate of the greater wing of the sphenoid, together with the orbital surface of the zygoma, make up the lateral wall of the orbit. It provides the surgeon with a constant and reliable landmark in the lateral orbit. The lateral wall is the strongest wall of the orbit.[6]

THE ORBITAL PLATE OF THE PALATINE BONE

This structure is a constant landmark in the deep orbit and lies medial to the junction of the infraorbital nerve and the inferior orbital fissure at the posteromedial aspect of the orbital floor. The orbital plate of the palatine bone is a relatively strong structure and provides the surgeon with a constant and reliable landmark in the medial floor. In cases of severe disruption of the orbital floor, this may be the only remaining intact bone of the floor and the landmark that will permit correct orientation and positioning of the reconstruction in this critical area of the orbit. Reconstruction of the floor of the orbit does not need to extend beyond this.[6]

The advantage of the 4 surgical landmarks of the deep orbit is that they are all present in virtually every case of nonpenetrating orbital injury, particularly in cases of high-energy injuries of the orbit. These landmarks are based on the relation between structures rather than absolute distances.

DIAGNOSIS AND INDICATIONS FOR SURGERY

Orbital fractures can occur in numerous patterns. They are often described by their location and the size of the defect. Three patterns of orbital fractures have been described: linear, blow-out, and complex. Linear fractures do not result in a defect, but they can result in an enlargement of the orbit. Blow-out fractures are the most commonly occurring injury and are limited to one wall with a defect of less than 2 cm in diameter, and they most commonly occur in the middle part of the floor. Complex fractures consist of extensive fractures that affect 2 or more orbital walls. They are usually associated with fractures of the facial skeleton (Le Fort II and III fractures).[4]

A systematic approach assessing both orbits will further define functional and anatomic defects associated with orbital injuries. The initial ophthalmologic evaluation should include periorbital examination, visual acuity, ocular motility, pupillary responses, visual fields, and fundoscopic examination. The eyelids and periorbital area should be inspected for edema, ecchymosis, lacerations, ptosis, asymmetric lid drape, and canthal tendon disruption. When traumatic forces have produced lid ecchymosis, there should be heightened awareness of the possibility of an occult ocular injury or an orbital wall fracture.

Extraocular movements are evaluated to rule out mechanical entrapment or paresis. Any diplopia and the field of gaze in which it occurs should be noted. Mild (<5°) restriction in extreme fields of gaze is common in the face of severe orbital edema. Pupillary size, shape, and symmetry should be evaluated, as well as light reactivity. The globe should also be evaluated for acute enophthalmos or proptosis, which can be ascertained by viewing directly from above or below. The vertical position of the globe should be also noted.

The bony orbital rim should be palpated for evidence of a bony step, bony crepitus, or mobility.

IMAGING TECHNIQUES

Noncontrasted computed tomography (CT) scan is the primary imaging modality currently used for evaluating injuries related to orbital trauma. Standard radiographs are inadequate in evaluating internal orbital fractures and soft tissues.[4,6]

The standard imaging approach for facial trauma is to obtain direct (not reformatted) 3 mm sections in the axial and coronal planes without IV contrast. Computer-generated three-dimensional CT images and sagittal plane cuts may provide additional information in more severe cases thus helping the treatment plan and reconstruction (**Figs. 1–4**).

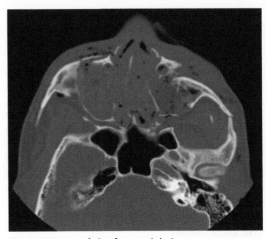

Fig. 2. CT scan of the face: axial view.

Despite the accuracy of modern imaging, the size of the defect on CT is often smaller than the size of the defect identified at the time of operation.[7]

Magnetic resonance imaging (MRI) has limited uses in orbital trauma and is less sensitive than CT in depicting fractures. MRI is useful for assessing soft tissue involvement, such as incarceration of extraocular muscles or orbital fat.[4]

Forrest and colleagues[8] reported the use of the ultrasound in the diagnosis of orbital fracture as a safe, inexpensive, noninvasive, portable, and readily available device that has been well documented in the diagnosis of orbital pathologic conditions. The advantages are decreased cost, portability, less patient positioning, less time required, and absence of radiation. The disadvantages are contraindication in suspected penetrating injuries, difficult examination in periorbital soft tissue injuries, significant learning curve (eye-hand coordination), no standard cross

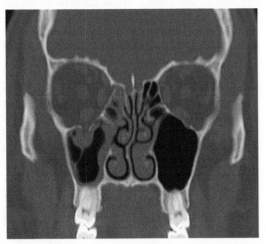

Fig. 1. CT scan of the face: coronal view.

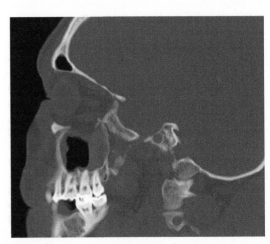

Fig. 3. CT scan of the face: sagittal view.

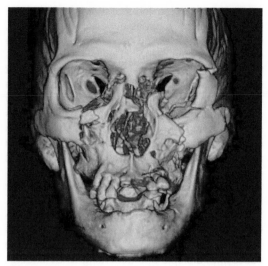

Fig. 4. CT scan of the face: 3-dimensional reconstruction.

section is available for easy reference, and it is uncertain whether ultrasound can adequately diagnose posterior defects (greater than 4 cm posterior to the orbital rim) or the presence of associated facial fractures.[8]

INDICATIONS FOR SURGERY

Several factors need to be considered in determining whether surgical intervention is indicated in patients with an orbital fracture. A careful history and a thorough physical examination are integral components in making decisions regarding the subsequent management of these patients.

OCULAR MOTILITY

Lack of ocular motility is an important consideration. Motility limitation can be graded on a scale from 0 to 4, whereby 0 equals no limitation (normal) and 4 equals no movement in the field of gaze. The most commonly accepted cause for limited motility is entrapment of the extraocular muscles (inferior rectus muscle) or their fascia into a gap in the orbital floor (**Fig. 5**).[3]

The herniation of orbital contents into the maxillary antrum can cause restriction of the affected globe in primary upward and lateral gaze resulting in diplopia in that quadrant. When the medial wall is ruptured, restriction in lateral gaze can result.[1]

De Man and coworkers[9] have suggested that young patients with severely restricted eyeball motility, an unequivocally positive forced duction test, and CT findings indicating a blow-out fracture of the orbital floor should undergo operative treatment as soon as possible after injury, whereas a

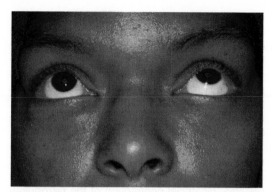

Fig. 5. Entrapment of the right extraocular muscle (inferior rectus muscle).

wait-and-see policy, keeping patients under observation, seems to be appropriate for blow-out fractures in adults.[9]

DIPLOPIA

Usually a consequence of muscle entrapment, diplopia or double vision can also result from muscle edema, hemorrhage in the orbital cavity, motor nerve palsy, and dystopia. It usually takes 7 to 10 days for the initial edema or bleeding, or both, to disappear and resorb. It is, therefore, difficult to ascertain during that period whether the diplopia noted is of a transitory nature.[1]

ENOPHTHALMOS

The underlying cause of enophthalmos is a discrepancy between the volume of the orbital soft tissues and the bony orbital cavity.[10] Enophthalmos greater than 2.0 mm typically indicates the need for surgical repair; however, factors such as globe tethering by entrapment, fat necrosis, and posterior soft tissue necrosis also may lead to enophthalmos (**Fig. 6**).

The ability to recognize enophthalmos is crucial for the surgeon. Ahn and coworkers[10] published a study related to orbital volume change and late

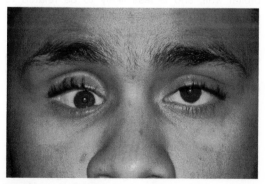

Fig. 6. Enophthalmos.

enophthalmos assessed by CT scanning. There seems to be a direct relationship between the increase of orbital volume and measured enophthalmos. In cases with an orbital volume increase of less than 1 mL, the extent of enophthalmos is around 0.9 mm, whereas the enophthalmos is 2.3 mm at a volume of 2.3 mL. For every 1-mL increase of volume, there is approximately a 0.9-mm increase in enophtalmos.[10]

Lew and colleagues[1] report that posttraumatic enophthalmos is a result of atrophy of orbital fat, enlargement of the bony orbit, dislocation of the trochlea, cicatricial contraction of the retrobulbar tissues, unrepaired fracture of the orbital wall, and displacement of the orbital tissue.

It is important to understand the relationship of the globe to the orbit, global axis, orbital volume, and osseous structures. The analogy is that the globe is a ball suspended in a box filled with foam and open anteriorly. The ball has a central axis; and if one were to add foam behind the axis, the globe or ball would move forward, whereas if foam were added in front of the axis, the ball would neither move backward nor forward but superiorly. Foam removed from the front of the axis would allow the ball to drop inferiorly.

This axis of the globe extends from the lateral orbital rim to the anterior portion of the lacrimal bone. Most of the fat along the orbital floor is extracoronal and is anterior to this and seldom causes enophthalmos. However, most of the lateral orbital wall is behind this axis; therefore, displacement of this osseous segment will increase the orbital volume in an exponential fashion, creating excessive volume expansion within the orbit and resultant enophthalmos. Comminuted fractures of the lamina papyracea on the posterior floor also lie behind the global axis. Intracoronal fat is found primarily behind the axis and its loss is also critical to the creation of enophtalmos.[1]

The cause of enophthalmos is the result of an increase in bony orbital volume by displacement of the medial orbital wall, posterior floor, or lateral orbital wall, and is less likely to be related to defects in the inferior orbital floor. Treatment should be focused on these 3 areas and, secondarily, the anterior orbital floor. Anterior orbital floor reconstruction should be limited to changes in the vertical relationship of the globe and not to the correction of the anterior/posterior problems.

TIMING OF ORBITAL FRACTURE SURGERY

Adequate surgical timing is of paramount importance in resolving clinical impairment, and it should be individualized according to patient age, fracture type, and clinical and radiographic findings.[11]

It has been suggested that there is an increase in complications, such as adhesions and fibrosis, with late or delayed surgery, which can lead to unsatisfactory outcomes. However, orbital fractures differ from all other facial fractures in that surgery does not typically attempt to achieve bone healing. The goal of surgery is simply to restore the preinjured form of the orbital walls. As such, delaying the operation for varying periods is often recommended. This delay is beneficial in allowing the orbital swelling to resolve, facilitating accurate diagnosis, and strengthening the indications for surgery. Rarely can orbital fracture repair be considered urgent.[3,12]

In 2002, Burnstine[13] presented a literature review regarding orbital floor fractures and recommended surgery within 2 weeks after trauma in cases with diplopia and according to CT findings of orbital fracture or orbital tissue entrapment.

Matteini and colleagues[11] studied 108 consecutive orbital fractures, and the timing of surgical treatment ranged between 1 hour and 12 days, with an average of 4 days. They suggested early treatment of floor fractures or roof fractures with diplopia as opposed to wall fractures without diplopia. Fractures with diplopia should be further differentiated according to patient age. The presence of functional impairments requires prompt surgical treatment, which should be performed within a week in adults and within a few days in children. Muscular entrapment in children needs to be corrected as soon as possible and earlier than that observed in adults so as to prevent the precocious fibrosis that can be observed in younger patients.[11] In their study, temporary persistence of diplopia was noted in 4 adult patients after surgery; in all cases, double vision spontaneously resolved within 2 weeks. All 4 cases of temporary postsurgical double vision received treatment after more than 7 days after trauma.

SECONDARY RECONSTRUCTION

Late orbital reconstruction is sometimes necessary for inadequate primary reconstructions, for severe injuries with adequate primary reconstruction, or for orbital injuries that were missed or for which no medical evaluation was sought. Healing and wound contracture make the identification and mobilization of orbital structures difficult in secondary reconstructions. As a result, secondary orbital reconstructions can be technically demanding, require more soft tissue dissection, and often produce compromised results. The types of deformities that can present secondarily include cosmetic ones, such as enophthalmos, hypo-ophthalmos, telecanthus, contour abnormalities, and eyelid deformities. Functional deformities, including restricted ocular motility and diplopia, may also occur. Late reconstruction is usually not undertaken until approximately 6 months after the primary repair to allow for adequate healing and neuromuscular recovery.[4]

After several weeks of enophthalmos, scar contracture can prevent the correction of the anteroposterior deformity. As a result, complete dissection into the posterior orbit is necessary to mobilize the soft tissues of the orbit and to locate stable bony landmarks for graft placement. Overcorrection of enophthalmos by 1 to 2 mm is often necessary to achieve the proper anteroposterior position postoperatively.

Raskin and colleagues[14] reported that enophthalmos after orbital blow-out fractures is linearly related to the volumetric expansion of the fractured orbits, with each 1 cm^3 increase in volume causing approximately 0.47 mm of enophthalmos. Based on their results, they proposed an algorithm to facilitate clinical decision making in the treatment of orbital fractures. Patients with less than 13% orbital expansion are selected for surgical management because of persistent motility deficits after a 7-day course of steroid therapy unless contraindicated. Patients with more than 13% orbital expansion are managed surgically after preoperative treatment with a 5-day course of steroids, systemic antibiotics, and decongestants.[14]

The timing for orbital fracture repair is controversial. The decision regarding surgical intervention in the management of orbital fractures is influenced by a variety of factors, including the presence and severity of ocular motility restriction and enophthalmos, estimated fracture size, and the surgeon's clinical judgment. Early surgical intervention may improve the ultimate outcome, but identifying patients at risk of late complications is often difficult.

MATERIALS FOR RECONSTRUCTION

Several different materials are available for restoration of the orbital walls, and there is no consensus about which is preferable; however, there is a general consensus that the ideal material for orbital floor repair should be strong enough to support the orbital contents, inexpensive, readily available, easy to contour, resorbable, and (most importantly) biocompatible.[3] Specific criteria for the ideal properties of a generic biomaterial include a material that is chemically inert, nonallergenic, and noncarcinogenic.[15] If alloplastic, it should be cost-effective and capable of sterilization without deterioration of its chemical composition. The material should be easily cut and sized in the operating room, and it should be able to be shaped to fit orbital contours and retain its new form without memory. It should allow fixation to host bone by screws, wire, suture, or adhesive. The material should be capable of removal without damage to surrounding tissues and radiopaque to allow radiograph.[16] So far, no single material has proved to be successful in meeting all of these criteria. It is the responsibility of the surgeon to understand the advantages and disadvantages of the available materials and to choose which one is the best for his or her patient.

A host of materials have been used to reconstruct the internal orbit, including autologous bone, autologous cartilage, allogeneic bone and cartilage, methyl methacrylate, silicone polymer, polyurethane, aluminum-oxide ceramic, Teflon (DuPont, Wilmington, Delaware; polytetrafluoroethylene polymer), gelatin film (Gelfoam, Pharmacia, Kalamazoo, Michigan), Supramid (S. Jackson Inc, Alexandria, Virginia), polyethylene, polyvinyl sponge, polydioxanone plates, polyglactin mesh or plates, polylactide plates, porous polyethylene, lyophilized dura, and metal sheets or mesh.[16]

Reconstruction of acute traumatic defects of the orbit may have different biomaterial requirements than defects restored later, after enophthalmos and/or hypoglobus has been established. A given biomaterial may, therefore, have properties that are ideal for the acute setting but not ideal for delayed reconstruction.[16]

There is a trend in our days that surgeons would rather like to have something off the shelf at hand for implantation and replacement of body substance than to harvest and graft an autologous tissue.[17]

Selection of the source of material has been and remains an ongoing debate. Autogenous bone remains the standard to which other materials are compared; but, in general, the material selected for orbital reconstruction is largely determined by the experience of the surgeon. Many investigators outlined the relative advantages and disadvantages of each class of material. These characteristics are based on concerns for donor-site morbidity, complication rates, availability of the material, operating room time, and stability of the material over time.[15]

AUTOGENOUS MATERIALS

The most common autogenous materials used are autogenous bone and autogenous cartilage. Autogenous materials require a second operative site, increasing patient morbidity, require increased operative time to harvest, are limited in quantity, and resorption is a concern for long-term success.

AUTOGENOUS BONE

Autogenous bone grafting has been the gold standard to provide framework for facial skeleton and orbital walls. There are 2 forms of free autogenous bone grafts: cortical and cancellous. The most common donor sites are calvarium, iliac crest, anterior wall of the maxillary sinus, and mandibular bone.[18]

The advantages of autogenous bone are its ability to form new bone (osteoinduction), its relatively good resistance to infection, its lack of host response against the graft, and its lack of concern for late extrusion. The disadvantages are donor site morbidity, variable graft resorption, and limited ability to contour some types of bone.[3,15,18]

The use of autologous bone for reconstruction of the orbital skeleton is best indicated for large, complex disruptions of the bony orbit. Resorption of graft volume is obviously a concern for the long-term success of reconstructions using autogenous bone. For this reason, the use of calvarial bone is the primary choice for autogenous bone. It has the advantage of being located in the same operative field and is mostly cortical bone (**Fig. 7**).[15]

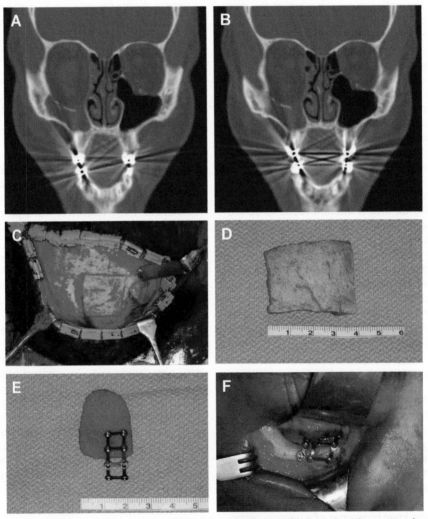

Fig. 7. (*A, B*) Coronal CT scan showing a 1-year-old right orbital floor fracture that the patient had never had treated. (*C, D*) Harvesting of the calvarial bone for reconstruction of the orbital floor. (*E, F*) The bone was prepared, shaped, and fixed to the inferior orbital rim with a 1.5-mm titanium miniplate. (*G, H*) Postoperative coronal CT scan showing the reconstruction of the orbital floor with the calvarial bone. (*I*) Preoperative photograph. (*J*) Six-week postoperative photograph.

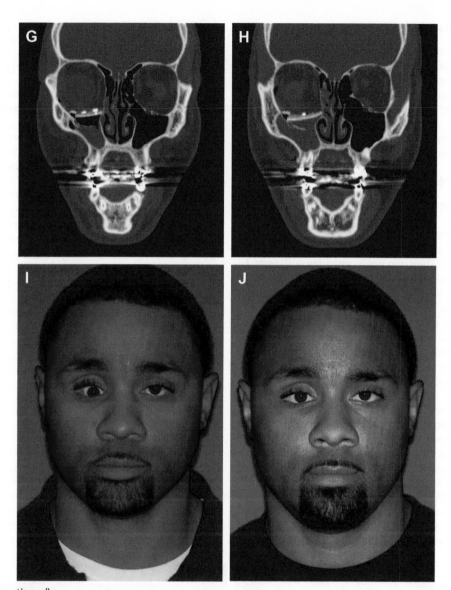

Fig. 7. (*continued*)

AUTOGENOUS CARTILAGE

Proponents of autogenous cartilage tout its ease of harvest, flexibility, and limited donor site morbidity as its main advantages.

The main sources of autogenous cartilages for orbital reconstruction are the cartilaginous nasal septum and conchal cartilage. In general, both of these require contouring for accurate reconstruction of the internal orbit, which is problematic because cartilage possesses inherent memory and a tendency to return to its previous shape. Progressive changes in the shape of the graft can alter support and volume within the orbit, causing increased likelihood of late complications.

ALLOGENEIC MATERIALS

Allogeneic materials (allografts, homografts, and xenografts) contain no living cells but, depending on the material, may possess osteoinductive and/or osteoconductive properties.

The use of allogeneic materials is marked by concern for antigenicity of the material and transmission of infectious disease. Both xenograft and allogeneic materials are processed by various methods to reduce antigenicity.

The most common allogeneic materials used for orbital floor reconstruction are lyophilized dura, homologous bone, homologous cartilage, and xenografts.[15]

ALLOPLASTIC MATERIALS

Alloplasts have been gaining popularity for reconstruction of the internal orbit because of their ease of use and elimination of donor-site morbidity. Other benefits of alloplasts include shorter operation times, the large variety of sizes and shapes available, and their seemingly endless supply. The alloplasts can be classified into those that are nonresorbable and those that are resorbable.[3]

TITANIUM

These materials are thin, easy to contour, easily stabilized, maintain their shape, and have the unique ability to compensate for volume when properly contoured without the potential for resorption. They can easily span large defects to provide rigid support, are visible on radiographs, and are sterilizable. Titanium has the further advantage of producing fewer artifacts on CT than other metals.[15]

In 2003, Ellis and Tan[19] compared the use of cranial bone versus titanium mesh for reconstruction of blowout fractures. Titanium mesh was found to more accurately reconstruct the orbital defects, especially in the posterior regions of the orbit.[19] The reason that titanium mesh provided more optimal reconstructions may be because of the ease with which titanium mesh can be contoured to adapt to the intricate contours of the internal orbit. Cranial bone is very brittle and cannot be as easily contoured. The ability of titanium mesh to conform to the contours of the orbit made it a more ideal material for reconstructing those defects that involved both the floor and medial wall. For isolated floor fractures, titanium mesh

reconstructions also proved to be better than those reconstructed with cranial bone (**Figs. 8** and **9**).[19]

HIGH-DENSITY POROUS POLYETHYLENE

Commercially available as Medpor (Porex Surgical, College Park, GA), it is a versatile material used as a substitute for both bone and cartilage as an alternative to silicone for facial reconstruction. It is insoluble in tissue fluids, does not resorb or degenerate, incites minimal surrounding soft tissue reaction, and possesses high tensile strength. The material is easy to shape, is strong yet somewhat flexible, is highly stable, and permits tissue ingrowth into its pores.[16] Its main disadvantage for reconstruction of the internal orbit is that it is not radiodense, so its position cannot be easily visualized on immediate postoperative CT scans.[15]

Other alloplastic materials are used for orbit reconstruction, but the indication is a lot more restricted. These materials include hydroxyapatite, silicones (Silastic; Dow Corning, Midland, MI), polytetrafluoroethylene (Teflon), polylactide (Lactosorb; Walter Lorenz Surgical, Inc, Jacksonville, FL), polyglactin (Vicryl), polydioxanone plates (PDS), and gelatin film (**Fig. 10**).

SECONDARY RECONSTRUCTION OF INTERNAL ORBIT

When treating an established enophthalmos and/or hypoglobus, one is dealing with a different problem than treating the acute injury. In the chronic case, the orbital soft tissues are in an abnormal configuration. Instead of being the shape of a modified pyramid, the shape of the soft tissue composite is more spherical, which means that to correct the

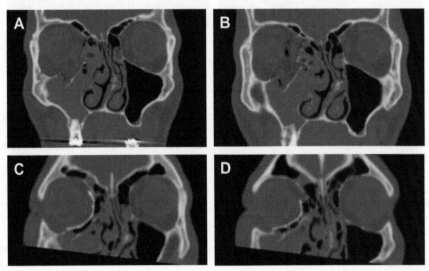

Fig. 8. (*A, B*) Coronal CT scans showing a right orbital floor fracture. (*C, D*) Postoperative coronal CT scans demonstrating excellent adaptation of the titanium orbital floor plate on the medial wall and orbital floor.

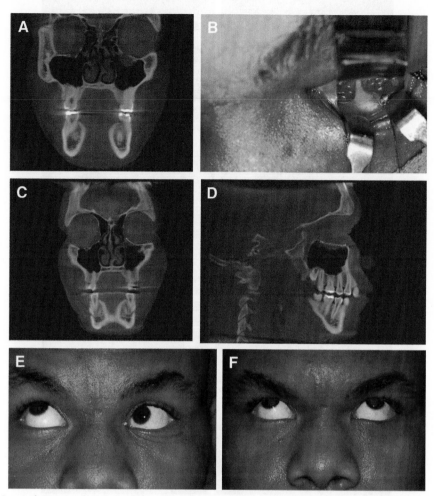

Fig. 9. (*A*) Coronal CT scan showing a left orbital floor fracture with orbital contents entrapped. (*B*) The orbital floor was repaired with titanium mesh. (*C*) Postoperative coronal CT scan showing the mesh adaptation and contour to the medial wall and orbital floor. (*D*) Postoperative sagittal CT scan showing the adaptation of the plate on the posterior ledge. (*E*) Preoperative photograph showing muscular entrapment at the left eye; the patient was complaining of diplopia on the superior field of gaze. (*F*) Six-week postoperative photograph; entrapment was corrected and the patient had no further complaints.

abnormal globe position, one must change the shape of the orbital soft tissue composite from spherical to pyramidal. Unfortunately, simply reestablishing the normal contours and volume of the internal orbit may not completely correct established enophthalmos. To do this, one must decrease the volume available of the orbital soft tissues in the posterior orbit, forcing the globe anteriorly. To decrease the volume of the posterior orbit, the desirable physical properties for a material include the following:

1. Nonresorbable
2. Can occupy different amounts of volume within the orbit (different thicknesses, shapes, and so forth)
3. Easy to position and stabilize

The best material for secondary reconstruction of internal orbit defects or the correction of enophthalmos/hypoglobus is high-density porous polyethylene (Porex Surgical Inc, College Park, GA). The main advantage for using this material as a secondary reconstruction is that it is volumetrically stable and does not resorb. The material is strong yet flexible and easy to contour and shape using scissors or a scalpel, and it can be molded into the desired shape. Despite its ability to be curved, it has surprisingly little memory. It comes in several different thicknesses, including 0.85-, 1.5-, and 3-mm sheets.[16]

The main disadvantage for reconstruction of the internal orbit with porous polyethylene is that it is not radiopaque, so its position cannot be easily visualized on immediate CT scans.

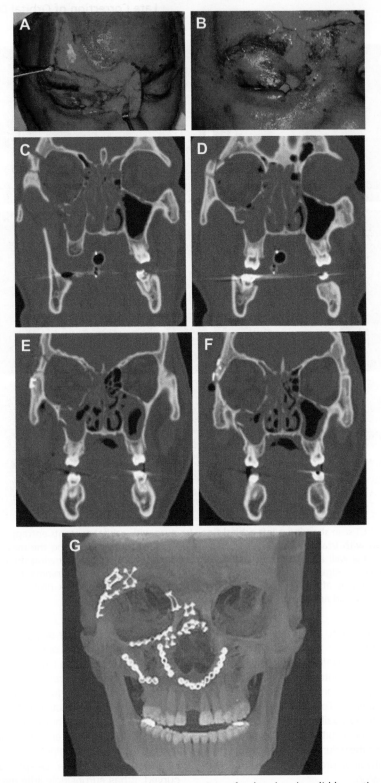

Fig. 10. (*A, B*) Preoperative photographs of a patient sustaining forehead and eyelid lacerations. (*C, D*) Preoperative coronal CT scans showing right ZMC and orbital floor fractures. (*E, F*) Postoperative coronal CT scans showing the ZMC fracture fixed; the orbital floor was left to be fixed as a second procedure. (*G*) Postoperative CT 3-dimensional reconstruction. (*H, I*) Orbital floor fracture was fixed in a second surgery using a titanium-embedded, high-density, porous, polyethylene plate to reconstruct the orbital floor. (*J, K*) Postoperative coronal CT scans showing the reconstruction of the orbital floor. (*L*) Six-week postoperative photograph after the floor reconstruction.

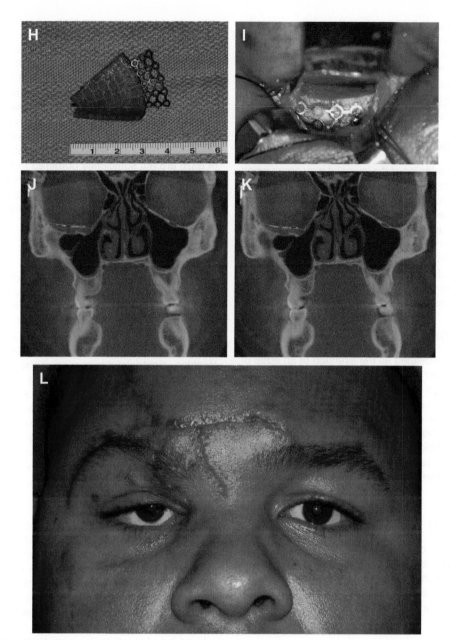

Fig. 10. (*continued*)

COMPLICATIONS

The most common complications after orbital trauma and surgery are diplopia, lid retraction, ectropion, entropion, ocular motility deficits, and enophthalmos.

Diplopia

Binocular diplopia is a common complication of the orbital fractures; it may be temporary or may become permanent if not treated. Initially, the binocular diplopia is most likely caused by edema or hematoma of one of the extraocular muscles or their nerves as well as by intraorbital edema or hematoma. Resolution of diplopia after fracture treatment usually occurs spontaneously within 5 to 7 days. Diplopia can also be caused by muscle entrapment, but this cause is usually evident on clinical examination with a forced duction test or by simple examination of extraocular movements.[4] CT scans using 2-mm coronal cuts of the orbit demonstrate entrapment of the inferior rectus muscle and can aid in differentiating between contused and entrapped extraocular muscles. A contused muscle appears round on the scan; the normal muscle appears flat. In the case of possible muscle entrapment, the results of a forced duction test provide evidence of the need to explore the orbital floor.

LID RETRACTION

Vertical shortening of the lower lid may occur when the scar contracts between the tarsal plate and the periosteum, thereby shortening the orbital septum. This complication can be prevented by providing superior support of the lower lid for several days after surgery.[4]

If retraction is appreciable in the early postoperative period, aggressive lower eyelid massage and forced eye closure exercises are instituted. This retraction resolves in most of the cases.[12]

ECTROPION

Ectropion is defined as the eversion of an edge or margin. Lower eyelid malpositions are graded mild when there is slight eversion of the cilia inferiorly with or without sclera show, moderate when the lid margin is everted with lower eyelid descent and sclera show, and severe when frank ectropion is present. Mild ectropion and moderate ectropion usually resolve over time with gentle massage of the lid. Severe ectropion may require surgical correction.[4]

ENTROPION

Entropion is defined as an inversion or turning inward of an edge. It is usually symptomatic with eye discomfort to the point of pain, tearing, photophobia, discharge, secondary infection, and various degrees of corneal surface breakdown (**Fig. 11**).

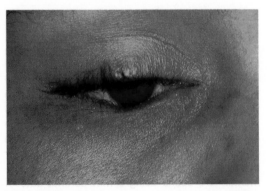

Fig. 11. Entropion.

OCULAR MOTILITY DEFICITS

Deficits in extraocular movements may be manifest as diplopia in the postoperative period. Although there is always concern regarding entrapment of these muscles, a normal forced duction test at the end of the procedure should rule this out. Frequently, periorbital swelling or muscular contusion and edema may be the underlying cause. Many patients with diplopia only at the extremes of gaze are not sufficiently bothered to seek intervention.[12] Typically, most patients complain when diplopia is in primary field or in down-gaze, which interferes with walking. The majority of these cases will resolve without intervention.

ENOPHTHALMOS

Enophthalmos is defined as recession of the globe within the orbit. It can result from an absolute reduction of orbital tissue, a relative reduction of tissue, or both. Posttraumatic enophthalmos has been attributed to atrophy of intermuscular fat, enlargement of the bony orbit, dislocation of the trochlea, cicatricial contraction of the retrobulbar tissues, unrepaired fractures of the orbital wall, and displacement of the orbital tissue.[4]

Failure to reconstruct the orbital walls results in disruption of the orbital ligaments. Such disruption causes the anterior support of the globe to be weakened and results in enophthalmos. Physical findings suggestive of enophthalmos include a deeper eyelid sulcus, eyelid position, eyelid asymmetry, or smaller eye.[1]

Blow-out fractures, either isolated or in conjunction with zygoma or rim fractures, must extend far enough behind the axis to the globe to create volumetric expansion that results in enophthalmos. This condition does occur, but the more logical diagnosis is that of medial wall fracture because this occurs completely behind the global axis and allows displacement and an increase in intraorbital volume.[1] It is essential to complete the infraorbital dissection far enough posteriorly to completely address the orbital floor injury that is posterior to the global axis. Failure to do this will result in later enophthalmos.

MISPLACED HARDWARE

The initial evaluation of postoperative orbital fractures should include a CT scan to determine implant location and to characterize intraorbital volume. Occasionally, an implant may have been unintentionally placed in a horizontal orientation into the maxillary sinus or too medial. The lack of good bony references (ledges) may lead the surgeon to an error when orienting the hardware position on the 3 planes of the space. In some cases, the existing implant may be repositioned, and the sooner one does it the better because scarring of the periorbita can impede removal and/or repositioning of the implant.

SUMMARY

Orbital fractures are some of the most challenging injuries the oral surgeon deals with on a daily basis. The treatment of orbital fractures includes repairing the bone anatomy, correcting functional disturbances, and restoring the cosmetics of the face. In some situations, the surgeon is obligated to delay the treatment; sometimes patients do not seek medical evaluation or the orbital injuries are missed at the time of consultation. Any delay of the treatment of orbital fractures will have an impact on the final result; for that reason, the diagnosis, timing, and treatment plan are critical to obtain an optimal result. Late orbital reconstruction is sometimes necessary for inadequate primary reconstruction or for severe injuries with adequate primary reconstruction. Healing and wound contraction will make secondary reconstruction even more difficult to restore the orbital contents back to normal. There are different materials available for orbital reconstruction, and there is no consensus about which is best. Early surgical intervention may improve the ultimate outcome, but identifying patients at risk of late complications is often difficult.

REFERENCES

1. Lew D, Sinn DP. Diagnosis and treatment of midface fractures. In: Fonseca R, Walker RJ, editors. Oral and maxillofacial trauma. St Louis (MO): Saunders; 2005. p. 653–709.
2. Ochs MW. Orbital and ocular trauma. In: Miloro M, editor. Peterson's principles of oral and maxillofacial surgery, vol. 1. Hamilton (Ontario): BC Decker; 2004. p. 463–90.
3. Kontio R, Lindqvist C. Management of orbital fractures. Oral Maxillofac Surg Clin North Am 2009;21: 209–20.
4. D'Addario M, Cunningham LL Jr. Management of zygomatic fractures. In: Fonseca R, Marciani R, Turvey T, editors. Oral and maxillofacial trauma. St Louis (MO): Saunders; 2009. p. 182–201.
5. Scolozzi P, Momjian A, Heuberger J, et al. Accuracy and predictability in use of AO three-dimensionally preformed titanium mesh plates for posttraumatic orbital reconstruction: a pilot study. J Craniofac Surg 2009;20:1108–13.
6. Evans BT, Webb AA. Post-traumatic orbital reconstruction: anatomical landmarks and the concept of the deep orbit. Br J Oral Maxillofac Surg 2007; 45:183–9.
7. Ilankovan V, Hadley DA, Moos K, et al. Comparison of imaging techniques with surgical experience in orbital injuries: a prospective study. J Craniomaxillofac Surg 1991;19:348–52.
8. Forrest CR, Lata AC, Marcuzzi DW, et al. The role of orbital ultrasound in the diagnosis of orbital fractures. Plast Reconstr Surg 1993;92:28–34.
9. De Man K, Wijngaarde R, Hes J, et al. Influence of age on the management of blow-out fractures of the orbital floor. Int J Oral Maxillofac Surg 1991;20: 330–6.
10. Ahn BA, Ryu WY, Yoo KW, et al. Prediction of enophthalmos by computer-based volume measurement of orbital fractures in a Korean population. Ophthal Plast Reconstr Surg 2008;24:36–9.
11. Matteini C, Renzi G, Becelli R, et al. Surgical timing in orbital fracture treatment: experience with 108 consecutive cases. J Craniofac Surg 2004;15:145–50.
12. Cole P, Boyd V, Banerji S, et al. Comprehensive management of orbital fractures. Plast Reconstr Surg 2007;120(Suppl 2):57S–63S.
13. Burnstine MA. Clinical recommendations for repair of isolated orbital floor fractures: an evidence-based analysis. Ophthalmology 2002;109:1207–11.
14. Raskin EM, Millman AL, Lubkin V, et al. Prediction of late enophthalmos by volumetric analysis of orbital fractures. Ophthal Plast Reconstr Surg 1998;14:19–26.
15. Potter JK, Ellis E. Biomaterials for reconstruction of the internal orbit. J Oral Maxillofac Surg 2004;62: 1280–97.
16. Ellis E, Messo E. Use of nonresorbable alloplastic implants for internal orbital reconstruction. J Oral Maxillofac Surg 2004;62:873–81.
17. Enislidis G. Treatment of orbital fractures: the case for treatment with resorbable materials. J Oral Maxillofac Surg 2004;62:869–72.
18. Kontio R. Treatment of orbital fractures: the case for reconstruction with autogenous bone. J Oral Maxillofac Surg 2004;62:863–8.
19. Ellis E, Tan Y. Assessment of internal orbit reconstructions for pure blowout fractures: cranial bone versus titanium mesh. J Oral Maxillofac Surg 2003; 61:442–52.

Aesthetic Surgery of the Orbits and Eyelids

Joseph A. Broujerdi, MD, DMD

KEYWORDS

- Aesthetic surgery • Orbits • Eyelids

KEY POINTS

- A complete evaluation of the patient for oculoplastic procedure is important.
- The paradigm in oculoplastic surgery has shifted to more conservative eyelid skin, muscle, and fat resection as well as more periorbital soft tissue lift, suspension, and volumization.
- The effects of facial aging are dependent not only on gravity but also on both intrinsic (gender, genetic) and extrinsic (environmental) factors.

INTRODUCTION

The term blepharoplasty derives from the Greek term *blephron* meaning eyelid and *plastos* meaning formed.[1] Ali ibn Isa (AD 940–1010) wrote[2];

> Gather a fold of lid skin between a couple of fingers, or raise it up with a hook, and lay the fold between two small wooden bars or rods as long as the lid and as broad as a lancet. Bind their ends very tight together. The skin between these small pieces of wood, deprived of nutrient, dies in about ten days, the enclosed skin falls off, leaving no scar.
> —*(The Tadhkirat of Ali ibn Isa of Baghdad)*

Reading this passage enlightens one that ancient humans' ideas were not far fetched compared with the modern-day search for the fountain of youth. Aesthetic surgery of the eyelids has advanced with new instrumentation, technology, innovation, research, and good practice of evidence-based medicine.

If the eyes are the window to the soul, then the periorbital tissue is the frame for this window. Aesthetic surgery of the eyelid and surrounding structures aims to keep a youthful frame for the soul. The practice of periocular rejuvenation has moved from skin, muscle, and fat resection of the eyelids only to incorporate a more complex lift, suspension, and volumization of the midface and brow structures. Our improved understanding of the anatomy and pathophysiology of the aging process has assisted in this paradigm shift. The demand from our patients to look natural and youthful has forced us to reevaluate our practice methods and incorporate new advances and techniques into our practice.

PERIORBITAL AND EYELID EVALUATION

A complete evaluation of the patient for oculoplastic procedure is the most important step. The initial conversation with the patient should access what their desires are, psychological readiness for cosmetic surgery (eg, acceptance of surgical downtime, risks, and finances), if the patient has realistic expectations, and any ophthalmologic conditions or past surgeries that might change management of the patient (eg, keratorefractive surgery, which may cause dry eyes syndrome after eyelid procedures). Have the patient present pictures of themselves at a more youthful stage in their life so you may evaluate the aging process that has taken place. The medical history should also identify any conditions that might place the patient at greater risks, such as coagulopathies, hypertension, thyroid disease, and neuromuscular conditions. Take into consideration that patients

Aesthetic Plastic Surgery Institute, 9401 Wilshire Boulevard Suite 1105, Beverly Hills, CA 90212, USA
E-mail address: jbplasticsurg@yahoo.com

Oral Maxillofacial Surg Clin N Am 24 (2012) 665–695
http://dx.doi.org/10.1016/j.coms.2012.07.005
1042-3699/12/$ – see front matter © 2012 Published by Elsevier Inc.

are in your office for consultations because they want to have elective cosmetic surgery not because they need to be at your office. You should also consider having an ophthalmologist and optometrist in your area to whom you can refer. Almost all patients in need of periorbital rejuvenation need a basic ophthalmologic evaluation and clearance before their surgery. Do not undertake unnecessary risks and perform your due diligences thoroughly.

An aesthetically pleasing object to the trained eye has symmetry and balance and is proportionate. On your initial evaluation of the patient, start with architectural framework of the orbitomaxillofacial structures, the position and fullness of the soft tissue, and the texture and quality of the periorbital skin.

A full surgical ophthalmologic examination is discussed elsewhere in this issue by Powell et al, but for the sake of completeness pertinent details are included in this article.

Examination of the Forehead and Eyebrow

The forehead is described with 3 major aesthetic subunits: the forehead, brows, and temples. In evaluating the forehead, start with hairline position. The forehead should on average measure 5 to 6 cm from the glabella to the trichion and should be one-third of the facial height. A patient with a low hairline is a good candidate for an open coronal or anterior hairline brow-lift procedure if there is brow ptosis (**Fig. 1**). A patient with a high hairline is a good candidate for an endoscopic, limited incision, direct or transblepharoplasty (palpebral) brow-lift procedure if there is a brow ptosis (**Fig. 2**). The forehead should have a natural curvature; consider autologous fat transfer if this curvature has been lost because of the aging process. Look for temporal hollowing with aging and consider autologous fat transfer as well.

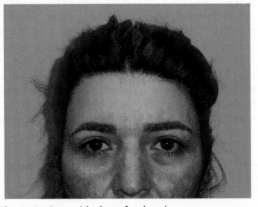

Fig. 1. Patient with short forehead.

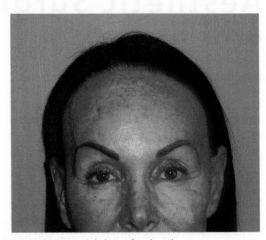

Fig. 2. Patient with long forehead.

Evaluate your patient for forehead rhytids and furrows and whether they are dynamic or static; consider toxins or endoscopically assisted or open partial muscle resection with your brow lift.

Normal brow position was described by Gunter and Antrobus[3]:

1. The medial brow is at or below the level of the orbital rim
2. The medial border of the eyebrow is above the medial canthus
3. The eyebrow should rise gently, with a gentle peak at least two-thirds of the way to its lateral end, and with this peak usually above the lateral limbus
4. The lateral tail of the brow should be higher than the medial end
5. The male brow is at the level of the supraorbital rim medially and below laterally.

The brow itself is divided into 3 subunits: lateral, medial, and central. The youthful lid-brow junction should have a natural convexity contour. This shape is in part because of the subgaleal fat as well as the retro-obicularis oculi fat (ROOF) pads. With age, there is loss of volume and descent of tissue. Gunter and Antrobus[3] also describe how the eyebrow and the nasojugal fold should create an oval, with the pupil at the center. If the distance of the brow to pupil is reduced, then there is brow ptosis, and if the distance between the pupil and nasojugal fold is increased, then there is midface ptosis or hypoplasia. In a normal head position with primary gaze, the distance between the central upper lid margins and the palpebral fold is one-third the distance from the lid margin to the eyebrow. A decrease in the distance of the eyebrow to the lid margin indicates brow ptosis, and an increase in the distance from the fold to the lid margin indicates eyelid ptosis.[4] One can also measure the distance between the central upper lid margin and the inferior edge of the central eyebrow in a normal gaze position called the brow upper lid; this distance is normally 10 mm. One can also measure the distance between the central inferior eyebrows and the inferior limbus (called the brow inferior limbus distance) in a normal primary gaze; this measurement is normally 22 mm.[5] Another method for measuring brow ptosis or asymmetry is to use the ocular asymmetry measuring device (Bausch and Lomb Storz Instruments) designed by Putterman and Chalfin.[6]

Examination of the Upper Eyelid

When one evaluates the upper eyelid, one should look for excessive skin (dermatochalasia), herniated orbital fat, prolapsed lacrimal gland, abnormal eyelid crease, blepharoptosis, and retraction (**Fig. 3**). Excessive skin of the upper eyelid is easily assessed, and herniated nasal and central fat pads are identified by lifting the skin and pushing the eye. This maneuver intensifies the herniation of fat pockets and distinguishes edema of the eyelid from herniation of orbital fat. The position of the lacrimal gland is identified by elevating the temporal eyebrow skin; if the gland is prolapsed, one notices the herniated position of the gland. The upper eyelid crease is identified by elevating the eyebrow and marking the central crease. One can intensify the crease by asking the patient to look up and down from a central gaze position. An upper eyelid creaser can be used to identify the position of or the new proposed position of the eyelid crease. The distance from the central upper eyelid margin to the upper eyelid crease is referred to as the margin crease distance.[7] This distance is measured to be from 8 to 10 mm. A lid ptosis should be suspected if the distance is decreased (**Fig. 4**). Also, identifying the upper lid crease

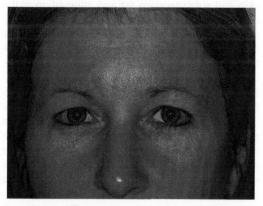

Fig. 3. Female patient with dermatochalasia and herniated orbital fat pads.

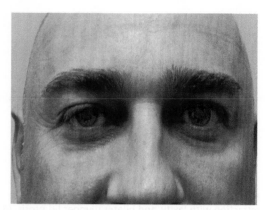

Fig. 4. Patient with right upper eyelid ptosis.

allows the surgeon to determine how much skin should be removed and if a brow-lift procedure needs to accompany a blepharoplasty.

Identifying ptosis preoperatively saves the surgeon and patient grief and potential litigations in the future. There are several methods to access ptosis. One method is by measuring the palpebral fissure width at a normal gaze, which is the distance from the central lower lid margin to the upper lid margin.[7] The normal distance is 10 mm and this measurement is not significantly specific but can identify ptosis. Margin reflex distance is measured by shining a light at the pupils at a normal gaze position and measuring the distance of the reflected corneal light reflex to the central upper lid margin.[7] This distance is usually between 4 and 4.5 mm. A distance less than that measurement determines the amount in distance required to elevate the upper lid during ptosis repair. Upper eyelid ptosis can also be identified by blocking the brow on the examined side, having the patient lift the opposite side, and asking the patient to look to the extreme down gaze from a normal gaze position.[8] If the distance between the lower and upper central lid margin is less than 2 mm, then a ptosis should be suspected. Patients with ptosis are not able to lift the upper lid because the forehead muscles are blocked.

Upper eyelid retraction could be a sign of thyroid disease. A palpebral fissure width test can identify an excessive distance between the eyelids. Prompt ophthalmologic and endocrine evaluation is recommended before proceeding to elective cosmetic surgery.

Examination of the Lower Eyelid

The lower eyelid examination should include evaluation for excessive skin (dermatochalasia), herniated orbital fat pads, lid retraction, and laxity (**Fig. 5**). Excess skin is evaluated by asking the

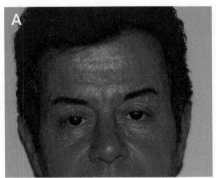 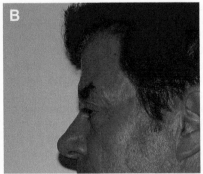

Fig. 5. (A) Frontal view, patient with bilateral lower lid dermatochalasia, herniated orbital fat pads, lateral lid retraction with laxity, and bilateral upper lid ptosis. (B) Left lateral view, patient with lower lid dermatochalasia, herniated orbital fat pads with inferior descent of lid-cheek junction, malar hypoplasia, and ptosis.

patient to look up, and the amount of excess skin is evaluated for either skin resection or laser resurfacing and tightening. The herniated orbital fat pads are evaluated in the nasal, central, and temporal positions by placing pressure over the eyelid and noting herniation of the fat in each position. This maneuver distinguishes edema versus herniated fat. The examiner should also consider hypertrophied obicularis oculi muscle.

Lower eyelid retraction is evaluated by having the patient and examiner at the same eye level and shining a light into the patient's pupil. The distant from the corneal light reflex to the central lower lid margin is measured. This distance is usually 5.5 mm and the lower lid is at the level of the lower limbus of the eye or just slightly below it. Any distance greater or below the lower limbus is an indication for lid retraction and the surgeon should be prepared for reconstruction. This examination is referred to as the marginal reflex distance 2.[9]

Lower lid laxity is evaluated with a snap back test. The lower lid is pinched between the 2 fingers and allowed to snap back into position. The laxity, the time it takes to snap back, and possible eversion of the lid are assessed. If there is any indication of lid laxity, one should consider a concomitant lower lid suspension procedure. The examiner should also assess the laxity of the lateral and medial canthal tendons by pulling on the canthal tendon; if the complex moves easily and lateral or medial fissures are rounded off easily, then a canthal tuck should also be considered as part of the treatment plan.

Examination of the Midface

The examination of the midface should start with a skeletal evaluation. Hypoplastic maxillary and zygomatic bones should be noted with a negative vector at the lid-cheek junction. If indicated, I obtain a cone beam computed tomography (CBCT) scan of the patient to analyze the facial skeletal pattern and distinguish whether skeletal augmentation is necessary. The position of the globe should also be determined with an exophthalmometry instrument to distinguish between a true negative vector or an exophthalmos. The amount and position of the midfacial fat compartments should be evaluated. The surface anatomy of the cheek forms a Y, where the center is the subobicularis oculi fat (SOOF). Above the SOOF is the lid-cheek junction formed by the orbital retaining ligament. Medial to the SOOF is the nasojugal groove (tear trough), which is formed by the junction of the levator labii superioris muscle fibers and the preseptal orbicularis oculi muscle fibers, with skin and subcutaneous fat overlying it. Recent anatomic studies by Haddock and colleagues[10] have shown that the tear trough is formed between the preseptal fibers of pars palpebrarum and pars orbitalis of the orbicularis oculi muscle and the levator labii superioris muscle is much inferior to the tear trough area. These investigators also explain that the tear trough deformity is the atrophy of the overlying skin and subcutaneous fat and attenuation of the orbital retaining ligaments in the valley of the orbicularis oculi muscle with bulging of the postseptal orbital nasal fat pads to exacerbate the deformity. Lateral to the SOOF is the palpebral-malar groove, which separates the malar fat pad and SOOF. Continuation of the nasojugal groove into the midface forms the midcheek furrow, which is the separation of the malar fat pad from the nasolabial fat pad. The presence of tear trough deformity with malar bags and festoons is an indication of hypoplasia, inferior descent, and separation of the midfacial fat compartments. There is always a combination of volume loss and separation with inferior descent of attached tissue. The tear trough deformity is classified as class I to III, class I being volume loss medially (loss of subcutaneous fat and herniation of nasal fat pad), class II volume loss medial and centrally (volume loss in SOOF and attenuation of the lid-cheek junction), and class III volume loss medial, central, and laterally (volume loss in the malar fat pads with inferior descent) with complete orbital hollowing.[11] The skin should also be evaluated for signs of aging, including atrophic skin changes, dyschromia, rhytids, and loss of skin elasticity (**Fig. 6**).

The Rest of the Examination

The visual fields, acuity, and ocular motility should be evaluated, as described elsewhere in this issue. The eyes should also be evaluated for tear secretion with a Schirmer test. Patients with low secretions are prone to postoperative complications. This test is also described elsewhere in this issue. The cornea should be evaluated and a test for Bell phenomenon performed. The eyelid is closed tightly by the patient, the examiner pries the lid open slightly, and the position of the iris is noted. If the iris has not elevated, then the test is abnormal and the patient is prone to postoperative irritation of the eye. Because the patient is not able to elevate the eyeball superiorly and protect it, the risk of postoperative irritation increases.

Photography

The standard photography for periorbital surgery is to obtain a frontal periorbital view in a normal, upward, and downward gaze as well as periorbital lateral and oblique views preoperatively and postoperatively. In addition, I also obtain a full-frontal, basal, bilateral oblique, and lateral views of the patient preoperatively, 1 week, 1 month, 3 months, and 6 months postoperatively. I also take a three-dimensional (3D) surface image of the patient before and after surgery via the 3dMDface system (3dMD, Atlanta, GA).The 3dMDface System

consists of 6 machine vision cameras synchronized to fire at the same time, within a 1.5-millisecond window. 3dMD systems are based on an advanced software technique called active stereo photogrammetry, which momentarily projects a unique light pattern on the subject while the image is taken. 3dMD software then identifies the same unique point from multiple images and uses simple geometry and complex algorithms to calculate the coordinates of the point and construct the 3D facial shape in a TSB file format. In certain cases, I combine DICOM (Digital Imaging and Communications in Medicine) files from a CBCT study with the TSB files to form a 3D surface image from a 3dMFface system using 3dMDvultus software to obtain a true skeletal facial image of a patient. These complete data assist me in preoperative planning, and the 3dMDvultus software allows me to perform virtual surgery on both skeletal and soft tissue components (**Fig. 7**).

RELEVANT SURGICAL ANATOMY OF PERIORBIT

Detailed orbital anatomy is described elsewhere in this issue, and only relevant surgical anatomy is discussed in this section. The 7 facial skeletal structures that form the orbital framework (maxilla, zygoma, ethmoid, frontal, lacrimal, palatine, sphenoid) provide a platform for the attachment of the soft tissue (**Fig. 8**). The main sensory nerves of the periorbital structures are branches of the trigeminal nerve (V2, V3) and exit the facial bones via foramina, notches, or along the bone to provide sensation. The supraorbital nerve exits the orbit via a notch or foramina on the frontal bone. The supratrochlear and infratrochlear nerves exit the orbit through a notch. The zygomaticofrontal nerves exit the frontal bone via its foramina, and zygomaticofacial nerves also exit the zygomatic bone via its foramina. The infraorbital nerve exits the maxilla

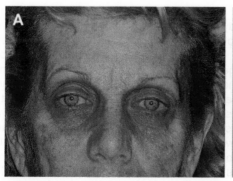
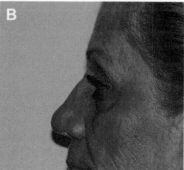

Fig. 6. (*A*) Frontal view, patient with periorbital hypoplasia, upper and lower lid dermatochalasia, tear trough deformity, and midface hypoplasia with ptosis. (*B*) Left lateral view.

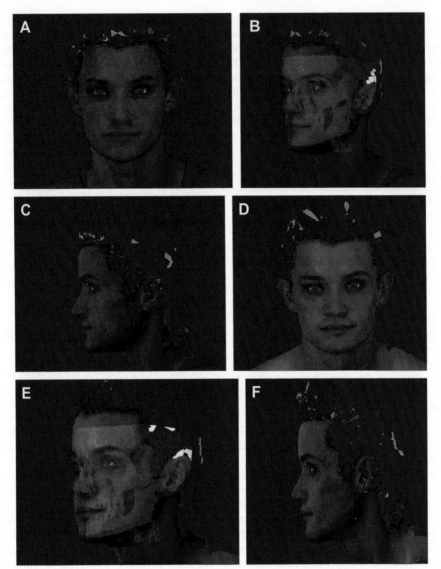

Fig. 7. (*A*) 3D surface image preoperative frontal view by 3dMDface system, patient with malar and paranasal hypoplasia and a negative vector. (*B*) 3D surface image fused with 3D computed tomography scan image, before left oblique view. (*C*) Before lateral view. (*D*) Frontal view, patient after malar and paranasal Medpore (Porex Surgical, Stryker) implant. (*E*) Postoperative left oblique view. (*F*) Postoperative left later view.

via its foramina. The motor nerve supply is mostly through the facial nerve and its branches (zygomatic and frontal).

On the frontal bone above the supraorbital ridge is the orbital ligamentous adhesion, where the deep galea aponeurotica adheres to the bone. This galea invests the frontalis with the procerus, depressor supraciliary, and corrugator muscles. Just above this ligamentous attachment and below the galea, the galeal fat pad exits, which allows for the smooth gliding of the muscles of facial expression. As we age, this fat pad atrophies and creates a flatness and droop to the appearance of the forehead. At the temporal crest, the orbital ligamentous adhesions become the temporal ligamentous adhesions and run superior-posterior to become the superior temporal septum, where the temporalis muscle and its fascia insert. Over the supraorbital ridge, the orbicularis retaining ligament exits where the orbital septum attaches to and it assists in the attachment of the obicularis oculi muscle. The preseptal fat in the lateral brow area between the orbital septum and the obicularis oculi is called the retro-obicularis oculi fat. This fat layer provides a lateral fullness to the brow, and with aging, the fat pad loses its volume and assists

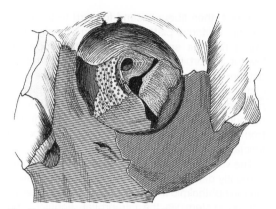

Fig. 8. Orbital anatomy, orbital bones.

in the dropping appearance of the brow. The obicularis retaining ligament also runs along the lateral orbital ridge and down to the inferior orbital rim. The lateral attachments are thick and are known as the lateral brow thickening and lateral orbital thickening. On the internal aspect of the orbital rim over the lateral orbital thickening is the site of attachment for the lateral canthal ligament. At the lateral brow area, the temporalis muscle with its deep fascia travels through the infratemporal fossa, and just above this, the sentinel vein pierces through the galea aponeurotic layer into the loose areolar fat and crosses over to the supraorbital ridge. Above the loose areolar tissue, the partial temporal fascia (superficial temporal fascia) houses the frontal branches of the facial nerve. The partial temporal fascia is also in continuation with the superficial musculoaponeurotic system (SMAS) layer in the face.

At the midfacial level just below the orbital retaining ligament, the zygomatic cutaneous ligament originates from the zygomatic bone and has attachments on the obicularis oculi muscle and on to the subcutaneous structures. Between these 2 ligaments, the SOOF resides, and above it are the pars orbitalis fibers of the obicularis oculi muscle. Between the SOOF and the preperiosteal fat and periosteum is the potential prezygomatic space. Just below the space laterally, the zygomatic major and zygomatic minor muscles originate and medially the levator labii superioris originates. These groups of muscles are deeper to the obicularis oculi muscle. Just inferior to the SOOF and superficial to the muscles are the malar fat pad medially and lateral-inferiorly the nasolabial fat pad.

The surgical zones of the eye and periorbit are divided into zones 0 to 6: zone 0 is the globe and all structures behind the orbital septum; zones I and II are the upper and lower eyelid and any structure to the orbital septum; zones III and IV are the

medial and lateral canthus and all structures posterior to the ligaments; zone V is all the contagious structures. The aperture of the eyelids measures 28 to 30 mm horizontally and 10 to 12 mm vertically. Both the horizontal and vertical aperture can decrease with aging because of laxity of the aponeurotic, canthal, tarsal, and retinacular attachments. The upper lid margin rests 2 mm below the upper limbus of the iris, and the lower lid margin rests at the lower limbus of the iris. The lateral commissure of the eyelid is positioned 2 mm higher than the medial side; with aging, there is definitive laxity of the canthal attachment apparatus and there are changes in the lateral commissure of the lid. The periorbital skin is thin, with minimal subcutaneous fat; this predisposes the skin to wrinkling, stretching, with age. The obicularis oculi muscle is a sphincter muscle divides into 2: the pars palpebrarum and pars orbitalis. The obicularis oculi muscle is innervated on its deep surface by the zygomatic branches of the facial nerve. The pars palpebrarum is further divided into the preseptal and pretarsal sections. The pars orbitalis is attached circumferential to the orbital retaining ligament superiorly and inferiorly and laterally to the lateral thickening ligaments. Inferiorly, this attachment is known as the lid-cheek junction. Medially the muscle fibers connect directly to the orbital wall and canthal tendon in a complex anatomic arrangement linked to the lacrimal sac.

The upper eyelid fold is created by the dermal attachment of the levator aponeurotic extensions through the obicularis oculi muscle (**Fig. 9**). These attachments start at the lid margin and terminate above the superior tarsal plate, which forms the

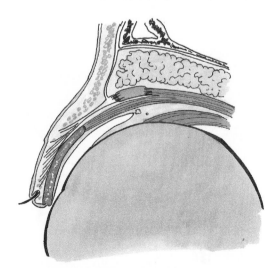

Fig. 9. Orbital anatomy, midsagittal section, upper eyelid.

supratarsal fold. The supratarsal plate is about 10 mm long and is suspended by the lateral and medial canthal tendons. Posteriorly, the supratarsal plate is suspended by the Whitnall ligament in the orbit. The lateral and medial extensions of the Whitnall ligament are known as the medial and lateral horns, which connect to the canthal tendons. Posterior to the Whitnall ligament and attached to the levator apo neurosis is the levator palpebral superioris muscle, which is innervated by the branches of the oculometer nerve. Just beneath the levator aponeurosis is the Müller muscle, which also attaches to the posterior border of the supratarsal plate. This muscle is innervated by the sympathetic nervous system traveling with arterial system. The superior septum orbitale at its inferior leg attaches to the levator aponeurosis at the superior tarsal plate junction and at its superior leg attaches to the orbital periosteum and arcus marginalis. Posterior to the septum are the fat pads. Medially, the nasal fat pad (pale yellow) is divided from the central fat pad (rich yellow) by the superior trochlear muscle, which rotates around the pulley attached to the orbital roof by the trochlea. There is no lateral fat pad. This space is occupied by the lacrimal gland.

The lower lid has 3 main layers: the anterior lamella is formed by the skin and obicularis oculi muscle (**Fig. 10**); the middle lamella is formed by the inferior tarsal plate (which is 2–5 mm high), the inferior orbital septum, and the orbital fat pads; the posterior lamella is formed by the capsulopalpebral fascia, which is an extension of the inferior rectus muscle, the counterpart to the levator aponeurosis and the palpebral conjunctiva. The capsulopalpebral fascia splints around the inferior oblique muscle and attaches to the Lockwood

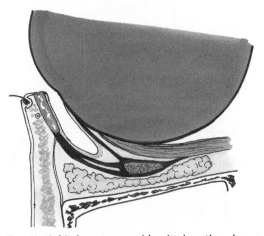

Fig. 10. Orbital anatomy, midsagittal section, lower eyelid.

ligament, then fibers ascend forward to attach to the inferior tarsal plate and septum orbitally. This fascia has the same function as the upper lid levator. The orbital septum joins the orbital rim periosteum and forms the arcus marginalis. There are 3 distinctive fat pads in the lower lid. The medial fat pad is divided from the central fat pad by the inferior oblique muscle and the central fat pad is separated from the lateral fat pad by the capsulopalpebral fascia.

The vascular supply to the periorbital structures is mostly derived from the internal carotid system via the ophthalmic artery and partly by the external carotid system via the infraorbital, angular, and superficial temporal artery. The ophthalmic artery gives off the lacrimal, supraorbital, and supratrochlear and dorsal nasal arteries. The upper and lower eyelids are supplied via the lateral palpebral artery (a branch of the lacrimal artery) and medial palpebral artery (a branch of the ophthalmic artery). The lateral and medial palpebral arteries anastamose to form the marginal arcade artery. The venous system parallels the arterial blood supply. The lymphatic drainage of the periorbital is in the inferior lateral direction to the preauricular, parotid, and submandibular lymph nodes.

THE AGING PERIORBIT

The effects of facial aging are dependent not only on gravity but also on both intrinsic (gender, genetic) and extrinsic (environmental) factors. The intrinsic component is a complex dynamic change that occurs over time in the hard tissue (bone, teeth) and soft tissue (eg, skin, ligaments, muscle, fat) of the face. At the skeletal level, there is a reduction of facial height and loss of bony prominences (convexity to concavity), most marked in the maxilla and mandible; this is strongly correlated with loss of teeth.[12–15] There is also a decrease in soft tissue thickness with age.[16] There are significant changes to the facial muscles with aging; morphologically, the muscle thins out, and histologically, there is an atrophy of muscle fibers and increase in intracellular matrix.[17] A recent morphologic study of the upper pretarsal obicularis oculi muscle[18] revealed that the muscle layer remained intact with aging; this be isolated to the eyelids. The facial fat compartments also go through an inferior migration and volume loss with the aging process.[19] The retaining fibers and ligaments of the face become attenuated and laxer with the aging process as well.[20] Histomorphometric analysis has revealed statistically significant thinning of the cutis. Elastic and collagen fibers in the cutis undergo degeneration processes during aging.[21]

The process of aging is interdependent of all components and affects the tissues at all levels. The process reveals the separate components of the periorbital structures with aging such as the brow ptosis, blepharoptosis, lateral commissure droop, lid-cheek junction, periorbital hallowing, tear trough deformity, malar bags, and nasolabial fold (**Fig. 11**).

The Forehead and Brow

The forehead forms redundant tissue with atrophic changes in the skin. The anterior hairline recedes. Deep furrows and rhytids form in horizontal and vertical directions. The subgaleal and ROOF fat pads lose their volume; this shows up as concavity in the central midforehead area. The ROOF also descends inferiorly because of loss of attenuation of the retaining ligaments. This change creates a brow ptosis, with loss of convexity of the supra-brow ridge and lateral hooding.

In the temporal area, the temporal fat pads loses its volume and creates a hollowing shape to the lateral forehead area. The bony ridges of the frontal bones undergo remodeling, with loss of convexity and formation of concavities with atrophy and thinning of the muscles.

The Upper Eyelid

The supratarsal fold loses its definition. If the fat pads are herniated, they stretch the skin and create dermatochalasia and push the lid fold inferiorly. If there is excessive atrophy of the fat pads, it pushes back the lid fold superiorly and gives the patient a hollow look. In the case of senile ptosis, the tarsal fold does move superiorly. The lacrimal gland can droop and create a ptotic look to the lateral lid-brow junction.

The Lower Eyelid

There is an atrophic change to the lower eyelid skin, with thinning of the dermis with rhytid formations and dyschromia. Both the lateral and medial canthal attachments become lax and stretch out with a decrease in the eyelid fissures, rounding, and inferior displacement of the lateral canthus. The tarsal plates become lax and create a lid droop, with entropion and occasionally ectropion. Herniated fat pads can create puffiness to the lower lids with dermatochalasia. Also fat pad atrophy can create hollowness to the periorbital, with retraction of the globe into the socket and lid laxity. The orbital retaining ligaments become attenuated and pull the lid-cheek junction inferiorly. This situation increases the distance between the lid margin and the lid-cheek junction, giving the appearance of tear trough deformity.

The Midface

The aging process works at all different layers of the midfacial tissues, starting with bony changes in the maxilla and zygoma, with a decrease in vertical height and loss of bony prominence in the midface. The retaining ligaments become attenuated and the fat pads atrophy. As a consequence, there is a vertical droop in the midfacial tissue and loss of volume and separation of midface fat pads, with formation of nasojugal, palpebral-malar, and naso-labial grooves. The buccal fat pad also goes through the same transformation, which leads clinically to the formation of frowns and marionette lines. The muscles of facial expression also become attenuated and stretched with the aging process, leading to downturning of the lip commis-sure and elongation of the upper lip with atrophic and hypoplastic changes.

THE BROW AND FOREHEAD IN PERIORBITAL REJUVENATION

The evaluation of the forehead unit was described earlier. There are multiple surgical options for brow and forehead rejuvenation in combination with eyelid procedures for obtaining an aesthetically natural and youthful appearance to the periorbital structure. According to the literature,[20] there is

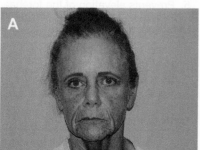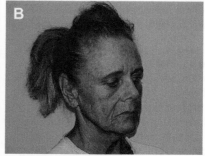

Fig. 11. (A) The aging face, frontal view. (B) The aging face, right oblique view.

no 1 single procedure favored for brow and forehead rejuvenation. In general, patients with brow ptosis with a low hairline are candidates for coronal or endoscopic brow lift and patients with a high hairline or prominent forehead are candidates for either anterior hairline, limited incision, or direct or transblepharoplasty (palpebral). Each technique has its indications, with its advantages and disadvantages, with no one technique superior to the others.[20] In general, open procedures allow for excision of redundant skin, whereas the endoscopic technique allows for repositioning of the redundant tissue. The selection of an appropriate technique is dependent on an accurate diagnosis, the patient's expectations, and the surgeon's skills.

With aging, not only is there a descent of the forehead and brow structures but also a loss of volume in the forehead and brow is apparent. The forehead loses its soft tissue convexity, with development of deep furrows, and at the forehead-brow-lid junction the loss of volume and convexity leads to brow ptosis and an aged look. One should also consider volume replenishment with autologous fat transfer with brow-lift procedures. This procedure restores the youthful and natural appearance to both forehead and brow.

Coronal Brow Lift

This technique has made a comeback after it lost popularity with the introduction of the endoscopic approach. The open approach allows for excision of redundant tissue and improved longevity.

Advantages:

1. Direct access to anatomic structures for resection and anchorage
2. Camouflage of scar in the hairline
3. Direct excision of redundant tissue
4. Longevity of the lift.

Disadvantages:

1. Long scar
2. Risk of alopecia
3. Elevation of the anterior hairline
4. Paresthesia of forehead and scalp.

The frontal incision is placed 5 cm posterior and parallel to the anterior hairline in a beveled direction to allow for hair growth into the scar. The temporal incision is designed in a zigzag fashion, starting with the first zigzag at the top of the superior sulcus of the ear, moving in an anterior direction and the third moving in an anterior direction and meeting the frontal incisions. This design allows for better camouflage and parting of the hair when wet. The temporal dissection is at the level of the glistening layer of the deep temporal fascia with release of the temporal and orbital ligamentous attachments as well as the lateral brow and orbital thickening ligaments. Preserving the sentinel vein reduces postoperative swelling and bleeding. This dissection preserves the fontal branches of the facial nerve. Interiorly, the dissection is in a subgaleal plane until 1 to 2 cm above the supraorbital rim, then it sharply dissects to a subperiosteal plane. With subperiosteal dissection release, the arcus marginalis with preservation and release of the supraorbital neurovascular bundle forms its foramina or notch. The galea is scored in a horizontal direction. The galea is meticulously incised and the muscle is partially resected without injuring the neurovascular bundle. The scalp flap is elevated and secured temporally with staples to verify the position of the brow, and the excess scalp is marked and excised. I recommend securing the temporal-parietal fascia to the deep temporal fascia in the temporal region with permanent sutures before layered closure of the scalp flap. I also advocate the use of drains and compression dressing to prevent hematoma formation.

Anterior Hairline Brow Lift

The major indication for this technique is a long (greater than 6–7 cm) forehead. The incision is placed along the hairline in a beveled fashion to allow hair growth into the scar line. Laterally, the incision is curved in to the temporal scalp. The remainder of the dissection is similar to the coronal brow lift. The excess skin is excised in a beveled fashion parallel to the initial incision.

Advantages:

1. Direct access to anatomic structures for resection and anchorage
2. Camouflage of scar in the hairline
3. Direct excision of redundant tissue
4. Longevity of the lift
5. Prevents elevation of the forehead.

Disadvantages:

1. Long scar
2. Risk of alopecia
3. Scar along the anterior hairline
4. Paresthesia of forehead and scalp.

Limited Incision Brow Lift

The limited incision brow lift is indicated for correction of brow ptosis without lifting the central forehead. The incisions are placed 2 to 3 cm behind the temporal hairline perpendicular to the vector of pull. The incisions are 3 to 5 cm as indicated. The dissection and release of attaching tissue in the temporal, lateral forehead, and periorbital region are similar to the coronal lift. The vector of lift is in a superior-posterior direction, and redundant tissue is excised in full thickness. Permanent sutures are placed between superficial fascia and the deep fascia for fixation and anchorage. Scalp closure is performed in a layered fashion (**Fig. 12**).

Advantages:

1. Direct access to anatomic structures for anchorage
2. May be combined with upper blepharoplasty and transpalpebral resection of the corrugators
3. Avoids injury to the deep division supraorbital nerve
4. Elevation of the lateral brow segment
5. No elevation of the forehead.

Disadvantages:

1. Limited access to the forehead muscles
2. Risk of alopecia along the scar
3. Difficulty in addressing deep forehead rhytids.

Endoscopic Brow Lift

The endoscopic brow lift has the ability to lift the brow, reposition the forehead, and address the deep forehead rhytids and minimize the complications of scalp paresthesia, alopecia, and a long scar. There is a need for additional endoscopic instrumentation (4 mm, 30° endoscope camera) and ability to create an optical cavity with the periorbital, forehead, and lateral brow structures. The incisions are 1 to 2 cm long in the hair-bearing scalp and 1 to 2 cm behind the hairline. A total of 5 incisions are recommended: 1 central, 2 lateral, and 2 temporal. The dissection is similar to the coronal lift, with use of endoscopic instrumentation and camera to create a surgical cavity and release adhering tissues. The vector of pull is in a superior-posterior and medial direction. The brow and forehead lift anchorage is provided by screw or cortical tunneling at 45° and suture fixation of the superficial fascia to the screw device as well as suture fixation of the superficial fascia to the deep fascia laterally in the temporal region for optimal results.[22] Drilling of the frontal bone should not exceed a depth of more then 3 to 4 mm because of risk of penetration of the inferior cortical layer and dural tear.[23] Mitek anchors (2 mm depth) with suture fixation can also be used. The periosteum needs 6 to 12 weeks for adhering back to the bone surface, and the fixation technique must provide anchorage until the periosteum fuses back to the bone.[21] Screw fixation is either by resorbable material or removable titanium screws that have holes to secure the superficial fascia to the screw for anchorage. The fixation screws can be removed in the office postoperatively with local anesthesia. Other types of resorbable screw have fixation prongs to the scalp, for example Endotine (Coapt System, Palo Alta, CA), which allows for rapid anchorage without suture material. This device has been reported to be palpable for up to 15 months and is recommended for patients whose scalp is thicker than 5 to 6 mm (**Fig. 13**).[24–26]

Advantages:

1. Direct visualization of forehead muscle
2. Minimal incision
3. Less chance for forehead and scalp paresthesia.

Disadvantages:

1. Technical learning curve
2. Additional cost
3. Need for fixation onto scalp.

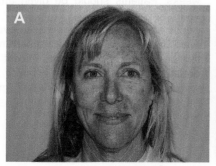 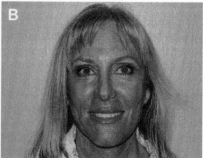

Fig. 12. (*A*) Preoperative frontal view, patient with age-related skin changes, periorbital hypoplasia, upper eyelid dermatochalasis with brow ptosis. (*B*) Postoperative frontal view, patient status after limited incision brow lift, upper blepharoplasty, autologous fat transfer to the periorbital soft tissue and erbium fractionated laser skin resurfacing.

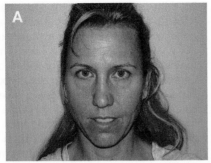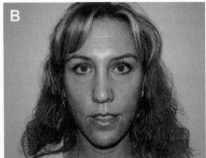

Fig. 13. (*A*) Preoperative frontal view, patient with brow ptosis. (*B*) Postoperative frontal view, patient status after endoscopic brow lift and sliding genioplasty.

Direct Brow Lift

The ideal candidate for a direct brow lift is a patient with deep forehead rhytids or male pattern hair loss or receding hairline. The incision is placed in the deep furrows of the forehead or superior brow margin. The dissection enters the subgaleal plane to release the attaching periorbital tissues and allow access to the forehead musculature. The forehead flap is redraped in a desired vector, redundant tissue is excised from the inferior flap, and the forehead flap is anchored with permanent sutures to the superior periosteum. The incision and dissection can be limited to the brow region only for brow elevation.

Advantages:

1. Ease of access to the brow structures and forehead muscles
2. Correction of brow asymmetry.

Disadvantages:

1. Visible scaring
2. Paresthesia of forehead and scalp.

Transpalpebral Brow Lift

Transpalpebral brow lift is performed through an upper eyelid blepharoplasty incision. A blepharoplasty may also be performed at the same time. The ideal candidate is a patient with high or receding hairline or who is balding.[27,28] This technique has been described in patients with recurrent brow ptosis or asymmetry after a brow-lift procedure. After the blepharoplasty incision is made, the obicularis oculi muscle is incised transversally and the dissection is in a submuscular plane carried in a superior direction above the supraorbital rim and lateral to the neurovascular bundle. Medially, the corrugators and procerus are excised. Browpexy is performed by fixating the undersurface of the obicularis oculi muscle to the periosteum with resorbable sutures in a desired vector. Care should be taken to prevent skin dimpling at the site of suture fixation. Meticulous hemostasis is required with this technique as well.

Advantages:

1. Ease of access to the brow structures and forehead muscles
2. Correction of brow asymmetry
3. Short operating time.

Disadvantages:

1. Highly vascularized surgical field
2. Paresthesia of forehead and scalp.

Postoperative Care and Complications

Scalp and hairline incisions are dressed with antibiotic ointment. If drains are used, they can be removed in 24 to 72 hours postoperatively. Paper tape is used on the forehead and lateral brow area to minimize edema, with a head wrap, which can be removed in 72 hours. Patients should sleep with their bedhead elevated for a minimum of 2 weeks. Patients should be given artificial tears and ophthalmic ointment in case dry eyes or lagophthalmos develops. Ice packs over the forehead and eyes should be used routinely to reduce postoperative edema. Patient should not participate in strenuous activity for the first 2 weeks. Any suture removal is performed after 7 days. The most common complications after brow lift are;

- Alopecia
- Dissatisfaction
- Scarring
- Asymmetry
- Sensory loss
- Infection

- Lagophthalmos
- Motor deficiency
- Abnormal contour
- Hematoma

REJUVENATION OF THE UPPER EYELID

The key to a successful surgical outcome is in preoperative diagnosis and planning your surgical technique. The natural youthful appearance of the upper eyelid was described earlier. The key components are:

1. Fullness, volume, and convexity of the lid-brow junction
2. The upper eyelid crease is more often in a low position

Routinely ask your patients to bring a photograph of themselves at a youthful stage that shows the periorbital area for comparison. Evaluate your patients for brow ptosis caused by either volume loss or a combination of volume loss and descent of soft tissue attachment. These patients develop flatness to the lid-brow junction or lateral hooding. This flatness can be addressed with brow volumization or lift at the same time as the upper blepharoplasty procedure. Look for abnormally high upper lid crease and ptosis. A patient with high upper lid crease has either had aggressive muscle and fat resection upper eyelid surgery or has congenital or senile ptosis. A patient with high lid crease position without ptosis needs volumization and lowering of the lid crease. Patients with ptosis excessively use their frontalis muscle and develop asymmetry of the brow position, forehead rhytids, and deep furrows. Evaluate your patient for concomitant blepharoplasty and levator aponeurosis repair or Müller muscle-conjunctival resection. A phenylephrine test with 2.5% strength identifies patients who benefit form Müller muscle resection. A levator suspension is usually performed under local anesthesia or intravenous (IV) sedation so that the patient can open and close the eyelid for repositioning of the lid during ptosis repair. If ptosis is not diagnosed in the initial evaluation, after eyelid surgery, ptosis becomes evident and can lead to an unhappy patient. Consult your ophthalmologist for a second opinion and work with an oculoplastic surgeon as needed. Description of ptosis repair is beyond the scope of this article, but its recognition is vital for proper surgical planning and achieving a natural youthful appearance after surgery.

There is a paradigm shift in aesthetic oculoplastic surgery in preservation of muscle and volumization. Fagien[29] describes preserving the preseptal obicularis oculi muscle during upper blepharoplasty by creating an accordion effect or bulking of the muscle during skin closure to create an improved supratarsal and lid-brow junction volume. Demasceno and colleagues[30] have found that muscle resection causes more postoperative symptoms and presents worse initial aesthetic outcome. However, the aesthetic outcome is the same when the preseptal orbicularis oculi muscle is excised or preserved. There is also a lack of consensus in the literature regarding preseptal obicularis oculi muscle resection during upper blepharoplasty, but most surgeons preserve muscle.[28]

Upper Blepharoplasty

Proper skin marking is essential for a good outcome. The inferior margin is marked at about 8 to 10 mm centrally, 6 to 8 mm medially (nasal), and 7 to 9 mm laterally from the lid margin paralleling the skin crease. The inferior margin should lie between the medial extent of the punctum and lateral extent of the lateral commissure of the eyelid. Excess skin is pinched with a forceps until 2 mm lagophthalmos is seen and then marked superiorly. The superior margin is parallel to the arch of the inferior extent of the brow, medially it curves inferiorly to meet the inferior margin, and laterally it extends out about 1 cm from the lateral commissure of the eyelid. The inferior and superior margins are connected with a curvilinear line mark laterally (**Fig. 14**). Sclera shields are used to protect the globe, and 1% xylocaine with 1/100,000 epinephrine is infiltrated with a 32-gauge needle for anesthesia and hemostasis. After waiting 10 minutes for hemostasis, incisions are

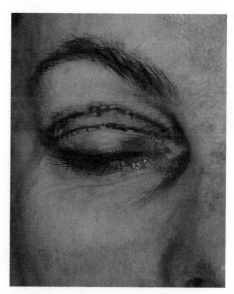

Fig. 14. Markings for upper blepharoplasty.

made with a 15-c blade. Hemostasis is achieved with electrocautery during each step throughout the procedure. The marked skin is excised via a de-epithelialization technique with a sharp blade. The excised skin should be saved for comparison. If preseptal obicularis oculi muscle excision is planned, Westcott scissors are used to remove a 1-mm-thick strip of muscle to expose the orbital septum. Digital pressure is placed over the orbit to identify the nasal and central fat pads. If muscle resection is not planned, Westcott scissors are used to make a buttonhole through the muscle and septum over the fat pads (**Fig. 15**). Each fat pad is teased out, clamped with a forceps, excised, and then cauterized. The fat should be saved for comparison with the contralateral side. Make sure that you have achieved meticulous hemostasis before moving to the next step. Next, the skin flaps are approximated with multiple interrupted 6-0 fast absorbing gut suture at high-tension areas. The skin is closed with a 6-0 nylon suture running in subcuticular fashion, with the ends sticking out for removal in 1 week (**Fig. 16**).

Revision Upper Blepharoplasty

Most patients who present for revision blepharoplasty are unhappy with their results for one of the following reasons:

1. Loss of periorbital volume with hollowing of the upper eyelid sulcus
2. High orbital lid crease
3. Dermatochalasia
4. Hypopigmentation of scar with marked transition between the upper lid and darker thick sub-brow skin.

Review operative records and photographs as part of your initial evaluation of the patient. Have your patient bring a photograph of them at a younger age as well. Evaluate your patient for

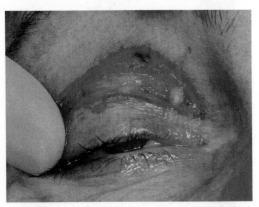

Fig. 15. Herniated nasal fat pad after gentle push on the globe.

brow ptosis, volume loss, and blepharoptosis. Have your ophthalmologist perform a routine eye examination and rule out ptosis of the lids. Be watchful of dry eye syndrome after surgery. The goals of revision blepharoplasty should include the following (**Fig. 17**):

1. Autologous fat transfer to the brow to volumize the lid-brow junction
2. Lowering of the lid crease by marking the inferior margin at about 8 mm from the lid margin
3. Minimal to no skin excision centrally and medially; skin excision mostly laterally to elevate the lateral hooding
4. Preserving preseptal obicularis oculi muscle and creating a bulking effect with skin closure
5. Autologous fat transfer to the nasal and central preseptal area as needed
6. Laser skin resurfacing or chemical peel of the subbrow skin after surgery can assist in smoothening the transition zone.

Asian Eyelid Surgery

The first description of Asian eyelid surgery dates back to the late nineteenth century in Japan by Mikamo, who used conjunctival-dermal suture ligation to create a supratarsal double eyelid fold.[31] By the early twentieth century, in Japan after World War I, Marou[32] described the first incisional Asian eyelid procedure. After World War II, in 1955, Millard's article subtitled "Oriental to occidental" coined the term "Westernization of the Asian eyelid".[33] Sayoc and Fernandez in the 1960s independently described suturing the dermis of the superior skin flap to the tarsal plate; Flowers later modified this technique and it has become a widely accepted and published technique for Asian eyelid surgery.[34–36]

The Asian eyelid blepharoplasty is not to westernize the Asian eye but to beautify oneself, have the ability to wear eye makeup without smudging and also to have aesthetically bigger eyes. The Asian cranium is a brachiocephalic to mesocephalic type, with flat and broad midface features with shallow orbits. These features give the eyes a puffy appearance compared with Whites.[37] The major anatomic difference between Asians' and Whites' upper eyelids are (**Fig. 18**A);

1. Point of fusion of the levator aponeurosis with orbital septum just above the tarsal palate in Asians as opposed to 5 to 10 mm above the tarsal plate in Whites[38]
2. Excessive orbital fat with distribution of the pre-aponeurotic fat compartment hanging over the fusion point of the aponeurosis and the septum

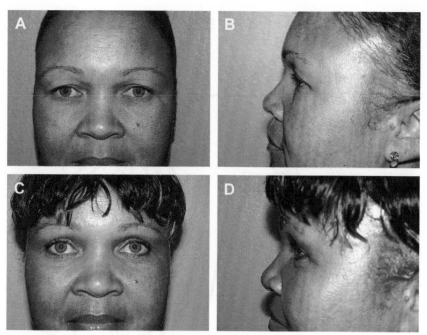

Fig. 16. (*A*) Preoperative frontal view, patient with dermatochalasia of the upper eyelid with herniated orbital fat pads. (*B*) Preoperative left lateral view. (*C*) Postoperative frontal view, patient status after upper blepharoplasty. (*D*) Postoperative left lateral view.

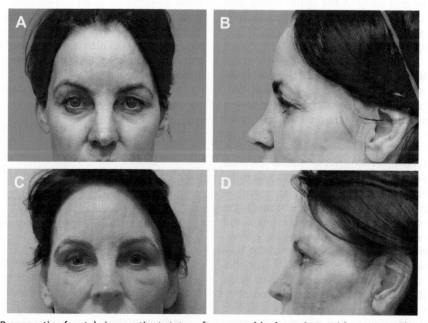

Fig. 17. (*A*) Preoperative frontal view, patient status after upper blepharoplasty with recurrent dermatochalasia. (*B*) Preoperative view, left lateral view. (*C*) Postoperative frontal view, patient status after revision upper blepharoplasty and cell-assisted fat transfer. (*D*) Postoperative left lateral view.

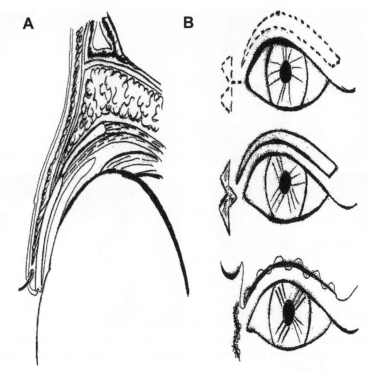

Fig. 18. (*A*) Midsagittal section of Asian upper eyelid with no crease. The orbital septum is not fused to the levator aponeurosis above the tarsal plate. (*B*) Medial epicanthoplasty as described by Flowers.[36]

3. Lack of fibrous attachments across the levator aponeurosis to the orbicularis oculi and the dermis of the eyelid
4. Excessive and laxity of the upper eyelid skin caused by overhanging of the preaponeurotic fat over the fusion point
5. Medial epicanthal folds.

The Asian eyelid and periorbita have been described as double eyelid folds, no eyelid fold, medial epicanthal folds, lateral hooding, or having high medial brows. The Asian medial epicanthal folds have been classified into 4 categories by Flowers [39]: type I, in which the medial canthus is exposed; type II, in which the medial canthus and fold form the same line; type III, in which the canthal fold covers the medial canthus completely; and type IV or pseudo I, in which the eyelid fold completely covers the lid margin, and a tight band of skin covers the medial corner. Flowers described a modified version of the V-W medial epicanthoplasty by Ochida[40] for the correction of the Asian medial epicanthal folds (see **Fig. 18**B). There are other description of Z-plasty or Y-V-plasty in the literature as well.[41,42] In the preoperative evaluation, pay close attention to the position of the medial brow in patients with blepharoptosis. It is common for Asian patients

with eyelid ptosis to develop a persistent medial brow elevation and lateral brow ptosis. This characteristic gives the appearance of a straight brow as opposed to an arched brow. A standard Asian blepharoplasty without correction of the eyelid ptosis, lateral brow ptosis with brow lift, and release of the medial insertions of the frontalis muscle leads to an unaesthetic outcome and an unhappy patient.

The goals in Asian eyelid surgery are outlined as follows (**Fig. 19**):

1. Create an upper eyelid crease that is lower in position relative to Whites'
2. Correction of the medial epicanthal canopy
3. Create a high arched lateral brow relative to the medial brow
4. Removal of excessive skin and fat.

The steps in Asian blepharoplasty are described as follows:

1. Skin markings in a lazy S-shape, the tip down medially and tip up laterally, vertical height centrally at 2 mm, the inferior margin of the marking at the level of the superior edge of the tarsal plate centrally
2. Skin excision with 2 to 3 mm of the pretarsal obicularis oculi muscle

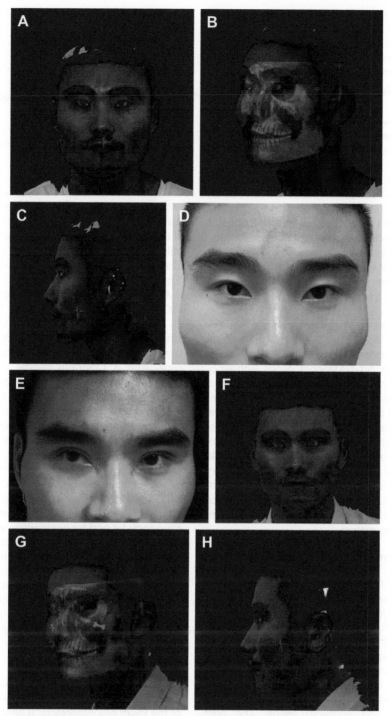

Fig. 19. (*A*) Preoperative 3D frontal view, Asian upper eyelid with medial epicanthal fold, malar, and mandibular angle hyperplasia. (*B*) Preoperative 3D fused left oblique view. (*C*) Preoperative 3D left lateral view. (*D*) Preoperative frontal view. (*E*) Postoperative frontal view, patient status after upper Asian blepharoplasty with medial epicanthoplasty, Malar and mandibular angle reduction. (*F*) Postoperative 3D frontal view. (*G*) Postoperative 3D fused left oblique view. (*H*) Postoperative 3D left lateral view.

3. Opening of the orbital septum in a horizontal fashion with excision of the preaponeurosis fat
4. Suturing of the dermis of superior margin to the levator aponeurosis and then to the dermis of the inferior margin
5. Skin closure.

Postoperative Care and Complications

Cold compresses are applied with a saline-soaked gauze and ice over the gauze for the first 48 hours on and off. This practice reduces the postoperative edema. Make sure the patient is able to count their fingers and is not complaining of severe pain, which are the signs for retrobulbar hemorrhage. If a patient is diagnosed with retrobulbar hematoma, a bedside opening of the incision should be performed immediately, diuresis is initiated with manitol, and IV steroids started to reduce edema and retinal and optic nerve damage. An emergent ophthalmologic consultation is required, and the patient should be taken to the operating room emergently for exploration and control of bleeding. If patients complain of dry eyes, initiate artificial tears as needed throughout the day and ophthalmic ointment during sleep. Patients may initially have lagophthalmos, with exposure keratitis. Patients should sleep with the head of their bed elevated and should not participate in strenuous activity for the first 2 weeks. Any suture removal is performed after 7 days. Antibiotic ointment over the eyelid incisions should be avoided because of possibility of granuloma formation. Reading should be minimized to no more than 5 to 10 minutes every hour to reduce eye strain and sclera edema formation. Other complications include wound dehiscence or infection, temporary eyelash eversion, and epithelial suture cyst formation.

REJUVENATION OF THE LOWER EYELID

In evaluating patients for lower lid blepharoplasty, you should also assess the position of the lower lids, degree of laxity of the lower lids, the position of the lid-cheek junction, and volume of midfacial tissue. There are multiple surgical approaches to the rejuvenation of the lower eyelid, including the transconjunctival or supraciliary approach and a combination as described by Fagien[43] with or without addressing the lateral suspension of the lower eyelids and midfacial tissue. The best approach is dependent on the effects of aging on the periorbital tissue and the surgeon's technical ability. Lateral canthal dystopia can be corrected with either canthopexy for mild to moderate dystopia and release of the canthal attachment with canthoplasty for moderate to severe dystopia.[44,45] The main goals in lower eyelid rejuvenation are:

1. Restore the horizontal length of the eyelid fissure
2. The position of the lower lid is restored at the lower limbus or just below it
3. The lateral canthal attachment is higher then the medial canthal attachment
4. There is a smooth transition between lower lid and cheek
5. The lid-cheek junction is elevated and the cheek develops a natural convexity.

Transconjunctival Approach

With the transconjunctival technique, the surgeon can address the herniated fat pads, resuspension of the lateral canthal tendon, excision of the lateral obicularis oculi muscle, elevation of the midfacial tissue, and restoration of the lower lid height with a graft.

After administration of 1% xylocaine with 1/100,000 epinephrine and waiting for 10 minutes for both hemostasis and anesthesia, a transconjunctival incision is made in the palpebral conjunctiva halfway between the fornix and inferior tarsal plate with a Colorado needle. The dissection should carry through the capsulopalpebral fascia and be retracted superiorly. Next, the fat pads are identified with digital pressure. The orbital septum is opened directly over each fat pad with Westcott scissors, and the nasal, central, and temporal fat pads are teased out, clamped, excised, and cauterized. Care should be taken not to injure the inferior oblique muscle, which separates the nasal and central fat pads. The amount of excised fat differs in each patient and the surgeon should save each fat pad for comparison with the contralateral side. Also, the excised fat pads can be used as autogenous fat transfer to the SOOF or tear trough area, with suture fixation or insertion into an elevated pocket.[46,47] Hemostasis is meticulously checked and the palpebral conjunctiva may be closed with a fat-absorbing gut suture, with the knots placed internally so as not to irritate the cornea (**Fig. 20**).

Canthoplasty

If a lateral canthal suspension is necessary as part of the lower blepharoplasty, a canthopexy or canthoplasty can be performed in conjunction with the transconjunctival approach. The canthopexy is discussed later with the subciliary and combination approach. A canthoplasty is performed by releasing the lateral canthal thickening attachment with a lateral canthotomy. A 0.8-cm to 1.0-cm incision is made in the lateral canthus and the skin flaps are elevated. Westcott scissors are used to

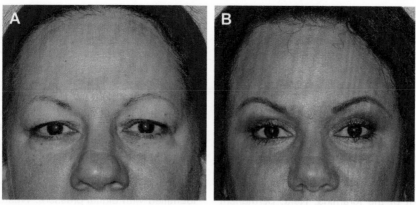

Fig. 20. (*A*) Preoperative frontal view, patient with upper and lower dermatochalasia and brow ptosis. (*B*) Postoperative frontal view, patient status after upper and lower blepharoplasty, limited incision brow lift and endonasal rhinoplasty.

sever the lateral canthus. The lateral retaining ligament is exposed for 0.5 to 1 mm by excising the conjunctival and skin epithelium depending on how lax and droopy the lower lid is. The lateral obicularis oculi muscle is incised elliptically, exposing the lateral orbital periosteum. A 4-0 polypropylene suture is used for a 3-point fixation from the inferior to the superior lateral retaining ligament then to the edge of the lateral orbital periosteum in a more posterior superior position relative to its insertion. Make sure your knot is buried and does not penetrate through the skin or conjunctiva. The edges of the obicularis oculi muscle are approximated with resorbable sutures and the skin closed with fast absorbing gut sutures (**Fig. 21**).

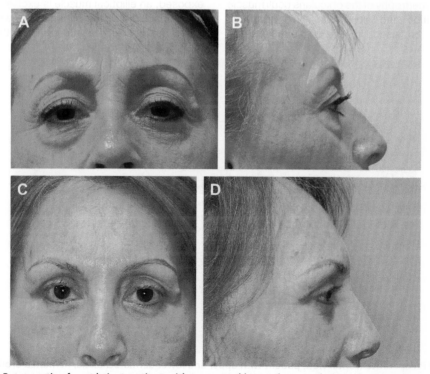

Fig. 21. (*A*) Preoperative frontal view, patient with upper and lower dermatochalasia, herniated orbital fat pads, lower lid laxity, brow ptosis, midfacial hypoplasia, and ptosis. (*B*) Preoperative right lateral view. (*C*) Postoperative frontal view, patient status after upper blepharoplasty, lower lid transconjunctival blepharoplasty with lateral canthoplasty, endoscopic brow and midface lift with autologous fat transfer. (*D*) Postoperative right lateral view.

If a midfacial lift is deemed necessary you may access the orbital rim and midface through your transconjunctival approach. After removal of the herniated fat pads, the capsulopalpebral fascia is retracted superiorly and the lid margin inferiorly. A malleable retractor is used to identify the inferior orbital rim. A Colorado tip is used to incise the periosteum 1 to 2 mm below the orbital rim in a preseptal fashion. A periosteal elevator is used to elevate the midfacial periosteum, including the attachments for the orbital retaining ligament, zygomatic ligaments, and soft tissue. Care should be taken to preserve the inferior orbital nerve and vasculature emerging out of the foramina. Next, permanent sutures such as 4-0 polypropylene are used to elevate the periosteum below the orbital retaining ligaments and suture fixated to the arcus marginalis of the inferior orbital rim. Autologous fat transfer can be performed to volumize the SOOF and the malar and nasolabial fat pads. If the midfacial descent is severe, consider performing an endoscopic midface lift with volumization in conjunction with your blepharoplasty (**Fig. 22**).

Subciliary Approach

The subciliary technique should be considered when the patient has formed excessive lower lid skin with hypertrophy of the obicularis oculi muscle or attenuation and elongation. This approach may also be used in conjunction with the transconjunctival approach. A lateral canthopexy may also be performed simultaneously.

After administration of 1% xylocaine with 1/100,000 epinephrine and waiting for 10 minutes for both hemostasis and anesthesia, an incision is made just below the lashes from medial to lateral then extending out to the lateral canthal skin. Dissection is carried down to the preseptal obicularis oculi muscle, and the skin flap is elevated in an inferior and lateral direction. Westcott scissors are used to penetrate the obicularis oculi muscle, and an incision is made along the incision line. The superior flap is elevated and the fat pads are identified with digital pressure. Westcott scissors are used to open the orbital septum and the fat pads teased out and clamped, cut, and cauterized. Next, a strip of the preseptal obicularis oculi muscle is excised from the inferior flap margin as deemed necessary. The skin flap is elevated in a superior lateral direction and marked. Excess skin is excised and the incision line closed with a 6-0 nylon suture in a running fashion (**Fig. 23**).

Canthopexy

Canthopexy may be performed simultaneously with the subciliary approach. After the skin flap is elevated and the lateral obicularis oculi muscle exposed, an elliptical muscle is excised, exposing the retinaculum at the commissure, which is just below the muscle. The inferior flap with obicularis

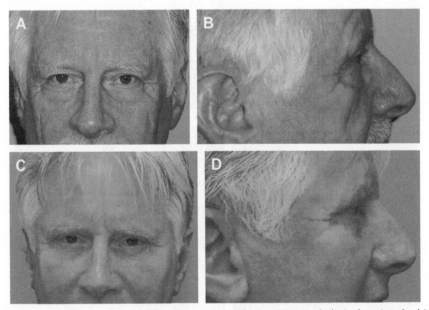

Fig. 22. (*A*) Preoperative frontal view, patient with upper and lower dermatochalasia, herniated orbital fat pads, lower lid laxity, lateral lower lid retraction, midfacial hypoplasia, and ptosis. (*B*) Preoperative right lateral view. (*C*) Postoperative frontal view, patient status after upper blepharoplasty, lower lid transconjunctival blepharoplasty with lateral canthoplasty, CO_2 fractionated laser resurfacing, endoscopic midface lift with autologous fat transfer. (*D*) Postoperative right lateral view.

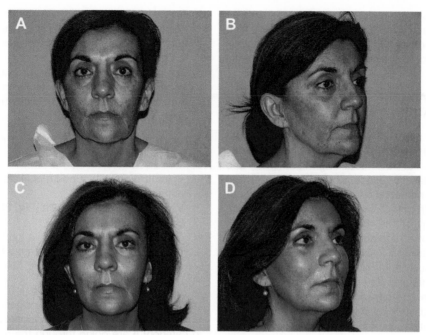

Fig. 23. (*A*) Preoperative frontal view, patient with lower lid dermatochalasia, herniated orbital fat pads, lower lid laxity, midfacial hypoplasia, and ptosis. (*B*) Preoperative right oblique view. (*C*) Postoperative frontal view, patient status after lower lid subciliary blepharoplasty with lateral canthopexy, endoscopic midface lift with autologous fat transfer. (*D*) Postoperative right oblique view.

oculi muscle is elevated from the retinaculum, which allows for the elevation of the muscle. A 4-0 polypropylene suture is used to elevate the superior obicularis oculi muscle to the incision and retinaculum at the commissure via a mattress suture in a superior lateral vector to the lateral orbital rim area. Next, the obicularis muscle inferior to the excision is elevated and sutured to its superior edge and the retinaculum ligament below it with a resorbable suture in a 3-point fixation technique. Excess skin is excised and closed as described earlier.

Combination of Transconjunctival and Subciliary Approach

A combination of the transconjunctival and subciliary approach has been described. This technique can be used when the patient requires a combination of midfacial lift, excision of obicularis oculi muscle, excision of excessive skin, or canthoplasty/canthopexy.

Postoperative Care and Complications

Cold compresses are applied with a saline-soaked gauze and ice over the gauze for the first 48 hours on and off. This procedure reduces the postoperative edema. Make sure the patient is able to count their fingers and is not complaining of severe pain,

which are the signs for retrobulbar hemorrhage. A lateral canthotomy is performed bedside if a patient is diagnosed with retrobulbar hematoma, diuresis is initiated with manitol, and IV steroids started to reduce edema and retinal and optic nerve damage. An emergent ophthalmologic consultation is required and the patient should be taken to the operating room emergently for exploration and control of bleeding. If patients complain of dry eyes, initiate artificial tears as needed throughout the day and ophthalmic ointment during sleep. The patient should sleep with the head of their bed elevated and should not participate in strenuous activity for the first 2 weeks. Any suture removal is performed after 7 days. Antibiotic ointment over the eyelid incisions should be avoided because of the possibility of granuloma formation. Reading should be minimized to no more than 5 to 10 minutes every hour to reduce eye strain and sclera edema formation. Homeopathic over-the-counter medications such as arnica gel and pills are recommended to reduce ecchymosis and its duration. Other complications that can occur are ectropion and lid retraction with an external approach. Careful preoperative evaluation for horizontal lid laxity and minimal skin excision are the best preventive measures. Immediate postoperative tarsorraphy suture and lid massage improve the outcome. If the patients continue to have problems, then skin grafting, tarsal strip procedures, cheek lift, and volumization may be necessary. Loss of eyelashes and suture cysts are also possible postoperatively.

THE MIDFACE IN PERIORBITAL REJUVENATION

The aging process affects the midfacial tissue by slight resorption of midfacial bone convexity, attenuation of the retaining ligaments and investing fascial tissue, loss of volume and atrophy of midfacial fat compartments, attenuation and atrophy of muscle of facial expression, and atrophy of the dermatocutis complex with formation of rhytids and furrows. Not all of these components are affected in the aging face simultaneously and to the same degree. Evaluate your patients and determine which components need to be addressed in your surgical plan. A natural and youthful midface has the following characteristics:

1. The transition point between the lower eyelid and cheek is at the lid-cheek junction, which is concave and smooth, with no hollowness or flattening.

2. The midface has a convex surface and its height of contour is located at the most superior and lateral point, where the malar complex and the arch transition.
3. The transition point between the cheek and the upper lip is at the nasolabial region, which is concave and smooth without furrows and deep grooves.

I have classified patients in need of midfacial procedures into 5 categories:

I. Volumization with subdermal fillers or autogenous fat (**Fig. 24**)
II. Volumization and fascial lift (**Fig. 25**)
III. Fascial lift
IV. Osteoplasty with implant augmentation or autogenous or cadaver bone (see **Fig. 7**)
V. Combination of volumization, fascial lift, and osteoplasty.

Patients in categories I and IV are generally young patients with congenital facial hypoplasia; patients in category II are going through the normal aging process; patients in category III are slightly obese or have hyperplastic tissues; and patients in category V are going through a normal or accelerated aging process and have facial bone hypoplasia.

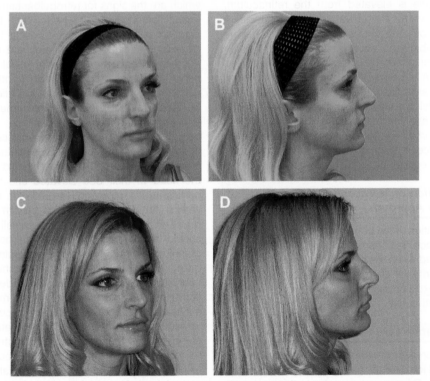

Fig. 24. (*A*) Preoperative right oblique view, patient with malar hypoplasia. (*B*) Preoperative right lateral view. (*C*) Postoperative right oblique view, patient status after subdermal fillers to the midface. (*D*) Postoperative right lateral view.

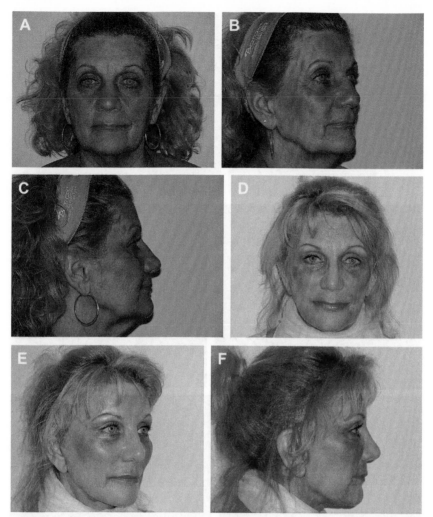

Fig. 25. (*A*) Preoperative frontal view, patient with periorbital, perioral, face, and neck age-related changes. (*B*) Preoperative right oblique view. (*C*) Preoperative right lateral view. (*D*) Postoperative frontal view, patient status after upper and lower lid transconjunctival blepharoplasty, endoscopic brow and midface lift, face and neck lift with SMAS and platysmal plication and autologous fat transfer. (*E*) Postoperative right oblique view. (*F*) Postoperative right lateral view.

For facial bone osteoplasty, I routinely use Medpor (Porex Surgical, Stryker) implants with fixation.[48] The orbital rim, malar, paranasal, or a combination of these anatomic implants can be used. Facial volumization is discussed in the following sections.

Endoscopic Midface Lift

The midface can be addressed simultaneously with lower blepharoplasty or brow-lift procedures. The endoscopic midface procedure addresses the following areas: lid-cheek junction, tear trough deformity, palpebral-malar groove, nasolabial folds, downturning of the commissure of the lip, central upper lip area, and alar base with nasal tip (**Fig. 26**). I perform a modification of Ramirez's endoscopic assisted midfacial lift.[49] I perform

a wider transvestibular incision, with wider dissection and incorporation of the alar base cinch suture with V-Y closure.[50] The technical steps are described as follows:

- Temporal brow incision as described for endoscopic brow lift
- Deep temporal fascial dissection with sentinel vein identification and preservation
- Release of zygo-orbicular ligament
- Forehead and brow dissection and muscle resection for a forehead and brow lift as needed
- Subciliary or transconjunctival incisions with removal of fat pads
- Release of arcus marginalis and orbital retaining ligaments

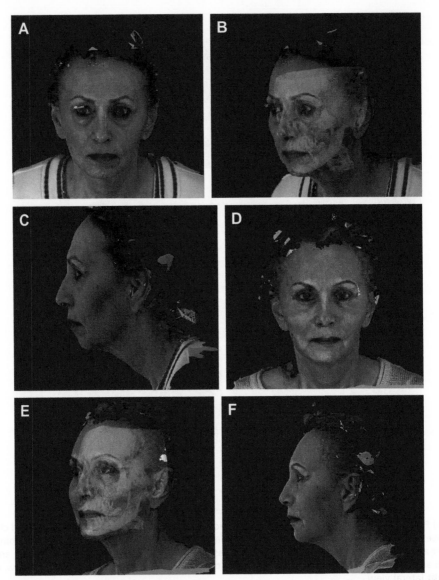

Fig. 26. (*A*) Preoperative 3D frontal view, patient with upper and lower lid dermatochalasia, lower lid laxity, brow ptosis, midfacial hypoplasia, ptosis, and retrogenia. (*B*) Preoperative 3D fused left oblique view. (*C*) Preoperative 3D left lateral view. (*D*) Postoperative 3D frontal view, patient status after upper and lower lid transconjunctival blepharoplasty, endoscopic brow and midface lift, autologous fat transfer, and sliding genioplasty. (*E*) Postoperative 3D fused left oblique view. (*F*) Postoperative 3D left lateral view.

- Maxillary vestibular incision from first molar to first molar with subperiosteal dissection
- Release of zygomatic and mesenteric ligaments with dissection of the buccal fat pads
- Connection of the temporal and zygomatic-maxillary pockets via subperiosteal dissection over the zygomatic arch
- Facial bone osteoplasty as needed
- Midface elevation and suture fixation of SOOF, malar fat pad, and buccal fat pad to the deep

temporal fascia in a superior-posterior vector with a 4-0 polypropylene suture
- Autologous fat transfer as needed
- Canthopexy or canthoplasty as needed
- Closure of temporal incision
- Closure of lower eyelid incisions with or without skin resection
- Alar base cinch suture and V-Y maxillary vestibular closure
- If combined with brow lift, drains are routinely used.

Postoperative Care and Complications

Scalp incisions are dressed with antibiotic ointment. If drains are used, they can be removed in 24 to 72 hours postoperatively. Paper tape is used on the midface and lateral brow area to minimize edema, with a head wrap, which can be removed in 72 hours. Drains are removed within 48 to 72 hours. Have patients sleep with their bedhead elevated for a minimum of 2 weeks. Patients should be given artificial tears and ophthalmic ointment in case dry eyes or lagophthalmos develops. Ice packs over the forehead, midface, and eyes should be used routinely to reduce postoperative edema. Oral rinse with cholorohexadine gluconate with strict oral hygiene and a soft diet are recommended. There should be no suction on straws for the first week. Patients may shower fully after 72 hours. Patient should not participate in strenuous activity for the first 2 weeks. Any suture removal is performed after 7 days. Postoperative complications of endoscopic midface lift are similar to the brow-lift procedure.

PERIORBITAL REJUVENATION WITH AUTOLOGOUS FAT TRANSFER

The use of autologous fat for correction of contour irregularities in reconstructive facial surgery dates back to the late nineteenth century.[51] The results were unpredictable, with fat resorption and local regional adverse effects such as cyst and fibrous tissue formation. The procedure fell out of favor until after the 1980s with the advent of liposuction.[52] The procedure was still unpredictable, with near-complete resorption of the fat, until Coleman[53] described the atraumatic technique of lipoaspirate harvest and injection techniques to preserve the fragile adipocytes. This technique has reduced the fat resorption rate and has made the facial volumization technique with autologous fat a more predictable procedure. The technique is described as:

- harvesting with low negative pressure
- purifying the lipoaspirate by washing out with normal saline and centrifugation
- placing minimal amounts of adipocytes in multiple tunnels.

Recent studies on fat tissue indicate that it contains not only adipocytes but also preadipocytes, endothelial cells, fibroblasts, and adipose-derived adult mesenchymal stem cells (ADSCs), which are multipotent cells that are capable of differentiating into neural, cartilage, bone, fat, and connective tissues.[54] Fat tissue contains the largest amount of multipotent and adult stem cells per area compared with bone marrow and other tissues. This finding indicates that isolated ADSCs from fat tissue can provide a basis for regenerative medicine. Scientific evidence suggest that ADSCs produce and secrete cytokines such as platelet-derived growth factor, transforming growth factor β, vascular endothelial growth factor, epidermal growth factor, and insulin-like growth factor. These growth factors induce autocrine and paracrine effects in their surroundings, promoting angiogenesis and wound healing. ADSCs can be isolated from lipoaspirate via an enzymatic digestion technique and centrifuged to separate the multipotent cells into stromal vascular fraction (SVF) cells.[55] In the laboratory, the SVF cells should adhere to a Petri dish, grow and replicate, and produce CD34 and CD 90 cell surface markers to identify as ADSCs. This technique can be performed in an accredited office-based outpatient surgical center under good manufacturing practice and must adhere to the Code of Federal Regulations (CFR) (US Food and Drug Administration [FDA] CFR title 21 part 1271) for use in a physician's practice. The SVF contains millions of isolated ADSCs that could be used for tissue regeneration. Studies have shown that enriched fat graft with SVF has increased adipose cell survival and retention of the graft via increased vascularization.[56] Other applications of ADSCs include direct injection of SVF into the dermis with increases in extracellular collagen, elastin production, and fibroblast, which reduce wrinkles and improve skin quality.[57] ADSCs are under investigation in the orthopedic, cardiovascular, urology, endocrinology, and neurology fields.

The latest technique in facial volumization with autologous fat transfer is cell-assisted lipotransfer (CAL). CAL is the enrichment of autologous fat graft with ADSCs. The technique involves removal of 300 to 500 mL of lipoaspirate via a tumescent suction-assisted liposuction technique. The harvested lipoaspirate is washed with normal saline through a filter and centrifuged. This procedure yields approximately 100 mL harvest lipoaspirate ready for use. Approximately 25 to 50 mL of the washed, filtered, and centrifuged lipoaspirate is treated with collagenase for enzymatic separation of the SVF cells from the adipose cells. The isolated SVF cells are then mixed with the remaining 50 mL prepared lipoaspirate for injections or directly injected into the dermis for aesthetic facial volumization or regenerative skin changes. The enriched lipoaspirate is injected via 1-mL Luer lock syringes and a blunt cannula into the forehead, temporal fat pads, ROOF, supraorbital rim, glabella, SOOF, malar and nasolabial fat pads, or other desired areas. Also, the SVF is injected directly into the dermis in an area approximately 1 cm^2 by creating a wheel under the skin (**Fig. 27**).

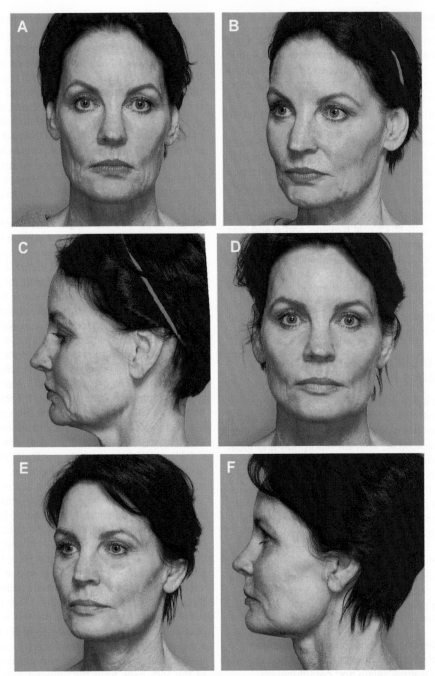

Fig. 27. (*A*) Preoperative frontal view. Patient status after upper blepharoplasty and neck lift presents with recurrent upper lid dermatochalasia, jowls, platysmal diastasis, age-related skin and soft tissue atrophy. (*B*) Preoperative left oblique view. (*C*) Preoperative left lateral view. (*D*) Postoperative frontal view, patient status after revision upper blepharoplasty, revision neck lift with suture suspension, cell-assisted fat transfer to the face. (*E*) Postoperative left oblique view. (*F*) Postoperative left lateral view.

THE ROLE OF SUBDERMAL FILLERS IN PERIORBITAL REJUVENATION

For any particular reason, patients might not choose autogenous volumization or might not be good or healthy candidates for aesthetic surgical rejuvenation. Subdermal fillers are alternative to autogenous volumization, and both patients and physicians may levitate toward them. The injectable industry is a billion-dollar market in the United

States and is growing daily. The number one procedure performed by aesthetic surgeons across the country is injectables. On the market there are multiple injectable products, and each subdermal filler has its advantages and disadvantages for use in a particular anatomic area. It is beyond the scope of this article to review all products that are FDA-approved in the market. Please review the insert in each product for indications, directions, and use. The products are divided into synthetic, nonsynthetic, resorbable, and nonresorbable. The resorbable nonpermanent nonsynthetic biodegradable fillers on the market and FDA-approved are bovine collagen (xenograft) (eg, Zyderm/Zyplast), porcine collagen (xenograft) (eg, Evolence), and human collagen (autologous graft) (eg, Dermalogen). The resorbable nonpermanent synthetic biodegradable fillers on the market and FDA-approved are hyaluronic acid (eg, Restylane or Juvederm), calcium hydroxylapatite beads (eg, Radiesse), and poly-L-lactic acid (eg, Sculptra). The permanent synthetic nonbiodegradable fillers on the market and FDA-approved are poly(methyl methacrylate) microspheres (eg, Artefill) and acrylic hydrogel (eg, DermaLive and DermaDeep).

The most common areas for subdermal filler injections are the temporal area, the brow, the tear trough, malar pads and the nasolabial folds, the nose, lips, marionette lines, prejowls, jaw line, and the chin. Each area has an ideal product for injection volumization depending on its properties; for example, hyaluronic acid is ideal for tear trough deformity because the material flows well, has a low viscosity, and the soft tissue is thin and unforgiving. Calcium hydroxylapatite is ideal for malar augmentation because the product is highly viscous, the tissues are thick, and longevity is needed (see **Fig. 24**).

The classification of complications of subdermal fillers include immediate, long-term, allergic reaction, and poor technique. After injection, patients may develop swelling, edema, erythema, and bruising immediately. This is a normal outcome after injection, and the recommended treatment is palliative care and use of homeopathic medications, gels, and creams. Long-term complications include dissatisfaction with results and granuloma formation, which could be caused by infection or foreign body reaction. The recommended treatment is steroid injection, antihistamines, and digital pressure.[58] Patients who develop an allergic reaction should be treated with steroids, antihistamines, and palliative care. Allergies should be reported and documented. For known products such as Zyderm/Zyplast, preinjection allergic testing should be performed. With poor injection techniques or using dermal filler for an anatomic area that is not recommended, a patient can develop beading, ridging, and nodule formation. Instruct patients to perform deep tissue massage immediately to disperse the product or use dissolving or digesting enzymes such as hyaluronidase (Vitrase) for hyaluronic acid.[59] Other complications such as intravascular and perivascular injections have been described. Patients may develop embolic events and skin necrosis. If embolic events with neurologic symptoms are present, immediate emergent evaluation and treatment are recommended. If a patient develops vascular insufficiency, the initial signs are poor capillary refill of the tissue followed by epidermolysis and hyperemia. Skin necrosis and scarring can ensue. The recommended treatment is recognition and treatment with enzymatic degradation intravascularly or vascularly if indicated, followed by aspirin therapy, nitropaste application, warm compresses, and local wound care as needed. If patients develop paresthesia after injection, enzymatic degradation if indicated followed by steroid therapy is recommended. The best method of prevention of neurovascular injury is to use a blunt syringe for injections and inject while moving forward to push away the neurovascular structure or advance aspirate, then inject in increments while pulling out.[60]

LASER SKIN RESURFACING IN PERIORBITAL REJUVENATION

Laser skin resurfacing can be used as an adjunct to periorbital rejuvenation. I routinely incorporate laser resurfacing with transconjunctival blepharoplasty to induce skin contractures as well as rejuvenation. This adjunct has allowed me to decrease the number of occasions for performing skin resection with lower blepharoplasty unless the patient presents with a significant amount of skin excess, laxity, and hypertrophic obicularis oculi muscle. I perform the laser skin resurfacing on the same surgical day or wait until the patient's edema and ecchymosis have subsided. The decision is based on the amount of swelling and bruising immediately after the treatment (see **Fig. 22**).

Whether a conservative treatment plan such as botulin toxin and dermal fillers is planned or complete surgical rejuvenation, laser resurfacing can be used to improve outcome and treat the atrophic changes in the skin. These age-related atrophic skin changes are (**Fig. 28**)[16]:

- Decrease in the thickness of the dermis with loss of type I collagen
- Decrease in elastin protein with loss of skin elasticity

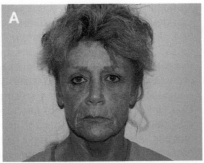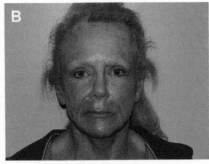

Fig. 28. (*A*) Preoperative frontal view, patient with age-related skin atrophy. (*B*) Postoperative frontal view, patient status after CO_2 fractionated laser resurfacing.

- Increase in the thickness of the epidermal layer with a decrease in the basal layer
- Discoloration of the skin (dyschromia) with increased rate of hyperpigmentation
- Sun damage with formation of actinic keratosis spots.

The 2 wavelengths of laser in common use for skin resurfacing are pulsed carbon dioxide (CO_2) at 10,600 nm and erbium:yttrium aluminum garnet (YAG) at 2940 nm. Laser physics are beyond the scope of this article, but both CO_2 and erbium:YAG laser are both absorbed by water molecules (chromophore) in the tissue and create selective photothermolysis.[61] These ablative lasers remove all of the epidermis and varying thicknesses of the dermis. Healing is from the skin appendages. Fractionated photothermolysis with ablation or ablation-fractionated laser (AFL) is the new treatment of skin rejuvenation.[62] AFL creates alternating columns of ablative photothermolysis of the epidermis and dermis called microthermal zones and nontreated columns. This selective treatment allows for faster healing from the side tissues and decreased complications of ablative lasers. This situation means less downtime and fewer complications, but results are comparable with the ablative lasers.

Patient selection, prelaser preparation, and postlaser follow-up of the patient are crucial in obtaining optimal results and avoiding unhappy patients and the risk of potential litigation. Patients with Fitzpatrick type I to III are the ideal candidates for laser resurfacing. I routinely pretreat my patients with 4% to 8% hydroquinone and Retin-A 0.025% cream for a minimum of 2 weeks before their ablative laser treatment. This strategy reduces postoperative hyperpigmentation and possible increase in healing potential and allows the skin to peel its dead, sun-damaged stratum corneum layer off for even penetration of the laser photons.[63,64] Orringer and colleagues[65] found no evidence of enhanced collagen formation, accelerated re-epithelialization, or quicker resolution of postoperative erythemia with tretinoin pretreatment before laser resurfacing. In my practice, I stop the creams 3 days before laser treatment to allow the inflammation to subside. Make sure your patients are not taking isotretinoin for 6 to 12 months before laser resurfacing, because it increases the risk of hypertrophic scarring by reducing the skin appendages for healing.[66] One can argue that with AFL treatment the healing is not completely dependent on the skin appendages but from the surrounding untraumatized epithelium. I routinely use antiviral antibiotics prophylactically against herpes simplex virus. Make sure your patients do not have active skin infection or multiple acne vulgaris lesions. Avoid smokers, because their healing potential is poor.

The procedure is performed under sedation or topical and local facial anesthetic block. I use nonreflective metal corneal shields to protect the eyes. Prevent oxygen pooling around your drapes with wet towels around the patient if supplemental oxygen is given in an open circuit. This strategy prevents laser fires. Use smoke evacuators with filters and a cooling device for patient comfort. Follow the American National Standard Institute and Occupational Safety Health and Administration laser safety standards.

Postoperatively, pain is generally not an issue with AFL treatments because the patient is not left with totally raw skin; patients complain of an intense burning sensation only after the first 2 hours. Immediately after treatment, apply Aquaphor cream mixed with small amounts of topical anesthetic on the treated areas. This strategy relieves the patient of the intense burning that ensues after laser treatment. Patients are instructed to keep a thin layer of Aquaphor continuously until the skin spontaneously peels off. This event usually happens within 3 to 7 days after laser depending on the intensity of the treatment.

Patients are given strict instructions to avoid sun and strenuous activity. Use of sun-blocking agents with zinc oxide and titanium oxide is crucial because theses agents block all ultraviolet rays. Patients are started on 4% to 8% hydroquinone with or without 1% hydrocortisone cream after they have peeled to reduce hyperpigmentation, inflammation, edema, and potential scarring. Patients with intense itching are prescribed 1% hydrocortisone cream with oral hydroxyzine. Patients are instructed to use skin moisturizers throughout the day to keep the skin hydrated after they have peels. Patients are also allowed to use mineral-based makeup several days after peeling.

REFERENCES

1. von Graefe CF. De rhinoplastic, P 13. Berlin: Reime; 1818.
2. Wood C. The Tadhkirat of Ali ibn Isa of Baghdad (trans). Chicago: Northwestern University; 1936. p. 98, 115, 118–9.
3. Gunter J, Antrobus S. Aesthetic analysis of the eyebrow. Plast Reconstr Surg 1997;99:1808–16.
4. Warren R. Non-endoscopic limited incision brow lift. In: Aston SJ, Steinbrech DS, Walden JL, editors. Aesthetic plastic surgery. Philadelphia: Saunders Elsevier; 2009. p. 263–73.
5. Putterman AM. Evaluation of the cosmetic oculoplastic surgery patient. In: Fagien S, editor. Putterman's cosmetic oculoplastic surgery. 4th edition. Philadelphia: Saunders Elsevier; 2008. p. 21–30.
6. Putterman AM, Chalfin J. Ocular asymmetry measuring device. Ophthalmology 1979;86:1203–8.
7. Putterman AM, Urist MJ. Müller muscle-conjunctiva resection. Arch Ophthalmol 1975;94:619–23.
8. Olson JJ, Putterman AM. Loss of vertical palpebral fissure height on downgaze in acquired blepharoptosis. Arch Ophthalmol 1995;113:1293–7.
9. Putterman AM. Basic oculoplastic surgery. In: Peyman GA, Sanders DR, Goldberg MF, editors. Principles and practice of ophthalmology. Philadelphia: WB Sanders; 1980. p. 2248–50.
10. Haddock NT, Saadeh PB, Boutros S, et al. The tear trough and lid/cheek junction: anatomy and implications for surgical correction. Plast Reconstr Surg 2009;123(4):1332–40 [discussion: 1341–2].
11. Flowers RS. Tear trough implants for correction of tear trough deformity. Clin Plast Surg 1993;20:403–15.
12. Levine RA, Garza JR, Wang PT, et al. Adult facial growth: applications to aesthetic surgery. Aesthetic Plast Surg 2003;27(4):265–8.
13. Bartlett SP, Grossman R, Whitaker LA. Age-related changes of the craniofacial skeleton: an anthropometric and histologic analysis. Plast Reconstr Surg 1992;90(4):592–600.
14. Farkas LG, Eiben OG, Sivkov S, et al. Anthropometric measurements of the facial framework in adulthood: age-related changes in eight age categories in 600 healthy white North Americans of European ancestry from 16 to 90 years of age. J Craniofac Surg 2004;15(2):288–98.
15. Vleggaar D, Fitzgerald R. Dermatological implications of skeletal aging: a focus on supraperiosteal volumization for perioral rejuvenation. J Drugs Dermatol 2008;7(3):209–20.
16. Kahn DM, Shaw RB. Overview of current thoughts on facial volume and aging. Facial Plast Surg 2010;26(5):350–5.
17. Penna V, Stark GB, Eisenhardt SU, et al. The aging lip: a comparative histological analysis of age-related changes in the upper lip complex. Plast Reconstr Surg 2009;124(2):624–8.
18. Lee H, Park M, Lee J, et al. Histopathologic findings of the orbicularis oculi in upper eyelid aging: total or minimal excision of orbicularis oculi in upper blepharoplasty. Arch Facial Plast Surg 2011. [Epub ahead of print].
19. Gierloff M, Stöhring C, Buder T, et al. Aging changes of the midfacial fat compartments: a computed tomographic study. Plast Reconstr Surg 2012; 129(1):263–73.
20. Elkwood A, Matarasso A, Rankin M, et al. National plastic surgery survey: brow lifting techniques and complications. Plast Reconstr Surg 2001;108: 2143–50.
21. Romo T, Sclafani AP, Yung RT, et al. Endoscopic foreheadplasty: a histologic comparison of periosteal refixation after endoscopic versus bicorporal lift. Plast Reconstr Surg 2000;105:1111–7.
22. Hönig JF, Frank MH, Knutti D, et al. Video endoscopic-assisted brow lift: comparison of the eyebrow position after Endotine tissue fixation versus suture fixation. J Craniofac Surg 2008;19(4): 1140–7.
23. Walden JL, Orseck MJ, Aston SJ. Current methods for brow fixation: are they safe? Aesthetic Plast Surg 2006;30(5):541–8.
24. Evans GRD, Kelishadi SS, Ho KU, et al. "Heads up" on brow lift with Coapt Systems' Endotine Forehead technology. Plast Reconstr Surg 2003; 113:1504–5.
25. Chowdhury S, Malhotra R, Smith R, et al. Patient and surgeon experience with the Endotine forehead device for brow and forehead lift. Ophthal Plast Reconstr Surg 2007;23(5):358–62.
26. Langsdon PR, Metzinger SE, Glickstein JS, et al. Transblepharoplasty brow suspension: an expanded role. Ann Plast Surg 2008;60(1):2–5.
27. Tyers AG. Brow lift via the direct and transblepharoplasty approaches. Orbit 2006;25(4):261–5.
28. Hoorntje LE, Lei B, Stollenwerck GA, et al. Resecting orbicularis oculi muscle in upper eyelid

blepharoplasty–a review of the literature. J Plast Reconstr Aesthet Surg 2010;63(5):787–92.

29. Fagien S. Upper blepharoplasty: volume enhancement via skin approach: lowering the lid crease. In: Fagien S, editor. Putterman's cosmetic oculoplastic surgery. 4th edition. Philadelphia: Saunders Elsevier; 2008. p. 87–103.

30. Damasceno RW, Cariello AJ, Cardoso EB, et al. Upper blepharoplasty with or without resection of the orbicularis oculi muscle: a randomized double-blind left-right study. Ophthal Plast Reconstr Surg 2011;27(3):195–7.

31. Mikamo K. A technique in the double eyelid operation. J Chugaishinpo 1896;17:1197.

32. Maruo M. Plastic reconstruction of a "double eyelid" operation in 1523 cases. Jpn J Ophthalmol 1929;24:393.

33. Millard R Jr. Oriental peregrination. Plast Reconstr Surg 1955;16:331.

34. Soyoc BT. Plastic reconstruction of the superior palpebral fold in slit eyes. Am J Ophthalmol 1954;38:556.

35. Fernandez LR. Double eyelid operation in the Oriental in Hawaii. Plast Reconstr Surg 1960;25:257.

36. Flowers RS. Anchor blepharoplasty. Clin Plast Surg 1993;20(2):193–207.

37. Onizuka T, Iwanami M. Blepharoplasty in Japan. Aesthetic Plast Surg 1984;8:97–100.

38. Kakizaki H, Leibovitch I, Selva D, et al. Orbital septum attachment on the levator aponeurosis in Asians: in vivo and cadaver study. Ophthalmology 2009;116(10):2031–5.

39. Flowers RS. Surgical treatment of the epicanthal fold. Plast Reconstr Surg 1983;73:751.

40. Uchida K. The Uchida method for the double eyelid operation in 1523 cases. Jpn J Ophthalmol 1926;30:593.

41. Park JI. Modified Z-epicanthoplasty in the Asian eyelid. Arch Facial Plast Surg 2000;2:43–7.

42. Kao YS, Lin CH, Fang RH. Epicanthoplasty with modified Y-V advancement procedure. Plast Reconstr Surg 1998;102:1835–41.

43. Fagien S. Lower blepharoplasty: blending the lid/cheek junction with orbicularis muscle and lateral retinacular suspension. In: Fagien S, editor. Putterman's cosmetic oculoplastic surgery. 4th edition. Philadelphia: Saunders Elsevier; 2008. p. 161–79.

44. Dailey RA, Chavez MR. Lateral canthoplasty with acellular cadaveric dermal matrix graft (AlloDerm) reinforcement. Ophthal Plast Reconstr Surg 2012;28(1):e29–31.

45. Lessa S, Nanci M. Simple canthopexy used in transconjunctival blepharoplasty. Ophthal Plast Reconstr Surg 2009;25(4):284–8.

46. Grant JR, Laferriere KA. Periocular rejuvenation: lower eyelid blepharoplasty with fat repositioning and the suborbicularis oculi fat. Facial Plast Surg Clin North Am 2010;18(3):399–409.

47. Momosawa A, Kurita M, Ozaki M, et al. Transconjunctival orbital fat repositioning for tear trough deformity in young Asians. Aesthet Surg J 2008;28(3):265–71.

48. Schendel SA, Broujerdi JA. Facial bone sculpturing. In: Ward Booth Peter, Hausamen Jarg-Erich, Schendel Stephen A, editors. Maxillofacial surgery. 2nd edition. St Louis (MO): Churchill Livingstone/Elsevier; 2007. p. 1404–22.

49. Ramirez OM. Three-dimensional endoscopic midface enhancement: a personal quest for the ideal cheek rejuvenation. Plast Reconstr Surg 2002;109(1):329–40 [discussion: 341–9].

50. Schendel SA, Williamson LW. Muscle reorientation following superior repositioning of the maxilla. J Oral Maxillofac Surg 1983;41(4):235–40.

51. Neuber G. Über die Wiederanheilung vollständig vom Körper getrennter, die ganze Fettschicht enthaltender Hautstücke. Zbl F Chirurgie 1893;30:16 [in German].

52. Illouz YG. The fat cell "graft". A new technique to fill depressions. Plast Reconstr Surg 1986;78:122–3.

53. Coleman SR. Long-term survival of fat transplants: controlled demonstrations. Aesthetic Plast Surg 1995;19:421–5.

54. Strem BM, Hicok KC, Zhu M, et al. Multipotential differentiation of adipose tissue-derived stem cells. Keio J Med 2005;54:132–41.

55. Yoshimura K, Shigeura T, Matsumoto D, et al. Characterization of freshly isolated and cultured cells derived from the fatty and fluid portions of liposuction aspirates. J Cell Physiol 2006;208:64–76.

56. Ma Z, Han D, Zhang P, et al. Utilizing muscle-derived stem cells to enhance long-term retention and aesthetic outcome of autologous fat grafting: pilot study in mice. Aesthetic Plast Surg 2011;36(1):186–92.

57. Kim JH, Jung M, Kim HS, et al. Adipose-derived stem cells as a new therapeutic modality for ageing skin. Exp Dermatol 2011;20(5):383–7.

58. Saylan Z. Facial fillers and their complications. Aesthet Surg J 2003;23:221–4.

59. Goodman GJ, Bekhor P, Rich M, et al. A comparison of the efficacy, safety, and longevity of two different hyaluronic acid dermal fillers in the treatment of severe nasolabial folds: a multicenter, prospective, randomized, controlled, single-blind, within-subject study. Clin Cosmet Investig Dermatol 2011;4:197–205.

60. Sclafani AP, Fagien S. Treatment of injectable soft tissue filler complications. Dermatol Surg 2009;35(Suppl 2):1672–80.

61. Papadavid E, Katsambas A. Lasers for facial rejuvenation: a review. Int J Dermatol 2003; 42(6):480–7.

62. Saedi N, Petelin A, Zachary C. Fractionation: a new era in laser resurfacing. Clin Plast Surg 2011;38(3): 449–61.

63. McDonald WS, Beasley D, Jones C. Retinoic acid and CO_2 laser resurfacing. Plast Reconstr Surg 1999;104(7):2229–35.

64. Goldman MP. The use of hydroquinone with facial laser resurfacing. J Cutan Laser Ther 2000;2(2):73–7.

65. Orringer JS, Kang S, Johnson TM, et al. Tretinoin treatment before carbon-dioxide laser resurfacing: a clinical and biochemical analysis. J Am Acad Dermatol 2004;51(6):940–6.

66. Ong MW, Bashir S. Fractional laser resurfacing for acne scars: a review. Br J Dermatol 2012;166(6): 1160–9.

Prosthetic Reconstruction of the Orbit/Globe

Ju Yon Sophie Yi, MD, DDS[a],*, Eric J. Dierks, MD, DMD[b,c,d],
Larry Michael Over, DMD, MSD[e,f], Matthew J. Hauck, MD[g]

KEYWORDS

- Ocular prosthesis • Orbital prosthesis • Orbital implants • Osseointegration • Reconstruction
- Exenteration • Enucleation • Evisceration

KEY POINTS

- When faced with devastating loss of orbital structures owing to tumor, trauma, burns, or congenital reasons, an implant-supported prosthesis is a viable option to an extensive and multistaged tissue reconstruction.
- Careful planning between the oral and maxillofacial surgeon and/or oculoplastic surgeon and the maxillofacial prosthodontist will result in a secure and accurate esthetic reconstruction using an implant-supported prosthesis.
- Osseointegrated implants have eliminated the need for adhesives while delivering superior mechanical support, vastly broadened the application, and increased patient acceptance of orbital and other facial prostheses.
- Long-term maintenance of implant sites and prostheses is critical to success.

MAXILLOFACIAL PROSTHETICS COMES OF AGE DURING WORLD WAR I

Varaztad Hovhannes Kazanjian (**Fig. 1**) was only 16 years old in 1895 when he fled the Armenian genocide to immigrate to the United States. After working in a wire mill in Worcester, Massachusetts, he studied dentistry at Harvard from 1902 to 1905, where he subsequently became an instructor in dental prosthetics. Kazanjian was already an accomplished and published maxillofacial prosthodontist when he joined the US Army for service with the "Harvard Unit" during World War I.[1] Trench warfare produced a staggering volume of horrific maxillofacial injuries and Kazanjian transitioned into the dual role of maxillofacial surgeon and prosthodontist. He became the most widely acclaimed dental and facial reconstructive surgeon of that war. He was referred to as the "Miracle Man of the Western Front" for his work at the first dental and maxillofacial clinic in Camiers, France.[2] Between 1915 and 1919, he reportedly treated more than 3000 cases of gunshot, shrapnel, and other severe wounds of the face and jaws. Much of that treatment involved innovative facial prosthetics.

All authors have nothing to disclose.
[a] School of Dentistry, Department of Oral and Maxillofacial Surgery, Oregon Health and Science University, 611 Southwest Campus Street SDOMS, Portland, OR 97239, USA; [b] School of Dentistry, Department of Oral and Maxillofacial Surgery, Oregon Health and Science University, 611 Southwest Campus Street SDOMS, Portland, OR 97239, USA; [c] Fellowship in Head and Neck Oncologic and Microvascular Reconstructive Surgery, Legacy Emanuel Medical Center, 2801 North Gantenbein Avenue, Portland, OR 97227, USA; [d] Head and Neck Surgical Associates, 1849 Northwest Kearney Suite #300, Portland, OR 97209, USA; [e] Private Practice, 911 Country Club Road, Suite #240, Eugene, OR 97401, USA; [f] School of Dentistry, Department of Oral and Maxillofacial Surgery, Oregon Health and Science University, 611 Southwest Campus Street, Portland, OR 97239, USA; [g] Casey Eye Institute-Marquam Hill, Oregon Health and Science University, 3375 Southwest Terwilliger Boulevard, Portland, OR 97239, USA
* Corresponding author.
E-mail address: sophieyi@yahoo.com

Oral Maxillofacial Surg Clin N Am 24 (2012) 697–712
http://dx.doi.org/10.1016/j.coms.2012.07.004
1042-3699/12/$ – see front matter Published by Elsevier Inc.

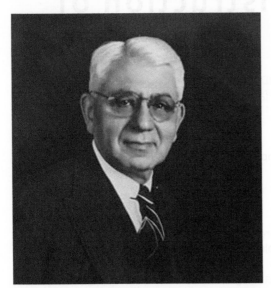

Fig. 1. Varaztad Hovhannes Kazanjian. (*From* http://www.trueknowledge.com/images/thumbs/180/250/ffb9534dfb8b319db28a6d82feec1a66.jpg. Accessed February 1, 2012.)

What set Kazanjian apart from his contemporaries was his integration of dental and maxillofacial prosthetics with surgery to produce optimal results for his disfigured patients. After the war, he went on to become Harvard's first professor of plastic surgery in 1922, where he continued to blend reconstructive surgery with his talent for prosthetics. He was termed a "magician" by Dr Sigmund Freud for his reconstructive and prosthetic efforts for Freud's oral cancer.

ADVENT OF MAXILLOFACIAL PROSTHESES

The facial prostheses of Kazanjian's era were made of vulcanized rubber, characterized by the addition of celluloid paints for coloring facial features, but the vulcanized rubber presented a problem because of its rigidity (**Fig. 2**).[3,4] Retention was a major obstacle to daily use and the design of these prosthetic artworks required a skillful blend of dental clasps, use of anatomic undercuts, and, later, tissue adhesives.

Latex rubber was introduced by Bulbulian[5] and Clarke[6] in 1939 and 1941, respectively. Acrylic resin later replaced vulcanized rubber for both intraoral and extraoral prosthetic use. Various modifications to acrylic resin helped overcome its rigidity and improved coloration techniques were developed.[7] Barnhart introduced the use of silicone elastomers in 1960.[8] Since then, improved materials have evolved, including polysiloxane, siphenylenes, RTV (room temperature vulcanization) silicones, HTV (high-temperature vulcanization) silicones, polyvinyl chloride (PVC), chlorinated polyethylene, and polyurethane. The most widely used materials today are the silicone elastomers, primarily the RTV silicone elastomers. Advances in polymer chemistry are being made continuously with regard to the potential for new silicones and other materials suitable for extraoral prostheses.

CRANIOFACIAL OSSEOINTEGRATION

A quantum leap in the design and comfort of facial prostheses occurred as a result of the introduction of titanium craniofacial implants for prosthetic reconstruction in the head and neck region. This arose in the late 1960s and early 1970s from the pioneering work of Brånemark, Briene, Adell, and Lindström, who demonstrated the success of implant-retained dental prosthesis.[9–12] In the late 1970s and early 1980s, Tjellström, Albrektsson, Brånemark and Lindström introduced the application of osseointegrated implants for bone-anchored conductive hearing aids and prosthetic auricular reconstruction.[13] In 1986, Granström reported 100 patients with craniofacial defects among whom endosseous implants were used for facial rehabilitation. The concept of anchoring craniofacial prostheses with osseointegrated implants was accepted by the Food and Drug Administration in 1985.[14] The first implants designed for facial prostheses were short 3 mm and 4 mm length titanium implants.[15] Because of the implants' success in reliable auricular reconstruction, a continuing stream of orbital, nasal, and frontal prostheses has been reported in the literature.[12,13,16]

Definitions

Orbital exenteration

Exenteration entails the complete removal of the entire orbital contents, including the globe, extraocular muscles, eyelashes, and part or all of the eyelids, orbital fat, and connective tissues, including the periorbita.

Orbital evisceration

Evisceration involves removing the interior contents of the globe, including all uveal tissue, with or without the cornea, and leaving the sclera and the attached extraocular muscles.

Orbital enucleation

Enucleation involves removal of the entire globe, including the cornea, sclera and a portion of the optic nerve.

Orbital prosthesis

A complex prosthesis that restores the exenterated orbit, including an immobile eye, eyelids,

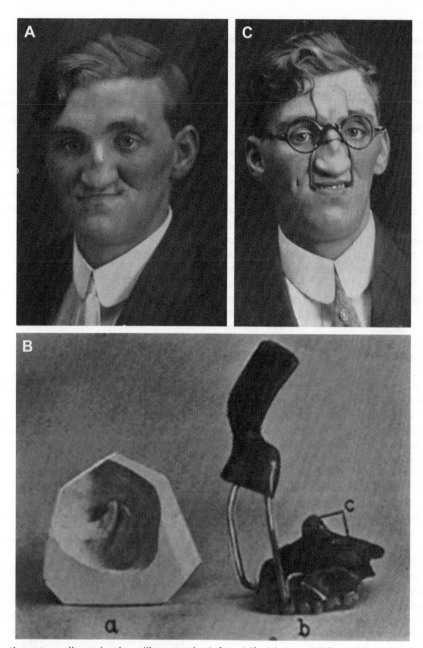

Fig. 2. Innovative extraorally retained maxillary prosthesis for midfacial wound defect, designed by Kazanjian in his 1915 article. (*A*) Midfacial defect, (*B*) prosthesis on the patient, and (*C*) impression model of defect (a) and prosthesis with external paddle, 8-gauge wire (b), palatal extensions (c) that provided anterior projection and stability.

and periorbital structures. Currently most are endosseous implant supported.

Orbital implant
Endosseous implant that is osseointegrated in the orbital/periorbital bony structures. This helps support and retain the orbital prosthesis.

Ocular implant
Spherical implant that replaces the globe and restores orbital volume following enucleation or

evisceration, and helps to impart movement to the exposed ocular prosthesis. These may be partially or completely implanted. These are available in a variety of sizes from various medical suppliers.

Ocular prosthesis
Prosthesis visible externally within normal, animated eyelids that accurately replicates the iris, pupil, and sclera. This is custom made, specific to the patient.

Scleral shell prosthesis

Small, thin variant of ocular prosthesis placed over blind deformed globe, to restore esthetic iris and pupil appearance. This is custom made, specific to the patient.

ORBITAL EXENTERATION

Exenteration of the orbit (**Fig. 3**) becomes necessary owing to malignant and extensive benign orbital pathology, orbital trauma, other acquired defects, or orbital radiation necrosis. Orbital pathology, such as squamous cell carcinoma, basal cell carcinoma, sebaceous gland carcinoma, conjunctival or uveal melanoma, sarcoma, and adenoid cystic carcinoma of the lacrimal gland will require exenteration to ensure complete removal of the diseased tissue. Ballistic trauma severe enough to cause gross dysfunction and deformity of the orbit will also require extensive removal of orbital contents to prevent further tissue necrosis and infection. The same principles apply to orbital radiation necrosis. Whatever the reason for orbital exenteration, the resultant deformity requires reconstruction to restore form, esthetics, self-confidence, and social acceptance.

An orbital exenteration prosthesis restores the form and shape, but not the function of the orbit. An exenteration prosthesis has an immobile, fixed globe, as well as immobile eyelids, and often requires complimentary camouflage, such as tinted eyeglasses. On the other hand, following enucleation, the globe is replaced by an alloplastic sphere implant, which supports and transmits motion to a prosthetic shell. This prosthetic shell restores the form of an iris and pupil, beautifully recreating ocular appearance. Enucleation prostheses are so lifelike in appearance and motion that many enucleation patients have a completely normal appearance without the need for camouflage eyeglasses. Evisceration and enucleation prostheses are covered later in this article.

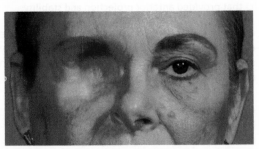

Fig. 3. Right orbital exenteration defect, lined with radial forearm flap.

ADVANTAGES OF PROSTHETIC REHABILITATION OF ORBITAL EXENTERATION DEFECTS

The importation of local, regional or distant autogenous tissue has been widely described and is highly successful for partial eyelid defects. Reconstruction of the complete loss of both upper and lower lids, when combined with loss of the globe and the rest of the orbit, presents an insurmountable challenge to the reconstructive surgeon. Because of the complex anatomy, accurate and comprehensive tissue reconstruction of these structures is not possible short of a facial transplant.

There are clear advantages to implant-supported orbital prostheses over reconstruction with autogenous tissue:

1. Cosmetically superior result
2. Excellent symmetry, color, texture, and anatomic detail
3. Allows direct access for surveillance for possible tumor recurrence
4. Vastly shorter and simpler operation, which lessens surgical morbidity
5. Obviates the need for a separate donor site, which carries its own set of morbidities

In his 1996 text, Beumer and colleagues thoroughly described the benefits derived from implant-supported prostheses over traditional prostheses[15]:

1. Improved retention and stability of the prosthesis
2. Elimination of occasional skin reactions to adhesives
3. Ease and enhanced accuracy of the prosthesis placement
4. Improved skin hygiene and patient comfort
5. Decreased daily maintenance associated with removal and reapplication of skin adhesives
6. Increased life span of the facial prosthesis
7. Enhance esthetics of the lines of junction between the prosthesis and the skin

DISADVANTAGES

Some disadvantages are inherent in implant-supported orbital prostheses:

1. Considerable cost of the implants and prosthetics, which is infrequently covered by insurance
2. Necessity of maintenance and replacement of prosthesis because of normal wear and discoloration
3. Necessity of peri-implant hygiene throughout the lifetime of the implant

4. Possible implant failure and need for replacement when indicated
5. Potential for prosthesis dislodgement at inopportune times, such as social events
6. Possible psychological issues related to the prosthesis

The literature has shown that auricular endosseous implants have highest success rate (90%) as compared with nasal or orbital implants (50%–70%).[16–18] This may be attributable to the difference in bone quality and quantity at the different regions that might dictate the primary stability of the implants. The average life span of a prosthesis has been reported to be in the range of 1.5 to 2.0 years.[19] Prostheses require periodic maintenance and replacement throughout the patient's life, as they are subject to discoloration, problems with attachment of acrylic resin attachment carrier to the silicone, rupture of the silicone, and/or bad fit.[19] The patient needs to understand these limitations and to appreciate that there will be ongoing costs.

PERFORMANCE OF ORBITAL EXENTERATION

Orbital exenteration is an inherently disfiguring procedure whose goal is to remove all orbital contents while maintaining a "negative space" or "negative volume" to receive a prosthesis. This negative space creates a concavity that fulfills 3 critical considerations:

1. It must provide enough surface area for multiple implant placement sites in different positional orientations within the orbital defect.
2. It must allow the orbital prosthesis to reside within the orbit in an inherently stable fashion.
3. It must provide for extension of the prosthesis to properly engage the implants, while avoiding the external appearance of an overly bulky reconstruction that does not match the contralateral orbital anatomy.

In concept, the exenteration technique entails a subperiosteal dissection around the bony orbital walls. Tissues entering the orbit from the superior and inferior orbital fissures and the optic foramen are divided with electrocautery. Classically, the exenterated socket is lined with a split-thickness skin graft, supported by a temporary bolster. Other methods of orbital defect reconstruction have been proposed, including temporalis muscle transposition, midline forehead flap, dermal graft, and dermis fat graft.[20] The use of a vascularized radial forearm or anterolateral thigh flap is a popular contemporary option. The orbital walls can heal via spontaneous granulation, but this has been associated with the development of sino-orbital fistulae through the paper-thin medial and inferior orbital walls.[21]

A thin layer of epithelized tissue covering the orbital walls is ideal for placement of an orbital prosthesis, as tightly adherent soft tissue creates a negative space, and provides enough room for implant placement and prosthetic material buildup. Reconstruction with a vascularized soft tissue flap avoids sino-orbital fistulae, but results in a bulky reconstruction, which requires a debulking procedure, described later in this article.

SOFT TISSUE SURGICAL PREPARATION: DEBULKING PREVIOUS RECONSTRUCTIVE FLAPS

The principles of soft tissue management regarding intraoral dental implant placement apply to orbital and craniofacial implant placement. Ideally, the peri-implant soft tissues should be thin, to allow a shallow cuff around the emerging fixtures that simplifies lifelong peri-implant hygiene.

A prior soft tissue flap reconstruction may have left behind bulky tissue or a "closed cavity," with an excess volume of tissue within the orbital structure (**Fig. 4**). In other patients, actual completion of the orbital exenteration may be necessary following the original partial resection or debridement. Either scenario creates a problem for

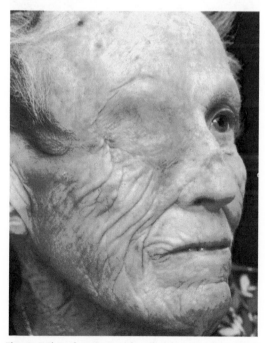

Fig. 4. "Closed cavity" with radial forearm flap reconstructing fronto-orbital resection defect.

receiving a prosthesis and for maintaining implant cleanliness (**Fig. 5**). A soft tissue debulking surgery may be required to

1. Establish an adequate negative volume or "open cavity" to receive an esthetically acceptable prosthesis
2. Provide ease of peri-implant hygiene and to prevent peri-implantitis

The final goal is a healthy, well-adhered, keratinized soft tissue covering of approximately 5 mm thickness or less, which is ideal for long-term implant health. Soft tissue reaction or "peri-implantitis" around percutaneous implants has been reported in between 3% and 7% of patients, with most being mild erythema or irritation.[22,23] Reyes and colleagues[18] reported that implant loss was primarily related to failure of osseointegration rather than skin reactions, but suggested that proper care and cleaning of implant sites is still mandatory for preventing infection. Although peri-implantitis has not been clearly related to the loss of percutaneous implants, its adverse effect on oral dental implants is widely accepted.

SOFT TISSUE SURGICAL PREPARATION: IPSILATERAL BALANCING BROW-LIFT

In general, any soft tissue healing is associated with variable degrees of wound and scar

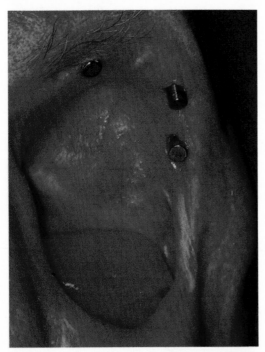

Fig. 5. Orbital implants with evidence of mild peri-implantitis.

contracture and the orbit, and periorbital tissues are not immune to this phenomenon. Following orbital exenteration, the healing of soft tissues in the upper aspect of the orbit may result in inferior contraction of the ipsilateral brow, producing an objectionable degree of brow ptosis. A balancing, ipsilateral brow lift may be an important component of the preprosthetic orbital soft tissue preparation (**Fig. 6**).

PLANNING: ROLE OF CT AND STEREOLITHOGRAPHIC MODEL

Computed tomography (CT) scanning provides an accurate representation of the orbital defect and a 3-dimensional (3D) reconstruction improves even better visualization and measurement of the defect. A stereolithographic (SLG) model made from a high-resolution 3D CT offers the surgeon a palpable model for surgical and prosthetic planning (**Fig. 7**). It enables the surgeon-prosthodontic team to identify sites around the orbital rim with adequate bone stock for placement of implants of adequate length and to plan optimal protection and avoidance of the adjacent frontal sinus and dura mater. It also allows the prosthodontist to create a 3-dimensionally accurate implant drilling guide. Clear communication between the maxillofacial prosthodontist and the maxillofacial surgeon is critical for treatment planning.

Implants for orbital prostheses are most commonly placed in the lateral and superior aspect of the orbital rim, into both the zygomatic and frontal bones (**Fig. 8**). In the frontal bone, SLG model surgery helps determine how far medially implants can be placed before entering the frontal sinus. The thick bone of the zygomatic body inferolaterally provides excellent bone stock for larger implants. Rarely is adequate bone present in the inferior or medial orbital rims. A minimum of 3 implants is needed, but 4 are preferred, ideally spaced with at least 5 mm between adjacent implants. If the patient has an associated maxillary defect requiring an obturator prosthesis below the orbital prosthesis, additional retention and/or connectors may be required in the form of magnets or mechanical attachments. The implants are oriented in an arc to allow better stress distribution and retention of the prosthesis. If possible, the implants are placed slightly behind the orbital rim to allow adequate prosthetic thickness and to provide camouflage for implant fixtures. The implant placement also should allow proper emergence profile for magnet placement or bar + attachment

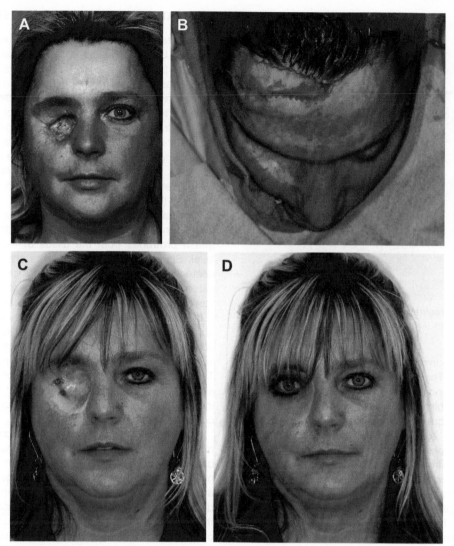

Fig. 6. (*A*) Brow ptosis following orbital exenteration. Note redundancy and thickness of the radial forearm flap. (*B*) Revision of brow ptosis with open brow lift. (*C*) Postoperative result following revision of radial forearm flap, brow lift, and implant placement. (*D*) Orbital prosthesis in place.

design without resulting in metal showing at the margin of the final prosthesis.

For implant-retained auricular prostheses, 3 implants are placed in the mastoid area using an acrylic resin surgical guide. The implants need to be placed in a position corresponding to the antihelix to esthetically conceal the implant attachments within the prosthetic auricle (**Fig. 9**).

Implants for a nasal prosthesis are ideally placed with paired implants in the nasal floor–piriform base that engage the maxilla and extend toward the palate, passing over the roots of the anterior maxillary teeth. An implant can also be placed in the glabella area of the frontal bone,

but poor success rates have been reported at this site (**Fig. 10**).[15]

IMPLANT PLACEMENT PROCEDURE

The implant preparation osteotomy is ideally done under general anesthesia within a sterile operating room environment. The surgical guide is used to mark the exact location of each implant site. To create an accurate transfer of the implant location from the surgical stent to the patient, methylene blue dye on a 1-mL tuberculin syringe on a small needle can be used to perforate the skin down to bone. The plunger is gently tapped to deliver

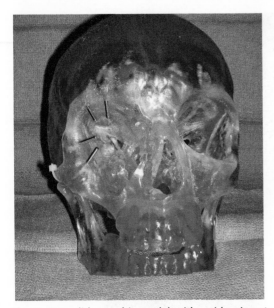

Fig. 7. Stereolithographic model with guide pins at implant sites.

a tiny amount of dye into and under the periosteum (**Fig. 11**). This will guide proper placement of the implants once reflection of the overlying skin is performed. Following exposure of the orbital rim, the drilling sequence to prepare the osteotomy site is the same as is used for conventional intraoral dental implants. Although not usually necessary, intraoperative navigation and/or intraoperative CT could be used as an adjunct to guide and assess the accuracy of implant position, angle, and depth. Implant placement can be done in either 1-stage or 2-stage fashion. The 1-stage method requires placement of temporary abutment and soft tissue adaptation around the exposed abutment, whereas the 2-stage technique allows initial soft tissue coverage of the cover screw and surgical exposure of implant is done later.

FABRICATION OF ORBITAL PROSTHESES

The orbital prosthesis can be connected to the implants by 1 of 2 methods. The original method entailed the fabrication of a metal framework, which was screwed to the implants and allowed either magnetic or mechanical connectors. This is similar to the design of an intraoral implant overdenture framework. Currently, most orbital prostheses are fabricated without a metal framework. This change evolved because of the use of longer implants, the hygiene problems associated with the framework, and the advent of much stronger magnets (**Fig. 12**).

The final abutment contains the titanium keeper and is torqued into the implant. Its length is such that it protrudes from the tissue at the desired level. Since the keeper abutments are not connected to other abutments, hygiene is greatly facilitated and the osseointegration of each implant can be readily rechecked should a question arise.

If the orbital defect is large, the magnets can be connected to an acrylic resin or fiber-reinforced composite resin subframework,[24] to which the eventual silicone orbital prosthesis is then bonded. This decreases the weight of the orbital prosthesis, strengthens it, and allows for more ideal processing of the silicone because the depth of the silicone can be controlled.

A master addition reaction silicone impression is made with the patient in an upright position to capture the natural facial contours. The impression needs to extend at least 3 cm past the desired eventual prosthesis border, which should be defined by the maxillofacial prosthodontist or prosthetist before fabricating the impression. A variety of individual patient-specific factors determine the prosthesis border, as well as the implant locations. These factors include the presence of adjacent thin mobile tissue, soft tissue clefts or the presence of orbito-nasal or orbito-antral fistulae,

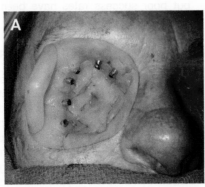
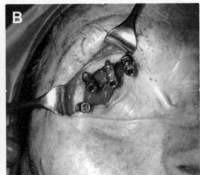

Fig. 8. (*A*) Prefabricated surgical guide. (*B*) Orbital implants placed at corresponding sites in lateral and superior rim.

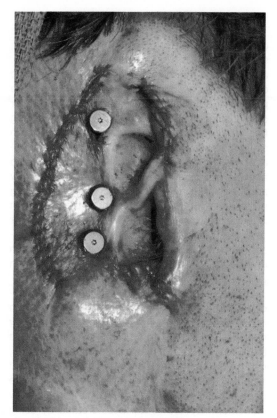

Fig. 9. Three implants placed at the position of the antihelix following burn injury to right ear.

the degree of facial muscle movement, and the natural angles of the face. Once the impression is obtained, the abutment analogs are placed on top of the magnets embedded into the impression and the impression is poured in dental stone.

The ocular prosthesis can be colored by artistic hand-painting as described later. An alternative is to have a custom-fabricated ocular prosthesis patterned after a photograph of the patient's normal opposite eye. The acrylic resin ocular can be modified in size, shape, and color if necessary.

The most difficult part of construction of the orbital prosthesis is accurate positioning of the

ocular prosthesis. Several measurements can be made of the position of the patient's normal eye to assist in the location of the "ocular." The frontal, sagittal, and horizontal planes must be checked to ensure that the ocular is in its proper position relative to the patient's normal eye. Once the ocular is placed in the orbital wax-up, the position of primary gaze must be verified in relation to that of the normal eye. When one looks at a patient's eye and views the pupil, there is a white square reflective area that can be oriented by the hands of a clock. In a patient with binocular vision, both eyes reflect the same "clock" orientation of this reflection. It is imperative that the ocular orientation gaze in the orbital prosthesis matches that of the patient's normal eye (**Fig. 13**). This can only be properly established by viewing the orbital wax-up within the patient. The eye position and gaze should be assessed repeatedly over the course of several appointments to ensure that the final position is accurate.

Details, such as the superior and inferior eyelids, medial and lateral canthi, wrinkles, skin folds, and facial contours, should be incorporated into the prosthesis. The patient's normal side is an excellent guide for the replication of these details in the orbital prosthesis, although modifications and compromises are often required, resulting in minor differences in symmetry.

Once the wax-up has been finalized, the margins of the prosthesis are thinned and adjusted to apply a gentle positive pressure on the margins of the orbital defect anatomy. This allows the prosthesis to conceal some normal functional tissue movement at the prosthesis margins. The prosthesis is then immediately removed from the patient, chilled in ice water and a new master cast poured. This technique optimizes the functional esthetics owing to the capture of the final margins in the second master cast impression (David Trainer, prosthotist, Naples, FL, personal communication 2010). Areas of the prosthesis that apply positive tissue pressure are trimmed back approximately 0.5 cm and the border of the

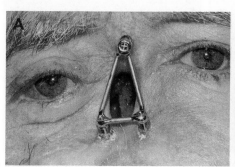
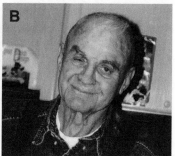

Fig. 10. (*A*) Peri-nasal implants and metal framework to support nasal prosthesis. (*B*) Nasal prosthesis in place.

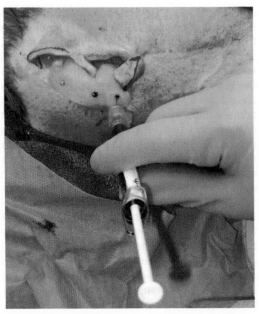

Fig. 11. As an example in this auricular implant case, a tuberculin syringe filled with methylene blue is gently tapped to mark the periosteum to accurately position the implants.

master cast is sanded and finely thinned to allow for very thin, translucent silicone margins. This design also places positive pressure on the tissue to help blend the margins to the patient's skin.

The ocular prosthesis is duplicated in clear acrylic and is processed in the mold. This will provide an ocular duplicate to be used if multiple colorations are needed, including the eventual remaking of the prosthesis in several years. This also allows the patient to continue to wear the existing orbital prosthesis during a remake procedure.

Most orbital prostheses will require 40 to 100 g of silicone. The presence of an "opaquer" agent, such as a standard cosmetic foundation makeup

color, is a vitally important addition to the silicone. The opaquer is added to the silicone until the desired opacity is obtained. Other colorants, such as dry earth pigments and flocking fibers, are mixed into the silicone as needed. This intrinsic coloration is performed in the presence of the patient to determine when the base shade color of the silicone has been reached. The flocking fibers help simulate the refraction and reflection of light as well as other elements of the micro-anatomy of the patient's skin. It is important to achieve a proper balance between translucency and opacity to arrive at a vital, lifelike-appearing prosthesis. The final component of the coloration is to coat the outer half of the mold with a thin layer of a clear silicone. Any features that can be represented by a different shade are colored on this thin outer edge, such as nevi, blood vessels, melanin pigmentations, and other skin color variances.

Once the tinting is completed, the colored silicone is poured into the halves of the mold, which is placed in a vise and is then processed in a dry heat oven at 82.2°C for 2 hours. The prosthesis is then cleaned and extrinsic coloration, if needed, can be added. It is then sealed with silicone and reheated to the same temperature. After 2 more heat cycles, it is ready for eyelash or eyebrow placement. Eyebrows are best created by using the patient's own hair (**Fig. 14**). Eyelashes are best duplicated using a more durable artificial lash. The final adjustment of the eyebrow and eyelashes should be done with the patient present.

HOME CARE OF THE ORBITAL PROSTHESIS

The patient is instructed to gently clean the prosthesis with antibacterial soap and hot water at least once per day, and care must be taken to ensure that the eyelashes and eyebrows are not damaged during this process. The prosthesis should be removed for sleep and can be kept in a refrigerator

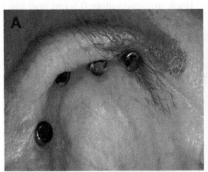
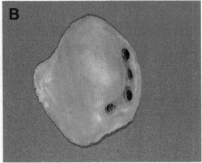

Fig. 12. (*A*) Orbital implants with magnet abutments. Note eyebrow ptosis in this patient managed with cosmetic eyebrow pencil application. (*B*) Implant-supported prosthesis.

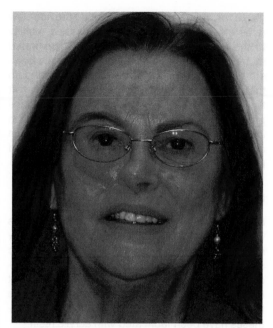

Fig. 13. Ocular orientation gaze matches that of patient's normal eye. Oversized eyeglasses provide excellent camouflage.

at night to prolong the life span of the silicone. The patient should be examined on a semi-annual to annual basis to evaluate the implants, tissue health, and prosthesis condition. Periodic reconstruction of the prosthesis is required.

THE ANOPHTHALMIC SOCKET

The removal of the globe alone or with additional orbital structures can be necessary for various reasons, including phthisis bulbi, malignancy, infection, or trauma and can present an indication for an operation of more limited extent than an exenteration. Removal of the eye can be a stressful undertaking for the patient and both physician and patient should be absolutely sure that the surgical

procedure is necessary. For example, globe removal may enhance patient comfort in the case of a blind, painful eye, and may protect the health of the fellow eye in the case of sympathetic ophthalmia, and may even save the patient's life in the case of malignancy. Whatever the reason for the removal of the eye, psychological issues may ensue. Even with a blind, disfigured but salvageable eye, a prosthetic scleral shell alone may provide excellent esthetics without an additional surgery.

EVISCERATION

Evisceration involves removal of the contents of the eye without removing the scleral shell, extraocular muscles, or optic nerve. Evisceration should not be performed in the case of intraocular malignancy.

The surgical procedure involves first dissecting the conjunctiva by performing a 360° peritomy. Next, the cornea is removed using scissors, although the corneal stroma may be retained in some cases. All intraocular contents including uveal tissue are then removed using an evisceration spoon. A spherical implant is then placed, and relaxing scleral incisions may be needed to facilitate the placement of the implant. The sclera is closed anteriorly over the implant. Tenon fascia and conjunctiva are then closed over the surgical defect. An acrylic or silicone conformer is placed within the conjunctival fornices to maintain space for the future prosthesis. The eyelids can be sutured together if they do not fully close to cover the conformer. Advantages of evisceration include less disruption of the orbital anatomy because of less extensive surgery, and improved esthetics and prosthesis motility.

ENUCLEATION

Enucleation involves removal of the entire globe, including the sclera and a portion of the optic

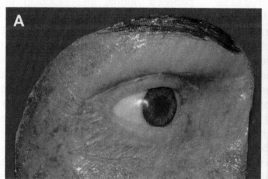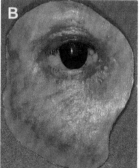

Fig. 14. (*A, B*) Eyebrow is patient's own hair, whereas the eyelashes are artificial lashes.

nerve. Care should be taken in eyes with endophthalmitis, as extraocular spread of infection is possible.

The surgical procedure involves dissection of the conjunctiva and Tenon fascia off of the globe via a 360° peritomy. The rectus muscles are secured with suture, then removed from the globe using scissors. The oblique muscles are severed, cauterized, and allowed to retract into the orbit. Alternatively, the oblique muscles can also be secured with suture for attachment to the ocular implant. Blunt dissection is performed in all quadrants to ensure that all attachments to the globe are severed. Next, the optic nerve is transected using scissors or a snare. The implant of choice is placed in the defect, the extraocular muscles are attached to the implant, and Tenon fascia and conjunctiva are securely closed. An acrylic or silicone conformer is placed within the conjunctival fornices to maintain a space for the future prosthesis. The eyelids can be sutured together if they do not fully close to cover the conformer.

DERMIS FAT GRAFT

If insufficient conjunctival surface area is present to allow the fornices to develop appropriately, a dermis-fat graft can be placed in the orbit to increase the restoration of orbital volume and create enough surface area for retention of the future ocular prosthesis. The dermis is sutured to the conjunctival edges in the orbit with the fat projecting posteriorly into the orbit. The goal is to increase the area of mucosalized lining. In adults, the volume of fat harvested must account for some expected postoperative atrophy. In children, the harvested fat has actually been shown to grow over time.[25]

OCULAR IMPLANTS

A spherical ocular implant is implanted at surgery to replace the globe following enucleation or evisceration, and can also be mistakenly referred to as an "ocular prosthesis." Its functions are to restore orbital volume and shape, and to transmit normal motion to the overlying ocular prosthetic shell located within the conjunctival fornices. Ocular implant size can vary depending on the patient; however, a large implant is usually preferred to maximize orbital volume. Most adult orbits can retain an 18-mm to 20-mm spherical implant. Appropriate implant size is especially important in children, as the development of the bony orbit depends on adequate orbital soft tissue volume.

Ocular implants can be classified as either inert or biointegrated. Inert materials include silicone, glass, or methylmethacrylate and provide low rates of extrusion, comfort, and passive motility to the overlying ocular prosthesis. Biointegrated materials include hydroxyapatite or porous polyethylene and allow for fibrovascular ingrowth into the implant with integration into the orbital soft tissues. Some implants have anterior surface projections or an option to drill a peg, which can improve the motility of the prosthesis, but can also increase the probability of exposure and possible extrusion.

HISTORY OF OCULAR PROSTHESES

Before World War II, virtually all ocular prostheses were made of glass. Because of the cutoff of raw materials from Germany for glass eyes, acrylic resin came into common usage following the development of the first acrylic resin ocular prosthesis at the Naval Hospital in Bethesda, Maryland.[26] Since then, ocular prostheses and scleral shell prostheses have been fabricated with acrylic resin.

FABRICATION OF THE OCULAR PROSTHESIS

The ocular prosthesis is fabricated by making a custom impression of the patient's anophthalmic socket under topical anesthesia. The materials most commonly used for this are an irreversible hydrocolloid or an addition reaction silicone used with a custom ocular impression tray. A 2-piece stone mold is made from this impression and a wax pattern blank is developed from the mold. This is adjusted as necessary to adapt to the extrinsic eye muscles as well as the anatomy of the upper and lower eyelids and the medial and lateral canthi. It is also adjusted for maximal contact with the orbital implant to allow optimal movement. The resulting processed acrylic resin scleral blank is then fitted to the patient's socket to determine if any further adjustments are needed.

The next step is to mark the center of the pupil in relation to the patient's normal opposite pupil. The patient's normal iris, including the limbus, is measured and a protractor is used to trace this diameter on the sclera blank. The blank is then ground down to allow for at least 2 mm of depth on the edges of the cutout where the iris will eventually meet the sclera. A watercolor paper disk that has been trimmed 1 mm smaller in diameter than the measurement of the patient's iris is used to paint the iris, including the collarette, pupil, and part of the limbus. This is painted with acrylic paints using a very small artist's brush to replicate the striations of the intrinsic iris muscle colorations (**Fig. 15**).[27] The pupil is approximated to the size that the patient's normal eye will exhibit most of the time.

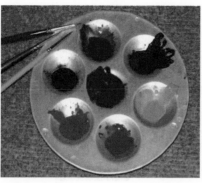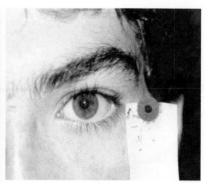

Fig. 15. Details of the pupil and iris intrinsic muscles are hand painted.

The gaze is then adjusted with a 1-cm peg protruding from the scleral blank. This is placed in the portion that has been hollowed out for the eventual iris. The patient is instructed to look straight ahead. The blank with the horizontal peg projection allows a 3D gaze evaluation in the horizontal, frontal, and sagittal planes. The inferior surface of the sclera that was hollowed out can be adjusted carefully with a bur or hand instrumentation to change the angulation of the patient's gaze until it is in the same three facial planes as the gaze of the patient's normal eye.

The completed iris watercolor disk is placed on the inside of the hollowed-out scleral blank. The edges and facial surface of the scleral blank are reduced so that only 0.2 mm of thickness is present at the edges of the iris depression. The edges are then sanded with fine sandpaper to replicate the fuzziness seen on the outer diameter of the limbus. The limbus is painted on the outer diameter of the hollowed-out iris depression projecting over the edge of the scleral blank. The remaining scleral surface is reduced 2 to 3 mm in depth to allow for coloration. Fine red and blue yarn are teased apart to simulate blood vessels. These can be affixed by a solution of acrylic resin. Blue tinting and fat pad replication are done with thin washes of acrylic paints. Once the external scleral anatomy is completed, the scleral blank and iris disk are placed in the mold and a clear acrylic resin is heat processed at 85°C to form the completed ocular prosthesis (**Fig. 16**). The process is similar for a scleral shell prosthesis, used for an ocular evisceration, where space is greatly reduced.

MAINTENANCE OF THE OCULAR PROSTHESIS

Patients are seen on a yearly basis to evaluate the mucosa of the socket to determine if any inflammation or pathology is present and to polish the ocular prosthesis. Ocular prostheses can demonstrate accretion of plaques, somewhat analogous to dental calculus, from a buildup of salt and protein

in tears. The patient is instructed to remove the prosthesis daily and clean it with an antibacterial soap. In addition, the prosthesis should be polished every 6 months by an ocularist or maxillofacial prosthodontist. This will minimize any irritation, ensure comfort, and increase life of the prosthesis.

POSTOPERATIVE CARE OF OCULAR PROSTHETICS

Complications of anophthalmic surgery may include infection, extrusion or exposure of the implant, contracture of the socket or fornices, the development of a superior sulcus defect secondary to decreased orbital volume, and eyelid malposition, such as blepharoptosis, ectropion, or entropion. Procedures to improve esthetics may involve orbital implants or dermis-fat grafts to increase orbital volume, mucus membrane grafts to increase conjunctival surface area, and eyelid procedures to improve prosthesis fit and facial symmetry.

In any case of evisceration or enucleation, patient rehabilitation is important to address any psychosocial issues as well as daily activities with monocular function. Polycarbonate spectacles in addition to monocular precautions should be used to protect the fellow eye. Cosmetic optics can also be considered to improve appearance of the prosthesis.

PARTIAL FACIAL TRANSPLANT VERSUS PROSTHESIS

The recent and well-publicized development of facial transplantation from a cadaveric donor has captured the imagination of surgeons and patients around the world. Facial transplantation has the capacity to replace multiple facial structures, or all of them, with perfect, uninjured tissue from another human being. Patients considering an extensive facial prosthesis that replaces one or both orbits plus adjacent tissues, such as the

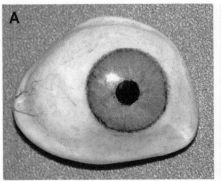
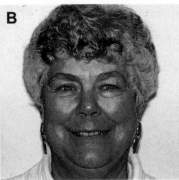

Fig. 16. (*A*) Ocular prosthesis and (*B*) prosthesis within the right orbit of the patient.

nose, might logically ask if they might be a candidate for facial transplant procedure (**Fig. 17**).

Prosthetic reconstruction provides superb restoration of form, color, and texture, but will neither restore animation or sensation, nor return vision. It is an adynamic, insensate reconstruction. Prostheses also deteriorate over time in response to normal wear and tear, and require maintenance and periodic replacement throughout the patient's life. Other disadvantages have been listed previously in this article.

In comparison with facial transplantation, prostheses do not require the availability of a suitable cadaveric donor or involve an extensive operation that is performed by only a few centers worldwide.

They do not require mandatory and costly lifelong antirejection medication, without which failure is both unavoidable and absolute. The implant placement itself is a much shorter and safer operation, especially with contemporary preoperative planning using 3D reconstruction via SLG models.

The time commitment of the prosthetic patient (4 months of osseointegration, an additional procedure for debulking soft tissue and/or brow lift, and several weeks of impression/prosthesis fabrication) is much less than that involved in careful planning, surgery, and rehabilitation of the patient who has had a facial transplant. The overall cost of an implant-supported maxillofacial prosthesis should also be considerably less than that of a transplant.

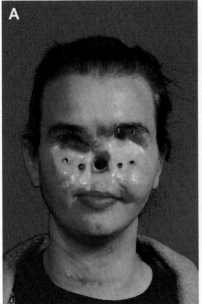
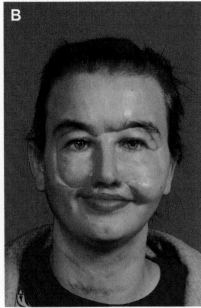

Fig. 17. (*A*) Extensive bilateral orbito-nasal defect with peri-orbital implants. (*B*) Magnet-retained prosthesis in place.

Facial transplantation enables multiple facial structures to be replaced, such as a complete nose plus lips, cheeks, and eyelids, as well as facial osseous architecture, all in one operation. It can result in the eventual return of function via nerve anastomosis to the transplant, which looks promising. Unfortunately, transplantation of a globe is not yet possible.

So what's the bottom line? Patients who require extensive replacement of multiple *mobile* facial structures, such as lips, cheeks, and eyelids, are probably better served with a transplant. If concomitant replacement of zygomatic, nasal, or jaw bony structure is also needed, this is all the more reason to consider a partial or total facial transplant. On the other hand, if facial tissue loss can be restored with an *immobile* reconstruction, such as an orbital, nasal, and/or auricular prosthesis, the prosthetic route is much more straightforward and far less expensive.

SPECIAL CONSIDERATION FOR RADIATED PATIENTS AND HYPERBARIC OXYGEN THERAPY

The literature has demonstrated a higher rate of implant failure in irradiated patients compared with nonirradiated patients.[13,28,29] Overall survival rate of irradiated patients with craniofacial implants range from 50% to 90% compared with nonirradiated patients, estimated to be about 70% to 100%, depending on years of follow-up. The role of hyperbaric oxygen (HBO) therapy is a controversial one, as there is mixed efficacy shown in the literature.[30–32] However, Granström demonstrated in the pooled data from various studies that adjunctive HBO therapy in irradiated areas had higher implant success than without HBO over time.[33] Therefore, when the option is feasible and available, HBO therapy should be considered.

SUMMARY

When faced with devastating loss of orbital structures because of tumor, trauma, or burns or for congenital reasons, an implant-supported prosthesis is a viable option to an extensive and multistaged tissue reconstruction. It will usually provide an esthetically superior orbital reconstruction compared with wearing an eye patch or receiving an autogenous tissue reconstruction. Osseointegrated implants have eliminated the need for adhesives while delivering superior mechanical support, vastly broadened the application, and increased patient acceptance of orbital and other facial prostheses. Long-term maintenance of implant sites and prostheses is critical to success.

REFERENCES

1. Kazanjian VH. Prosthetic restoration of acquired deformities of the superior maxilla. J Allied Dent Soc 1915;10:14–23.
2. Deranian HM. Miracle man of the western front. Worcester (MA): Chandler House Press; 2007.
3. Upham RH. Artificial noses and ears. Boston Med Surg J 1901;145:522.
4. Kazanjian VH, Rowe AT, Young H. Prostheses of the mouth and face. J Dent Res 1932;12:651.
5. Bulbulian AH. An improved technique for prosthetic restorations of facial defects by use of a latex compound. In: editor. 1. Proc Staff Meetings, Rochester, MN. Mayo Clinic 1939;14:721–7.
6. Clarke CD. Moulage prostheses. Am J Orthod Oral Surg 1941;27:214–25.
7. Tylman SD. Resilient and elastic resins: techniques for their use in maxillofacial prostheses. Dental Digest 1944;50:p. 260.
8. Barnhart GW. A new material and technique in the art of somato-prosthesis. J Dent Res 1960;39:836.
9. Brånemark PI, Adell R, Breine U, et al. Intra-osseous anchorage of dental prosthesis. I. Experimental studies. Scand J Plast Reconstr Surg 1969;3:81–100.
10. Adell R, Hansson BO, Brånemark PI, et al. Intraosseous anchorage of dental prosthesis. II. Review of clinical approaches. Scand J Plast Reconstr Surg 1970;4:19–34.
11. Brånemark PI, Breine U, Hallen O, et al. Repair of defects in mandible. Scand J Plast Reconstr Surg 1970;4:100–8.
12. Brånemark PI, Breine U, Adell R, et al. Experimentella studier av intraosseal forankring av dentala proteser. Rsbok/Goteborgs Tandlakare-Sallskaps 1970;0:9–25 [in Swedish].
13. Parel SM, Tjellström A. The United States and Swedish experience with osseointegration and facial prosthesis. Int J Oral Maxillofac Implants 1991;6:75–9.
14. Granström G. Invited review: craniofacial osseointegration. Oral Dis 2007;13:261–9.
15. Beumer J, Curtis TA, Marunick MT. Maxillofacial rehabilitation, prosthodontic and surgical considerations. St. Louis: Ishiyaku EuroAmerica; 1996. p. 436, 443.
16. Abu-Serriah MM, McGowan DA, Moos KF, et al. Outcome of extraoral craniofacial endosseous implants. Br J Oral Maxillofac Surg 2001;39:269–75.
17. Jacobsson M, Tjellström A, Fine L, et al. A retrospective study of osseointegrated skin-penetrating titanium fixtures used for retaining facial prostheses. Int J Oral Maxillofac Implants 1992;75:523–8.

18. Reyes R, Tjellström A, Granström G. Evaluation of implant losses and skin reactions around extra-oral bone anchored implants: a 0 to 8 year follow-up. Otolaryngol Head Neck Surg 2000; 122:272–6.

19. Visser A, Raghoebar GM, van Oort RP, et al. Fate of implant-retained craniofacial prostheses: life span and aftercare. Int J Oral Maxillofac Implants 2008; 23(1):89–98.

20. Rahman I, Cook AE, Leatherbarrow B. Orbital exenteration: a 13 year Manchester experience. Br J Ophthalmol 2005;89(10):1335–40.

21. Mohr C, Esser J. Orbital exenteration: surgical and reconstructive strategies. Graefes Arch Clin Exp Ophthalmol 1997;235:288–95.

22. Karakoca S, Aydin C, Yilmaz H, et al. Survival rates and periimplant soft tissue evaluation of extraoral implants over a mean follow-up period of three years. J Prosthet Dent 2008;100(6):458–64.

23. Roumanas ED, Freymiller EG, Chang TL, et al. Implant-retained prostheses for facial defects: an up to 14-year follow-up report on the survival rates of implants at UCLA. Int J Prosthodont 2002;15(4): 325–32.

24. Kantola R, Lassila L, Vallittu P. Adhesion of maxillo-facial silicone elastomer to a fiber-reinforced composite resin framework. Int J Prosthodont 2011;24: 582–8.

25. Heher KL, Katowitz JA, Low JE. Unilateral dermis-fat graft implantation in the pediatric orbit. Ophthal Plast Reconstr Surg 1998;14(2):81–8.

26. Murphy PJ, Schlossburg L. Eye replacement by acrylic maxillofacial prosthesis. US Naval Med Bull 1944;43:1085.

27. Haug SP, Andres CJ. Fabrication of custom ocular prosthesis. In: Taylor TD, editor. Clinical Maxillofacial Prosthetics. Chicago: Quintessence; 2000. p. 265–76.

28. Wolfaardt JF, Wilkes GH, Parel SM, et al. Craniofacial osseointegration: the Canadian experience. Int J Oral Maxillofac Implants 1993;8:197.

29. Tolman DE, Taylor PF. Bone-anchored cranio-facial prosthesis study. Int J Oral Maxillofac Implants 1996;11:159.

30. Ueda M, Kaneda T, Takahashi H. Effect of hyperbaric oxygen therapy on osseointegration of titanium implants in irradiated bone: a preliminary report. Int J Oral Maxillofac Implants 1993;8:41–4.

31. Keller EE. Placement of dental implants in the irradiated mandible: a protocol without adjunctive hyperbaric oxygen. J Oral Maxillofac Surg 1997;55:972–80.

32. Wagner W, Esser E, Ostkamp K. Osseointegration of dental implants in patients with and without radiotherapy. Acta Oncol 1998;37:693–6.

33. Granström G. Radiotherapy, osseointegration, and hyperbaric oxygen therapy. Periodontol 2000 2003; 33:145–62.

Index

Note: Page numbers of article titles are in **boldface** type.

United States Postal Service

Statement of Ownership, Management, and Circulation
(All Periodicals Publications Except Requestor Publications)

1. Publication Title — Oral and Maxillofacial Surgery Clinics of North America

2. Publication Number — 0 0 6 - 3 6 2

3. Filing Date — 9/14/12

4. Issue Frequency — Feb, May, Aug, Nov

5. Number of Issues Published Annually — 4

6. Annual Subscription Price — $355.00

7. Complete Mailing Address of Known Office of Publication (Not printer) (Street, city, county, state, and ZIP+4®)
Elsevier Inc.
360 Park Avenue South
New York, NY 10010-1710

Contact Person — Stephen R. Bushing

Telephone (Include area code) — 215-239-3688

8. Complete Mailing Address of Headquarters or General Business Office of Publisher (Not printer)
Elsevier Inc., 360 Park Avenue South, New York, NY 10010-1710

9. Full Names and Complete Mailing Addresses of Publisher, Editor, and Managing Editor (Do not leave blank)

Publisher (Name and complete mailing address)
Kim Murphy, Elsevier, Inc., 1600 John F. Kennedy Blvd. Suite 1800, Philadelphia, PA 19103-2899

Editor (Name and complete mailing address)
John Vassallo, Elsevier, Inc., 1600 John F. Kennedy Blvd. Suite 1800, Philadelphia, PA 19103-2899

Managing Editor (Name and complete mailing address)
Barbara Cohen-Kligerman, Elsevier, Inc., 1600 John F. Kennedy Blvd. Suite 1800, Philadelphia, PA 19103-2899

10. Owner (Do not leave blank. If the publication is owned by a corporation, give the name and address of the corporation immediately followed by the names and addresses of all stockholders owning or holding 1 percent or more of the total amount of stock. If not owned by a corporation, give the names and addresses of the individual owners. If owned by a partnership or other unincorporated firm, give its name and address as well as those of each individual owner. If the publication is published by a nonprofit organization, give its name and address.)

Full Name	Complete Mailing Address
Wholly owned subsidiary of	1600 John F. Kennedy Blvd., Ste. 1800
Reed/Elsevier, US holdings	Philadelphia, PA 19103-2899

11. Known Bondholders, Mortgagees, and Other Security Holders Owning or Holding 1 Percent or More of Total Amount of Bonds, Mortgages, or Other Securities. If none, check box — ☐ None

Full Name	Complete Mailing Address
N/A	

12. Tax Status (For completion by nonprofit organizations authorized to mail at nonprofit rates) (Check one)
The purpose, function, and nonprofit status of this organization and the exempt status for federal income tax purposes:
☐ Has Not Changed During Preceding 12 Months
☐ Has Changed During Preceding 12 Months (Publisher must submit explanation of change with this statement)

PS Form 3526, September 2007 (Page 1 of 3 (Instructions Page 3)) PSN 7530-01-000-9931 PRIVACY NOTICE: See our Privacy policy in www.usps.com

---

13. Publication Title — Oral and Maxillofacial Surgery Clinics of North America

14. Issue Date for Circulation Data Below — August 2012

15. Extent and Nature of Circulation

		Average No. Copies Each Issue During Preceding 12 Months	No. Copies of Single Issue Published Nearest to Filing Date
a. Total Number of Copies (Net press run)		1697	1583
b. Paid Circulation (By Mail and Outside the Mail)	(1) Mailed Outside-County Paid Subscriptions Stated on PS Form 3541. (Include paid distribution above nominal rate, advertiser's proof copies, and exchange copies)	1254	1191
	(2) Mailed In-County Paid Subscriptions Stated on PS Form 3541 (Include paid distribution above nominal rate, advertiser's proof copies, and exchange copies)		
	(3) Paid Distribution Outside the Mails Including Sales Through Dealers and Carriers, Street Vendors, Counter Sales, and Other Paid Distribution Outside USPS®	184	211
	(4) Paid Distribution by Other Classes Mailed Through the USPS (e.g. First-Class Mail®)		
c. Total Paid Distribution (Sum of 15b (1), (2), (3), and (4))		1438	1402
d. Free or Nominal Rate Distribution (By Mail and Outside the Mail)	(1) Free or Nominal Rate Outside-County Copies Included on PS Form 3541	61	66
	(2) Free or Nominal Rate In-County Copies Included on PS Form 3541		
	(3) Free or Nominal Rate Copies Mailed at Other Classes Through the USPS (e.g. First-Class Mail)		
	(4) Free or Nominal Rate Distribution Outside the Mail (Carriers or other means)		
e. Total Free or Nominal Rate Distribution (Sum of 15d (1), (2), (3) and (4))		61	66
f. Total Distribution (Sum of 15c and 15e)		1499	1468
g. Copies not Distributed (See instructions to publishers #4 (page #3))		198	115
h. Total (Sum of 15f and g)		1697	1583
i. Percent Paid (15c divided by 15f times 100)		95.93%	95.50%

16. Publication of Statement of Ownership
If the publication is a general publication, publication of this statement is required. Will be printed in the November 2012 issue of this publication. — Publication not required

17. Signature and Title of Editor, Publisher, Business Manager, or Owner

Stephen R. Bushing – Inventory Distribution Coordinator

Date — September 14, 2012

I certify that all information furnished on this form is true and complete. I understand that anyone who furnishes false or misleading information on this form or who omits material or information requested on the form may be subject to criminal sanctions (including fines and imprisonment) and/or civil sanctions (including civil penalties).

PS Form 3526, September 2007 (Page 2 of 3)

Moving?

Make sure your subscription moves with you!

To notify us of your new address, find your **Clinics Account Number** (located on your mailing label above your name), and contact customer service at:

Email: journalscustomerservice-usa@elsevier.com

800-654-2452 (subscribers in the U.S. & Canada)
314-447-8871 (subscribers outside of the U.S. & Canada)

Fax number: 314-447-8029

Elsevier Health Sciences Division
Subscription Customer Service
3251 Riverport Lane
Maryland Heights, MO 63043

*To ensure uninterrupted delivery of your subscription, please notify us at least 4 weeks in advance of move.

Printed and bound by CPI Group (UK) Ltd, Croydon, CR0 4YY

03/10/2024

01040332-0015